EPIDEMIOLOGY IN NURSING PRACTICE

EPIDEMIOLOGY IN NURSING PRACTICE

Gail A. Harkness, DrPH, RN, FAAN

Professor
University of Connecticut School of Nursing
Storrs, Connecticut;
Assistant Professor
University of Connecticut School of Medicine
Farmington, Connecticut

Mosby

St. Louis Baltimore Berlin Boston Carlsbad Chicago London Madrid
Naples New York Philadelphia Sydney Tokyo Toronto

Mosby
Dedicated to Publishing Excellence

Publisher: Nancy L. Coon
Managing Editor: Loren Stevenson Wilson
Senior Developmental Editor: Laurie Sparks
Project Manager: Gayle May Morris
Production Editor: Mamata Reddy
Manufacturing Supervisor: Kathy Grone
Design Manager: Susan Lane
Artwork: Karen L. Merrill
Cover Design: GW Graphics

Printed in the United States of America

Composition by International Computaprint Corporation

Printing/binding by R. R. Donnelly & Sons Company

Mosby-Year Book, Inc.
11830 Westline Industrial Drive
St. Louis, Missouri 63146

International Standard Book Number 0-8016-2052-X

94 95 96 97 98 / 987654321

Contributors

Henrietta Bernal, PhD, RN
Associate Professor
University of Connecticut
School of Nursing
Storrs, Connecticut
Center for International Community Health Studies
Farmington, Connecticut

Sandra Blake, MS, RN
Infection Control Nurse
Loyola University Medical Center
Maywood, Illinois

Elizabeth O. Dietz, EdD, RN, CS
Professor
San Jose State University
School of Nursing
San Jose, California

Edna E. Johnson, MS, RN
Assistant Professor
University of Connecticut
School of Nursing
Storrs, Connecticut

Carol Love, PhD, RN
Professor and Director,
Graduate Nursing
Simmons College
Graduate School for Health Studies
Boston, Massachusetts

Michael D. Merrill, MJ
Research Assistant, Technology Assessment
Health Care Plan
Buffalo, New York

Eileen Murphy, DNSc, RN
Assistant Professor
University of Connecticut
School of Nursing
Storrs, Connecticut

Marie V. Roberto, DrPH, RN
Chief, Office of Health Policy Development
Department of Health and Addiction Services
State of Connecticut
Hartford, Connecticut

Foreword

Like many life cycles that wax and wane, perspectives in the health care arena are shifting. At the turn of this century, focus was on public health, hygiene, and controlling epidemics. Over the decades, the primary setting for care moved from the community to the acute care institution; emphasis shifted from meticulous cleanliness and personal ministration for the sick to administration of drugs and "high tech" care.

From health status indicators, such as infant mortality rates and immunization statistics, it seems apparent that in the United States, the pendulum has swung so that great efforts and vast resources are expended on individuals (for example, repeat organ transplants, guaranteed dialysis treatment for all individuals with end stage renal disease, and dramatic efforts to save a child with severe immunologic disease), while at the same time, the population as a whole goes underserved in minimal preventive services.

This is not to suggest that we ought to react by putting a halt to technologic advances or reducing our concern for the individual in need of intensive medical intervention, but rather that it is time for the pendulum to swing back for balance. Once again, there is a shift from an institutional to a community location for care, a focus on primary rather than specialized care, movement from curative to preventive care, and emphasis on population-based rather than individual-based decision-making.

Epidemiology derives from the terms, EPI (upon), DEMOS (people), and OLOGY (study). It is the study of events occurring in groups of individuals and a search for the etiology and predictors of these events. Thus, epidemiology focuses on populations. This text is timely. No single nurse has enough experiences on which to base sound clinical decisions. While nurses are and will continue to be the traditional care-givers of individual patients, they must also take a more population-based approach to practice. That is, they must increasingly apply epidemiologic principles to professional practice.

In Chapter 1, the author describes epidemiology as a set of methods or tools as well as a body of knowledge. The contribution of this book is not just that it is a comprehensive and clear presentation of the body of epidemiologic knowledge and methods but that it provides the context necessary to apply epidemiology to the practice of nursing. Each chapter includes clinical applications that illustrate the principles and techniques described as well as supportive tables and figures. These examples not only facilitate learning but also bring the content to life. It is fascinating, for example, to read of the contributions of such historical figures as Farr and Nightingale to the burgeoning sciences of statistics and epidemiology. Their thought processes that went into solving disease mysteries are traced—the same thought processes necessary for clinical problem solving today.

There are other epidemiology texts written for the professional nurse. However, most of these have a specific focus, such as epidemiologic methods in infection prevention and control or in community health, for example. This text is unique in that its scope is comprehensive and the relevance of epidemiology to all aspects of practice is clear. This is a book whose time is now and whose place is with the professional nurse.

Elaine Larson, PhD, RN, FAAN, CIC
Dean and Professor
School of Nursing, Georgetown University
Washington, D.C.

Preface

A characteristic of this era of health care reform is an increased need for nursing care in the community setting. This is and will continue to be a challenge to the problem-solving skills that are fundamental to competent nursing practice. When caring for individual patients or clients, nurses use the nursing process to guide their problem-solving activities. In a similar way, the epidemiologic process should guide problem-solving activities when focusing on groups of people or the aggregate.

Nurses use the body of epidemiologic knowledge about various states of health and illness in clinical decision-making; in assessing individuals and populations at risk; and in planning, implementing and evaluating nursing care and health services. Nurses can also engage in the epidemiologic process as they examine the outcomes of their practice, institute surveillance and screening programs both within and outside of health care institutions, and monitor the quality of nursing care delivered.

The purpose of this book is to provide the background necessary for nurses to integrate principles of epidemiology into practice. The first objective is to present the classic principles of epidemiology from a nursing perspective. A second objective is to explore how nurses can use the body of epidemiologic information about various states of health and illness. The third objective is to demonstrate how nurses can use epidemiologic investigative methods to enhance and evaluate their practices.

Part I presents basic principles of epidemiology, with examples from nursing practice and nursing research whenever possible. A unique feature of this book is the demonstration of concepts through the use of studies in which nurses were often principal investigators or members of the research teams. Chapter 1 introduces the epidemiologic process from a historic perspective and defines the similarities and differences between the nursing process and the epidemiologic process. Chapter 2 presents various conceptual models of epidemiology, along with an explanation of the natural history of disease. Epidemiologic techniques that describe the distribution of health events, such as rate calculations and descriptors of person, time, and place, are discussed in Chapters 3 and 4. A discussion of epidemiologic research methods that are instrumental in identifying determinants of specific health problems follows in Chapters 5 and 6. These include cross-sectional, case-control, cohort, and intervention research study designs. Chapters 7, 8, and 9, focusing on infectious processes, noninfectious processes, and surveillance and screening, help synthesize the content of the first few chapters and provide the introduction for the content in Part II.

In Part II, each chapter demonstrates the extensive use of epidemiologic data; primary, secondary, and tertiary prevention strategies; and epidemiologic research methods in planning, implementing, and evaluating health care. The contributing authors in Part II have had extensive experience in integrating principles of epidemiology into their practice. Their practice sites are diverse, including nurse-managed centers, community health, infection control, occupational health, and health planning and health policy development.

Many people contributed to *Epidemiology in Nursing Practice* in a variety of ways. Heartfelt thanks belong to:

My aunt, *Arla Harkness MacDonald*—for guiding me forward at an early age and stimulating my first interest in sleuthing.

My parents, *Doris and Ronald Kerbs*—for their unfailing support and encouragement.

My children, *Michael and Karen*—for understanding my ambivalent affair with the computer.

My special friends—for picking up the pieces when the going got rough.

Robert Northrop, Paul Levy, Henry Gelfand, and Dale Mattson at the University of Illinois School of Public Health—for cultivating a fledgling epidemiologist.

The contributing authors—for accepting the challenge of explaining how epidemiologic principles are used in practice.

All the students and faculty members at the University of Connecticut, whose reviews and comments contributed to the clarity of the text.

Gail A. Harkness

Contents

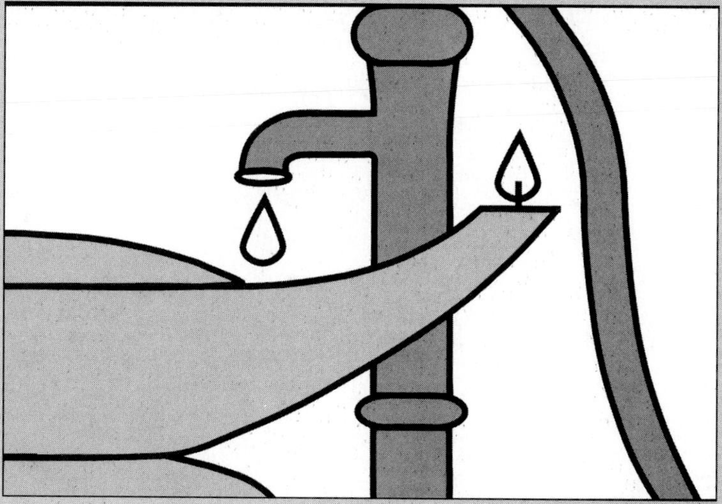

Part I
Epidemiologic Concepts and Nursing Practice

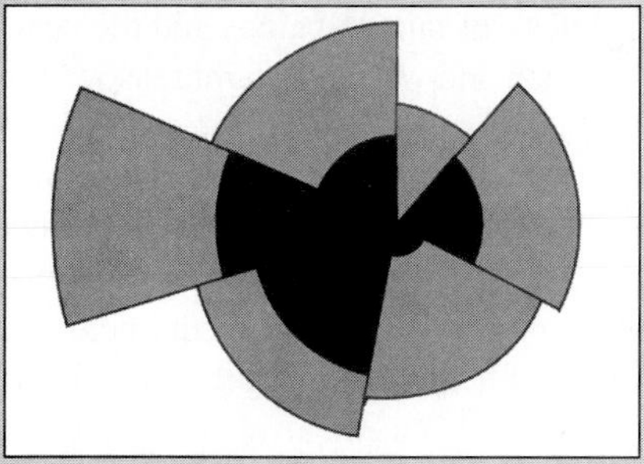

1

Epidemiology as a Basis for Nursing Practice

Objectives

1. Define the basic principles of epidemiology.
2. Explain the evolution of epidemiology from its origin to present time.
3. Describe the contributions of Florence Nightingale to epidemiology.
4. Comprehend the scope of epidemiology.
5. Contrast the epidemiologic process and the nursing process.
6. Interpret the use of epidemiology in nursing practice.
7. Identify sources of epidemiologic data.

Key Terms

body of knowledge
demos
descriptive epidemiology
epi
epidemiologic process
epidemiology
health-event data
logos
methodology
nursing process
polar-area diagram
population-based data
risk
risk factor

The origin of epidemiology lies in the curiosity of human beings and the need to explain the unknown. In ancient times, men and women sought reasons for their illnesses and pursued those activities that were believed to be sources of good health. Cave dwellers experimented with the effects of medicinal plants, and the Egyptians treated crocodile bites with herbal remedies (Davis, 1990). Amulets were used to ward off the worst of fears from wrinkles and impotence to the evil eye and the plague. Health was perceived as something holy in most societies. Healers looked to the spiritual world as a source of healing, uniting the sacred and secular in treating the human being as a whole. Advancement of these ancient healing arts was accomplished through a combination of observation, instinct, inquisitiveness, common sense, and chance.

Men and women today still search for reasons that will explain their illness and pursue those activities and events that they believe will bring them good health. The search for solutions to health problems and for the truth remains, but on a different plane. Today, as we approach the year 2000, scientific knowledge of human physiology has provided an understanding of the complex mechanism that is the human body and has provided the means for modifying and repairing its deficiencies. The application of the scientific method to the study of health events in groups of people using epidemiologic techniques has produced both a comprehensive understanding of the types of health problems that plague many communities and the ability to identify factors that put individuals at risk for certain illnesses. Although the knowledge and technical ability to prevent many health problems now exist, many barriers still remain in the delivery of preventive measures to groups in need.

EPIDEMIOLOGY: ITS DEFINITION

The science of epidemiology emerged from the study of illness in groups of people. *Epidemiology* is defined as the study of the distribution and determinants of states of health and illness in human populations. It is derived from the Greek word meaning epidemic: *epi,* upon; *demos,* people; and *logos,* thought. The goals of epidemiology are to prevent or limit the consequences of illness and disability in humans and maximize their state of health.

Through study of health problems as they occur in groups or populations, many characteristics of specific illnesses or disabilities can be identified that may not be evident in the study of individuals. For instance, the relationship between lung cancer and smoking would probably not have been ascertained by the study of individual people with lung cancer. Many smokers never develop lung cancer, and some nonsmokers do develop lung cancer. However, groups of people with lung cancer have been compared with groups of people without lung cancer. It has been demonstrated clearly that more people with lung cancer had smoked cigarettes than those without lung cancer.

It is only by observing large groups that similarities and differences between people who have, or do not have, a particular condition can be identified. Often people have certain characteristics or engage in specific activities that increase their potential for becoming ill or for developing a health problem. When these associations are found, preventive health measures can be instituted for those populations at high risk, even if the physiologic or environmental causes have not yet been identified.

The clinical practice of nursing, medicine, and other health professions focuses primarily on the health care of individuals. Health care professionals are assisted in their care delivery not only by information about the individual, such as the findings from physical examinations or screening results, but also by knowledge of the distribution of states of illness or wellness according to age, sex, socioeconomic factors, ethnicity, or other factors. Epidemiologic studies provide information about the distribution of illness and wellness, and that information can be used to investigate the factors that determine why that particular state of health exists. In epidemiology the individual patient is replaced by the community as the primary focus of concern (Mausner and Kramer, 1985).

HISTORICAL BACKGROUND

Two epidemiologic concepts that can be traced to ancient times are the influence of the environment on the occurrence of disease and the contagious nature of many diseases (Lilienfeld, 1980). Hippocrates, considered to be the father of modern medicine, was the first to record the concept that the development of illness in humans might be related to external factors in the environment as well as the internal composition of the individual. In the fifth century BC, he urged those who wished to investigate medicine to consider the seasons of the year, winds, waters that people used, origin of those waters, and characteristics of the ground. Hippocrates also addressed life-styles by encouraging the study of the way people live, " . . . and what are their pursuits, whether they are fond of drinking and eating to excess, and given to indolence, or are fond of exercise and labor" (Hippocrates, 1938).

John Graunt

For more than 2000 years, causes of disease in individuals were contemplated, but patterns of disease in populations were not considered. In 1662, John Graunt, a London haberdasher, analyzed the weekly reports of births and deaths (Graunt, 1939). By comparing numbers of men and women, he noted that more male babies were born than female babies and more men died than women. Graunt observed that infant mortality was high and seasonal variations in mortality occurred. He also attempted to statistically assess the impact of the black plague on London's population. Through these activities, Graunt demonstrated the value of examining routinely collected data for clues to human illness and formed the basis for modern epidemiology (Hennekens and Buring, 1987).

William Farr

It was a physician from London nearly 200 years later who established the field of medical statistics. In 1839, William Farr was appointed to the Office of the Registrar General for England and Wales. He recognized, as did John Gaunt, that studying the data from populations of people would provide much information

Table 1-1 Death rates from cholera in London from 1853–1854

Water company	Population in 1851	Cholera deaths in 1853–1854	Deaths per 100,000 living
Southwark and Vauxhall	167,654	192	114
Both companies	301,149	182	60
Lambeth	14,632	0	0

From Snow J: *On the mode of communication of cholera,* ed 2, London, 1855, Churchill.

about human disease. By setting up a system for consistent compilation of the numbers and causes of deaths, Farr was able to compare such events as the death rates of workers in different occupations, the differences in mortality between men and women, and the effect of imprisonment on mortality. He also identified an inverse association between deaths from cholera and sea level—deaths from cholera decreased with an increase in elevation above sea level (Humphreys, 1885).

Farr and his predecessors contributed significantly to the understanding of the frequency and distribution of illness and death. In doing so, they contemplated many methodologic issues that concern epidemiologists today. For example, Farr recognized (1) the necessity for a precise definition of both the onset of the health event and the population that was susceptible to, or at risk for, the health event, (2) the importance of choosing an appropriate comparison group, and (3) that factors existed that could confound the results of statistical studies, such as age, health status, or environmental exposure (Hennekins and Buring, 1987).

John Snow

It was the availability of routinely collected population data that allowed another British physician, John Snow, to investigate the epidemic of cholera that took place from 1848 through 1854. A contemporary of William Farr, Snow used population data along with his own observations to study the epidemic. He noticed that deaths from cholera were particularly high in those areas of London that were supplied by two water companies, the Lambeth Company and the Southwark and Vauxhall Company. The two companies served about two thirds of London's residents, and their water mains were often interwoven in such a manner that houses on the same street or even next door to each other were receiving water from different sources. Both companies obtained water from an area of the Thames River heavily polluted with sewage. However, at some time between 1849 and 1854, the Lambeth Company changed its source of water to a part of the Thames River that was less contaminated. The rates of cholera declined in those areas that were supplied by the Lambeth Company, but rates of cholera remained the same in those areas supplied by the Southwark and Vauxhall Company.

Snow demonstrated these findings clearly in his investigation of a particularly severe cholera outbreak between August 1853 and January 1854. During that period, he calculated the number of deaths from cholera according to the companies that supplied the water in the subdistricts of London (Table 1-1). The areas of London supplied by Southwark and Vauxhall had 114 cholera deaths per 100,000 people, while the area supplied by Lambeth Company had no deaths from cholera. In those areas supplied by both companies, there were 60 deaths per 100,000 people. The most severe outbreak occurred in the area of Broad Street, Golden Square, where more than 500 people died from cholera within 10 days. Believing contaminated water to be the source of the epidemic, John Snow was successful in removing the handle from a contaminated pump and "staying the epidemic." Today, a plaque near the John Snow Tavern, on the corner of Broad Street in Soho, London commemorates this event (Figs. 1-1 and 1-2).

Snow recognized the opportunity to test his hypothesis that contaminated water was related to cholera by making use of the natural experiment that existed.

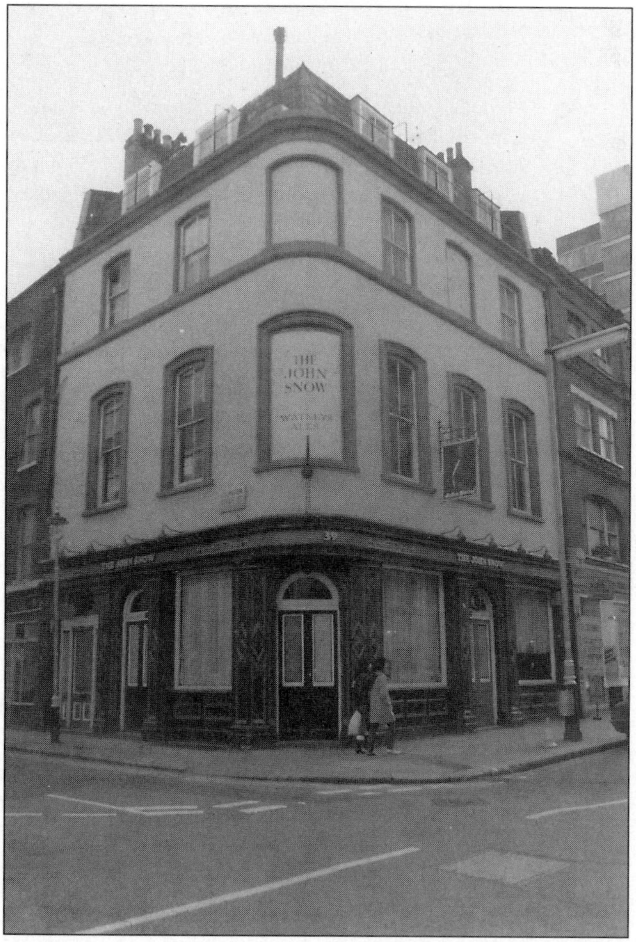

Fig. 1-1 The John Snow Tavern, London.

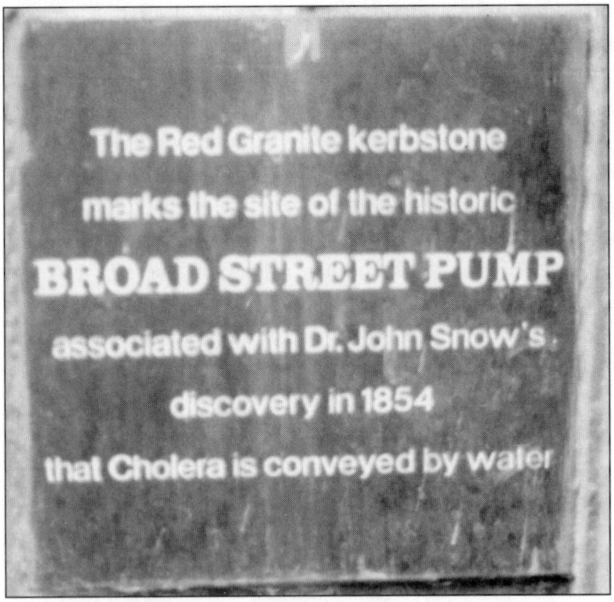

Fig. 1-2 Commemorative plaque honoring Dr. John Snow's discovery that cholera was associated with contaminated water.

He actually walked from house to house in the area served by the two water companies and was able to determine the source of water for every dwelling. He noted that no experiment could have been devised that would test the relationship between cholera and the water supply more thoroughly. More than 300,000 people of each sex and every age, occupation, and socioeconomic group were divided into two groups without their choice and, often, without their knowledge. One group received water contaminated with the sewage of London, and the other group did not. The results were dramatic (Table 1-2). However, Snow also was aware that it was possible that many other factors could account for the differ-

Table 1-2 Death rates from cholera by house in London from 1853–1854, (according to the water company supplying the individual house)

Water company	Number of houses	Deaths from cholera	Deaths per 10,000 houses
Southwark and Vauxhall	40,046	1263	315
Lambeth	26,107	98	37
Rest of London	256,423	1422	59

From Snow J: *On the mode of communication of cholera,* ed 2, London, 1855, Churchill.

ences in cholera rates, and he investigated variations in the data as possible clues to further understanding of the epidemic. Snow's achievements were remarkable for the times. As one of the first epidemiologists, he outlined the frequency and distribution of cholera and found evidence of a cause or determinant of the outbreak. Snow logically organized data, recognized and analyzed a natural experiment, and did so prior to the era of bacteriology.

Florence Nightingale

Florence Nightingale was also a contemporary of William Farr and John Snow. The daughter of a wealthy British landowner, she devoted her life to the prevention of needless illness and death with fierce determination. Many of her compelling arguments, which were ultimately successful in bringing about health care reforms, were based on her pioneering use of statistics. She is best known as both a reformer of hospital care and the founder of professional nursing.

At the age of 33 and despite family protests, Florence Nightingale was able to start her chosen career of nursing. Not only was the pursuit of a career a radical step for a woman of her social class, but at that time, nurses were also perceived as coarse, ignorant, and promiscuous. In 1853, she became superintendent of a London hospital. She supervised nurses and the operation of the physical plant and was responsible for the purity of the medicines. A year later, the British and French troops invaded the Crimea on the north coast of the Black Sea in support of Turkey in its dispute with Russia. Nightingale volunteered her services. Accompanied by 38 nurses, she left for the Crimea with official backing of the government (Cohen, 1984).

When Nightingale arrived at the British military hospital in Scutari, near Constantinople in Turkey, she was appalled by the conditions of the hospital barracks. The buildings were infested with fleas and rats, an open sewer ran under the buildings, facilities were over-crowded, linen was filthy, and essential supplies were missing. As well as suffering from wounds, the British army was ravaged by dysentery, malnutrition, frostbite, and diseases, such as cholera, typhus, and scurvy. The mortality rate was 42.7% of the cases treated at the hospital (Cohen, 1984).

At Scutari, Nightingale not only initiated sanitary reforms but also systematized record-keeping. Until that time, the number of deaths had not been recorded accurately. The polar-area diagram found in Fig. 1-3 was designed by Florence Nightingale to dramatize the needless deaths in the British military hospitals during the Crimean War. The size of the wedges, colored in her original diagrams, is proportional to the statistic represented. Here, the white wedges represent deaths from wounds, the gray wedges represent preventable deaths, and the dark wedges represent deaths from all other causes. Deaths peaked in January 1855 when 2700 soldiers died from infectious disease; only 83 soldiers died from wounds. Based on the average army population of 32,393 during that month, Nightingale calculated an average mortality rate of 1174 per 1000 soldiers. If the dead soldiers had not been replaced, the entire British army in the Crimea would have been wiped out by infectious disease (Aiken, 1988; Cohen, 1984).

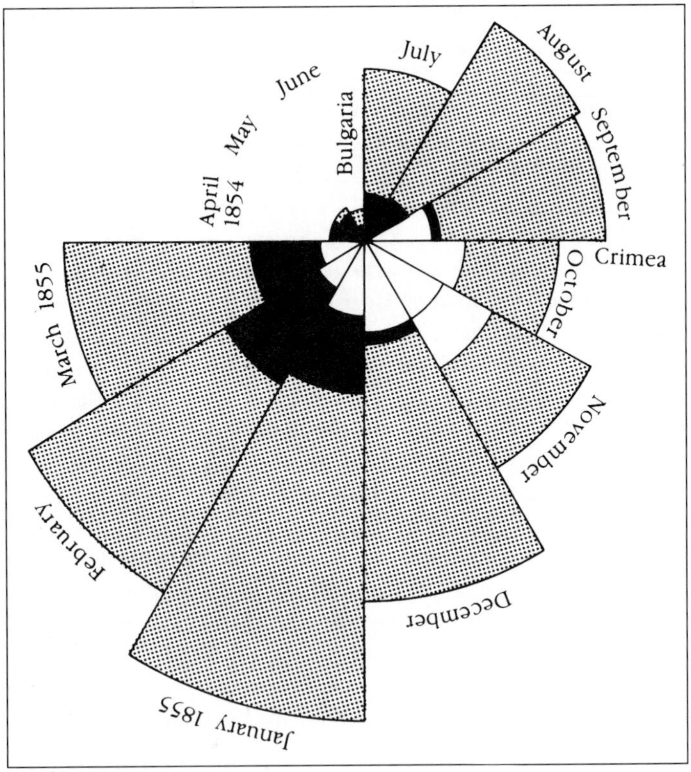

Fig. 1-3 Nightingale's polar-area diagram. The polar-area diagram was invented by Florence Nightingale to dramatize the extent of needless deaths in British military hospitals during the Crimean War (1854-1856). She called these diagrams "coxcombs." The area of each colored wedge, measured from the center, is proportional to the statistic being represented. Gray wedges represent deaths from preventable or mitigable zymotic diseases (contagious diseases such as cholera and typhus). White wedges represent deaths from wounds and dark wedges represent deaths from all other causes. Mortality in the British hospitals peaked in January, 1855, when 2761 soldiers died of contagious diseases, 83 of wounds and 324 of other causes for a total of 3168. Based on the army's average strength of 32,393 in the Crimea that month, Nightingale computed an annual mortality rate of 1176 per 1000. The diagram is taken from Nightingale's book, *Notes on Matters Affecting the Health, Efficiency and Hospital Administration of the British Army* (1858). Half of the diagram, representing the period from April, 1855, to March, 1856, does not appear. (From Aiken L: Assuring the delivery of quality patient care, *State of the Science Invitational Conference: Nursing resources and the delivery of patient care,* NIH Publication No. 89-3008: 3-10, Washington, DC, 1988, US Department of Health and Human Services, Public Health Service; Cohen B: Florence Nightingale, *Sci Am* 250(3):129, 1984.)

Another example of Nightingale's proficiency for using statistics to illustrate her concerns is a diagram of mortality rates both before and after her sanitary reforms were instituted in the military hospitals (Fig. 1-4). This diagram reflects both the impact of disease and the effects of the improved sanitary conditions. In

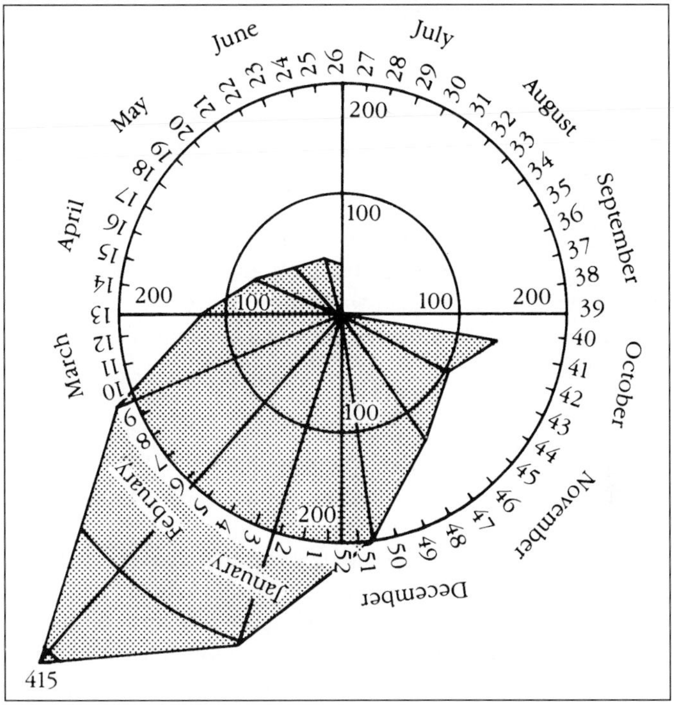

Fig. 1-4 Mortality rate as calculated by Nightingale. Mortality rate at Scutari, the main British hospital in the Crimean War, declined sharply after sanitary improvements were made under Nightingale's influence. In the winter of 1854-1855 the British was besieged by army malnutrition, exposure, and infectious disease, including dysentery, cholera, typhus, and scurvy. The death rate at Scutari, calculated here by Nightingale on an annual basis as a fraction of the patient population, reached 415% in February. Sanitary reforms began in March. This diagram is taken from the report of a Royal Commission set up after the war to investigate sanitary conditions in the army. (From Aiken L: Assuring the delivery of quality patient care, *State of the Science Invitational Conference: Nursing resources and the delivery of patient care,* NIH Publication No. 89-3008: 3-10, Washington, DC, 1988, US Department of Health and Human Services, Public Health Service; Cohen B: Florence Nightingale, *Sci Am* 250(3):131, 1984.)

February 1855, the death rate reached 415% but dropped dramatically during the following months. By the end of the war in 1856, the death rate among British soldiers in the Crimea was less than that of the troops at home (Cohen, 1984).

Florence Nightingale met William Farr soon after her return to England in 1856. With his help, she quickly recognized the potential of the statistics she had gathered at Scutari and of medical statistics in general. She compared the mortality among civilians to that among soldiers and found that in peacetime, soldiers in England had a mortality rate nearly twice that of civilian males. Nightingale argued that these unnecessary deaths could only be prevented by instituting the same sanitary reforms that were shown to be effective in the Crimea. Farr was impressed with her observations, calling them a "light shining in a dark place"

(Cope, 1958). She asked for and received a formal investigation of military health care, and eventually, her sanitary reforms were implemented.

During this period of time, there was a controversy among professionals in London between the contagionists and the noncontagionists. Contagionists believed that diseases such as smallpox, measles, scarlatina, whooping cough, typhus, syphilis, and particularly cholera could be communicated from one person to another and therefore believed that quarantine was the best means of control of these illnesses. Noncontagionists did not believe in the direct communication of these diseases or quarantine, but they advocated for sanitary measures to control these illnesses. Nightingale was a firm noncontagionist, believing that evil had been done to people in the name of contagion and through the use of quarantine. As a result, she held the work of her contemporary John Snow in low esteem. The literature indicates that Dr. Farr corresponded with her about this issue, attempting to induce her to be less dogmatic and more open-minded on issues that were still unproven (Cope, 1958). We now know that the beliefs of the contagionists and the noncontagionists were not mutually exclusive and that arguments on both sides of this issue were correct.

Florence Nightingale continued her lifelong career devoted to health-care reform, and much of her work was shared with William Farr. She studied the health of soldiers in India, investigated mortality in British hospitals, studied mortality following surgery, and developed a system for gathering data in hospitals. She experimented with graphs and diagrams so that everyone could understand her views and struggled to introduce statistics into higher education. Florence Nightingale effectively demonstrated that statistics provide an organized way of learning from experience, and as a pioneering epidemiologist, she used the concept of rate calculation (see Chapter 3) to emphasize her major points.

THE SCOPE OF EPIDEMIOLOGY

Since the techniques of epidemiologic investigation were first developed in the mid-nineteenth century when cholera and the plague were still killing much of the population of Europe, epidemiology has traditionally been associated with the study of infectious diseases. Similarly, measures for prevention and control have centered on altering the characteristics of the infectious agent, host, or environment (see Chapter 2).

The scope of epidemiology has been expanded and changed in recent years. Not only are the distribution and determinants of disease studied, but variables that contribute to the maintenance of health are also studied. Epidemiologic techniques have been used to identify the characteristics of people at high risk for noninfectious diseases, such as cancer and stroke and determine the factors that contribute to their cause. The distribution and determinants of psychosocial problems, such as alcoholism, drug abuse, child abuse, and suicide have been investigated. The epidemiologic literature addressing occupational injuries and diseases has expanded in recent years along with studies of environmental problems. Epidemiologic methodology is widely accepted in planning and evaluating health services.

Table 1-3 Comparison of the leading causes of death in the United States between 1900 and 1990

1900	1990
1. Major cardiovascular-renal diseases	1. Diseases of the heart
2. Influenza and pneumonia	2. Malignant neoplasms
3. Tuberculosis	3. Cardiovascular accidents
4. Gastritis, duodenitis, enteritis, and colitis	4. Accidents
5. Accidents	5. Chronic obstructive pulmonary diseases
6. Malignant neoplasms	6. Pneumonia and influenza
7. Diphtheria	7. Diabetes mellitus
8. Typhoid and paratyphoid fever	8. Suicide
9. Measles	9. Chronic liver disease and cirrhosis
10. Cirrhosis of liver	10. HIV infection
11. Whooping cough	11. Homicide and legal intervention
12. Syphilis and its sequelae	12. Nephritis, nephrotic syndrome, and nephrosis

*Excludes fetal deaths

Data from: US Bureau of the Census: *Historical statistics of the United States, colonial times to 1970, bicentennial edition, Part 2,* Washington, DC, 1975, US Government Printing Office; US Bureau of Census, *Statistical abstracts of the United States: 1993,* ed 113, Washington, DC, 1993, US Government Printing Office.

The evolving changes in patterns of disease, methods of control, prevention of health problems, and the need for maintaining wellness have contributed to this shift in the scope of epidemiology. Improved public health practices, such as maintenance of uncontaminated water supplies, provision for waste disposal, and the availability of a variety of food, lead to the decline in deaths from communicable diseases in the early twentieth century. Consequently, life expectancy has risen, and the United States and other developed countries are facing a change in the types of health problems affecting their populations. Noninfectious diseases and chronic degenerative conditions have increased (Table 1-3). At the same time, there have been changes in diagnostic practices, advances in treatment methodology, shifts in the demographic characteristics of the population, and an increased complexity of life associated with a technologic society. In order to meet the present and future health care needs of society, (1) problems and needs should be identified, (2) data should be collected and analyzed to identify factors that influence those problems or needs, and (3) plans for prevention and control should be implemented and evaluated. These steps form the basis of epidemiologic investigation (Hood, 1985).

THE EPIDEMIOLOGIC PROCESS AND THE NURSING PROCESS

Both the *epidemiologic process* and the *nursing process* have evolved from the problem-solving process. Both are designed to provide a framework for investi-

Table 1-4 Comparison of the nursing process and the epidemiologic process

Nursing process	Epidemiologic process
Assessment Establish data base about client	Establish nature, extent, and scope of problem by defining problem and gathering information from reliable sources
Diagnosis Interpret data, identify health care needs, select goals of care	Describe problem by person, place, and time Formulate tentative hypothesis Analyze detailed data to test hypothesis
Planning Select process for achieving goals	Plan for control or prevention of the condition or event
Implementation Initiate and complete actions to achieve goals	Implement plan
Evaluation Determine extent of goal achievement	Evaluate plan Prepare appropriate report Conduct further research

*Adapted from Anderson JE, Yoder KK, Daufman JS: In Phipps WJ, Long BC, Woods NF: *Medical surgical nursing, concepts and clinical practice,* ed 3, St Louis, Mosby, 1987.

gating health-related problems, obtaining new knowledge, and planning, implementing, and evaluating specific interventions (Table 1-4). Each process requires abstract, critical-thinking skills and complex reasoning abilities. Nurses use the nursing process to assess, diagnose, plan, implement, and evaluate care for individuals with specific problems or to plan for maintenance of wellness. The epidemiologic investigative process can be used in the same fashion to assess community (group) needs, identify factors that influence those needs, plan and implement prevention and control measures, and evaluate outcomes.

In any investigative process, the nature, extent, and scope of the problem must be clearly defined. This requires gathering data that will be carefully assessed, interpreted, and used to define the problem. In the epidemiologic process, data about the problem are then described by the characteristics of person, place, and time. This is termed *descriptive epidemiology.* When as much information has been obtained as possible, critical-thinking and reasoning skills are used to formulate tentative hypotheses, or probable assumptions, that may explain the occurrence of the problem. The detailed data are then analyzed to test the hypothesis. Depending on the nature of the problem, formal analytic epidemiologic research studies may be undertaken. The results of the analysis, whether it is descriptive, analytical, or both, are then used to plan, implement, and evaluate measures to control the condition or event. Results of the investigative process must be communicated appropriately, and often, this will lead to further research of the problem (Fig. 1-5).

USING EPIDEMIOLOGIC PRINCIPLES IN PRACTICE

Epidemiology emerged as a discipline because of the need to determine the etiology of disease conditions so that prevention and control measures could be instituted. Epidemiologic data supply information about the natural history of the disease. This includes the process by which it occurs, how it progresses within the population, and what outcomes may be expected (see Chapter 2). This basic use of the principles of epidemiology is still essential to the practice of health professionals.

Epidemiology can be considered both as a *methodology* used to study human health conditions and as the *body of knowledge* that results from the study of a specific health condition. The practice of nurses and other health care professionals can be enhanced by both approaches. However, rather than focusing on the investigation of the etiology or the natural history of a disease, nurses and other health care professionals most often use principles of epidemiology to (1) enhance the clinical decision-making process, especially as a foundation for choosing appropriate interventions, (2) identify people and populations at risk for threats to health, and (3) plan, implement, and evaluate health services.

Clinical decision-making

Altered states of health create problems that reflect a discrepancy between what exists and what could or should exist. In turn, these problems present the need for

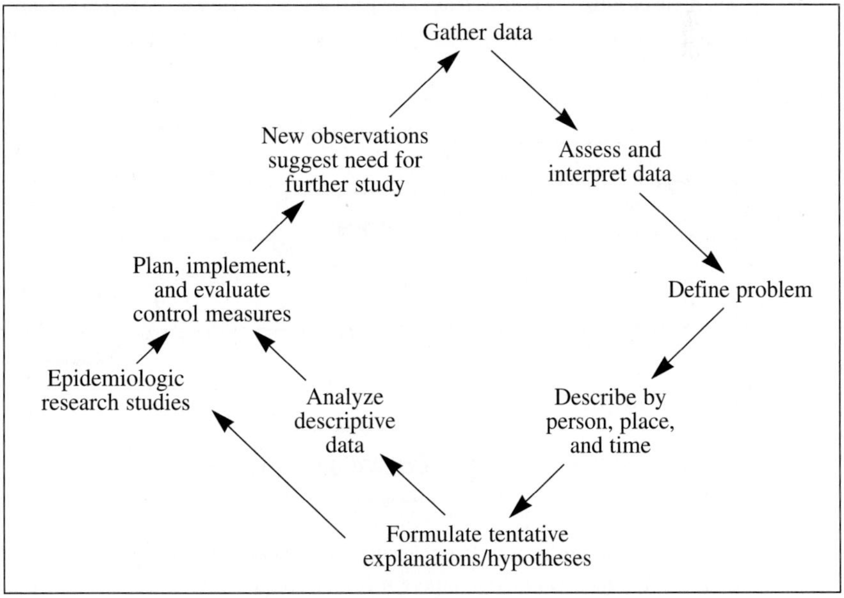

Fig. 1-5 Model of the epidemiologic process

making decisions about actions that may modify those problems. Nursing by definition is the diagnosis and treatment of human responses to actual or potential health problems (American Nurses' Association, 1980). Therefore nursing practice is based on clinical decision-making skills. These decision-making skills underlie the choice of nursing interventions that hopefully will provide optimal outcomes for patients or clients with actual or potential health problems.

Decision-making is a process that requires sufficient knowledge of the problem, the patient, and his or her environment. Critical-thinking skills are then used for appropriate analysis of this information. Although optimal decision-making is more likely to occur when done in a logical, sequential manner, a systematic method for making decisions was not often taught to clinicians in the past. Many clinicians, although benefiting from a knowledge base in health care, still rely on intuition and past experiences in their decision-making. However, the nursing process provides us with systematic observational and problem-solving techniques involving a dynamic process of continuous assessment, diagnosis, planning, intervention, and evaluation (Fig. 1-6). The effectiveness and efficiency of nursing interventions depend on the accurate use of the nursing process (Carpenito, 1989). The ability to make rational decisions that lead to optimal outcomes is a primary characteristic of an expert nurse clinician.

The epidemiologic body of knowledge that results from the study of specific conditions contributes significantly to the development of the knowledge base that is necessary for competent and successful clinical decision-making. It is particularly helpful in the initial assessment of a person's health status but can be used in all stages of the nursing process. Additional epidemiologic information also can be obtained at each stage using appropriate epidemiologic methodology.

Assessment. On entering a health facility, whether it be a community clinic, long-term care institution, or an acute care hospital, the nurse is usually the first

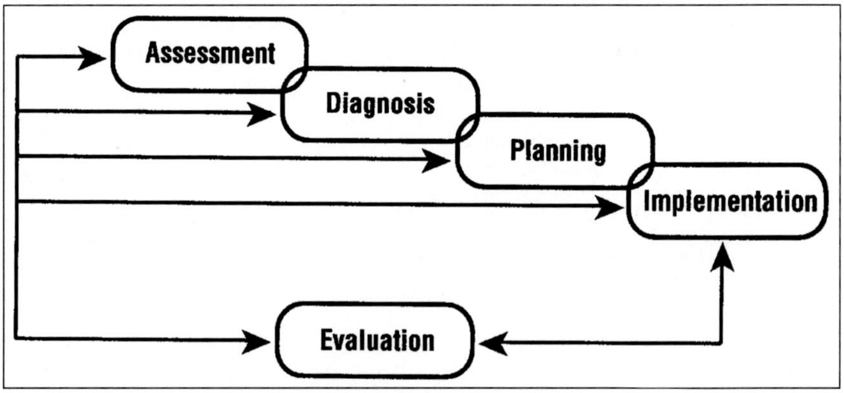

Fig. 1-6 Interrelationships between the steps of the nursing process. (Adapted from Alfaro R: *Application of the nursing process: a step-by-step guide,* Philadelphia, 1986, JB Lippincott.)

to assess the patient. This assessment includes systematically observing the patient, performing a nursing physical assessment, and differentiating between cues or observable findings and inferences or interpretations (Carpenito, 1989). One of the first decisions that is made in an assessment is whether the person is well or ill. The nurse should identify where the person is in relation to the full spectrum of health and identify his or her problems and needs. Planning and intervention are based on this assessment. Often, the clinical significance of an observation can be determined by comparing the characteristics of the person to the characteristics of similar people in the general population. For instance, a blood pressure of 140/90 may be abnormal and require treatment in a 25-year-old person but may be normal in a 70-year-old person. Knowledge of the natural progression of an illness is also provided through epidemiologic studies. The characteristics, frequency, and timing of signs and symptoms is essential information for client assessment and subsequent decisions regarding planning and intervention.

Diagnosis. Similarly, epidemiologic information is helpful to nurses in deriving diagnoses. In many community settings, such as industry, nurse-managed clinics, and private practice, nurses function autonomously in the delivery of health care. Nurses in advanced practice (1) infer and classify the status of the patient based on available data, (2) make medical diagnosis judgments about patients' pathophysiologic health status, (3) obtain clinical laboratory data, (4) prescribe intervention measures, and (5) follow patient progress. Knowledge of risk factors predisposing to illness and an understanding of the natural progression of illnesses are essential components of these activities.

Nursing diagnosis involves critical-thinking skills and focuses on identifying patterns, validating findings, and arriving at conclusions. Many nursing diagnoses use the concept of risk in identifying potential problems. For example, using knowledge of specific risk factors, the nurse is diagnosing a state of risk when the following nursing diagnosis is made: "Potential Altered Health Maintenance, related to lack of knowledge of adequate diet and daily nutritional requirements and living alone" (Carpenito, 1989). The diagnosis of potential altered health maintenance is based on epidemiologic knowledge about the influence of diet and socioeconomic factors on health.

Planning and implementation. Knowledge of the normal progress of an altered state of health that results from epidemiologic studies provides information that is useful in predicting patient outcomes. Therefore this information is helpful in planning for and choosing interventions. Advantages and disadvantages of specific actions can be weighed, and a course of action for an individual can be chosen. For example, epidemiologic data can help nurses in decisions to initiate a specific type of decubitus care to a diabetic patient, counsel an adolescent clinic patient regarding HIV exposure, or recommend a hospice referral. Nursing interventions that are chosen for each individual are usually intended to change patient outcomes, and therefore must be evaluated carefully for their benefit versus potential harm.

Evaluation. The epidemiologic body of knowledge that exists about specific states of health is also helpful in evaluating patient progress and patient outcomes and determining the effects of interventions for people at specific stages of illness. Data regarding the distribution and determinants of a patient's status at specific stages of treatment are a basic component of critical pathways that have been developed by many acute care hospitals and home health care facilities for evaluation purposes.

These critical pathways, developed jointly by physicians and nurses, reflect both scientific knowledge about patients' conditions at specific treatment stages and professional consensus. The expected progression of patients are outlined on a daily basis. Using a patient with a coronary artery bypass graft as an example, criteria are presented for evaluating patients preoperatively, the day of surgery, and 7 days postoperatively according to their educational needs, activity level, nutritional status, medications, diagnostic criteria, and treatment expectations. Each patient's progress is evaluated daily based on these average expectations. Nurse researchers should now use the developing data bases to evaluate the effects of specific nursing interventions.

Epidemiologic methodology can also be used to determine the frequency and reasons for specific patient outcomes. Differences in the frequency of specific outcomes for different groups can be studied using descriptive and analytic techniques. For instance, the characteristics of patients who have a high postoperative infection rate could be described and compared with those patients who are free of infection postoperatively.

Identification of people and populations at risk

Using an epidemiologic body of knowledge regarding specific health problems is more common than often realized. One of the most common ways is to assess individuals according to risk factors that have been associated with a health event through prior research. *Risk* refers to the probability or likelihood that a health event will occur in a group of people currently free of the problem. *Risk factors* are those characteristics or events that have been shown to increase the probability of developing a health event. While risk factors are indicators of an increased probability of a specific outcome, they may or may not be directly related to the cause of the health problem. For example, socioeconomic status or ethnicity may be risk factors for some conditions, but they are not directly related to the cause of the problem. However, exposure to an infectious agent is directly related to the cause of an infectious disease.

Usually a combination of risk factors can be identified that place people at high risk. These combinations may include the biologic characteristics of individuals, their behavior, stressful life events, or environmental exposure. Knowledge of the combination of factors that place people at particularly high risk for detrimental outcomes, such as coronary artery disease, can be applied to individuals during a health-risk appraisal. Some risk factors are modifiable, and some are not. Interventions that focus on reducing an individual's modifiable risk factors, such as encouraging changes in life-style, can alter outcomes, possibly preventing the onset of coronary artery disease in this example. Risk of coronary artery disease is associated with a sedentary life-style, smoking, obesity, hypertension, and other modifiable risk factors. Knowledge of these cardiac risk factors is the basis for promotion of exercise as a component of healthy life-styles, smoking-cessation clinics, weight-loss programs, and emphasis on the need to control blood pressure. As a result, life-style changes and health monitoring have been successful in preventing acute, premature heart attacks.

Using appropriate epidemiologic methodology, nurses can investigate or determine the factors that combine to place patients or clients at high risk for specific outcomes of care. For example, in the acute care setting, a clinical specialist in a surgical intensive care unit could gather data on patient characteristics and the surgical intervention to look for factors associated with the development of postoperative pneumonia. In an ambulatory setting, a nurse could examine the treatment and characteristics of clients who were or were not successful in controlling their hypertension. Information from both of these studies could lead to the development of alternative intervention strategies targeting high-risk people.

Epidemiologic methodology also can be used in identifying populations at risk. This is a primary role of the public health nurse. Epidemiologic surveillance of populations includes the investigation and description of who is involved (age, socioeconomic group, etc.), what the nature of the problem is, where it is occurring geographically, when it is manifest in time, and how health events occur (see Chapters 4 and 9). Careful monitoring of this information alerts health officials of emerging problems, such as disease outbreaks or community problems.

Planning, implementing, and evaluating health services

Using the data provided by epidemiologic surveillance of community health, health services can be planned to meet the needs of the community. Health planning is essential prior to services being implemented, and measures for evaluation of cost-effectiveness should be developed prior to implementation (see Chapter 14). Early detection methods, screening sessions, or preventive programs can be designed to control or prevent the problem. For example, statistics that indicate an increase of breast cancer, hypertension, and influenza in a community may result in breast self-examination education programs (early detection), vans that provide blood pressure monitoring (screening), and influenza immunization programs for the elderly and other high-risk groups (prevention). Communities characterized by a high birth rate and few financial resources will have need for family planning clinics, well-child clinics, and prenatal care facilities. Other communities with a high proportion of elderly people can be expected to have high rates of cardiovascular disease and other chronic conditions. Access to health care may be a problem, and resources for health monitoring, home care, meals, and transportation may be needed.

Epidemiologic data that are used to establish the need for health services can also be used to evaluate those services. The only way to demonstrate that a health problem was prevented or controlled is to compare epidemiologic statistics before and after the implementation of the health service. Planning and evaluation is a continuous process. As new data become available, modifications in health services can be made, and those modifications require evaluation.

SOURCES OF EPIDEMIOLOGIC DATA

Any health-related information that has been compiled about a group of people can be a source of data used to describe the distribution and determinants of states of health. Traditional sources of epidemiologic data are those collected routinely by national or state governments that are *population-based data.* Other sources of epidemiologic data regarding health-related events include the records of disease registries, health care institutions, insurance companies, industries, private physician offices, accident and police records, surveys, and any other place where statistics are gathered about people and factors that influence health. These sources are based on *health-event data.*

Population-based data

Epidemiologic data based on population statistics include the census, vital-statistic records of births (natality) and deaths (mortality), and morbidity records. The importance of data about the population is recognized by governments throughout the world. Population statistics form the basis for accurate description of the health status of the population and are the principle source of the denominator data required for the calculation of incidence and prevalence of health problems (see Chapter 3).

Many countries perform a population census every 10 years. In the United States, the Census of the Population has been taken every 10 years since 1790. While the original purpose of the census was to count people for equal representation in the House of Representatives, through the years, the census has expanded. Demographic data and some characteristics about housing are gathered from all people. Nativity, migration, education, employment status, income, and other characteristics are obtained from a random sample of the population. This census data is essential for health planning but is currently limited by the fact that it is conducted on a decennial basis and is not available for several years following its collection. The ever-growing, increasingly mobile world community requires more frequent enumeration of the population.

Health-event data

Beginning with the efforts of John Graunt in 1662, records of vital events, such as births and deaths, have become a primary source of information about the health of a population. In the United States, this is a function of state governments. In 1979, a National Death Index was established by the federal government to centralize and index the information. Mortality statistics are compiled from the information found in death certificates and are regularly published by all nations (Last, 1988). Often, mortality statistics are broken down by age, sex, ethnicity, cause, and other descriptors of person, place, and time. Rates of death in various populations are commonly calculated for public health purposes and provide indices of the health of communities. Also, many traditional epidemiologic studies have been based on the mortality data of a population. Mortality statistics are further described in Chapter 3.

Morbidity is defined as an objective or subjective departure from a state of physiologic or psychologic well-being (Last, 1988). Morbidity statistics may or may not be population-based. Governments usually require that the morbidity of certain communicable diseases, such as childhood diseases or sexually transmitted diseases, be routinely reported. The Centers for Disease Control (CDC) of the US Department of Health and Human Services collects data about reportable diseases and also monitors the health of the population. Through its surveillance functions, the CDC investigates many conditions that place people at high risk for illness or disability and therefore might be prevented. Examples include alcohol and drug abuse, tobacco use, accidents, suicides, drownings, fertility, congenital malformations, and occupational injuries and diseases. Morbidity and mortality statistics are published weekly in the *Morbidity and Mortality Weekly Report* prepared by the CDC.

Morbidity statistics from reportable diseases are population-based, but other morbidity statistics may be based on survey data or data obtained from institutional records. These data are not based on the total population and therefore may provide a biased view of the illness in a community. This must be taken into consideration when studies of the determinants of specific health problems are undertaken. Morbidity statistics are discussed in more detail in Chapter 3.

Nurses use existing epidemiologic data in critical decision-making, identifying people or populations at high risk, and planning, implementing, and evaluating health programs. Nurses also can gather epidemiologic data to describe a wide variety of problems, from investigating outbreaks of hospital-associated infections to studying the factors related to readmission of patients with congestive heart failure. Medical records are often used for this purpose. Through calculation and comparison of rates, people can be identified who are at risk for specific outcomes of care. Descriptive and analytic epidemiologic techniques can then be used to study determinants of these outcomes.

SUMMARY

Epidemiology is defined as the study of the distribution and determinants of states of health and illness in human populations. The science of epidemiology emerged from the need to determine the cause of disease conditions so that prevention and control measures could be implemented. By observing groups of people rather than individuals, similarities and differences between people who have or do not have health problems can be identified. The scope of epidemiology, while focused initially on the investigation of infectious diseases, has expanded and changed in recent years. The study of the distribution and determinants of noninfectious disease, psychosocial problems, occupational injuries, and environmental problems are examples. In addition, principles of epidemiology are used in planning and evaluating health services.

Both the epidemiologic process and the nursing process have evolved from the problem-solving process and provide a framework for investigating health-related problems, obtaining new knowledge, and initiating interventions. Nurses and other health professionals engaged in clinical practice use principles of epidemiology primarily in clinical decision-making, identifying people and populations at high risk, and planning, implementing, and evaluating health services. Epidemiologic data can be obtained from population statistics, notification systems, such as diseases reportable to the Centers for Disease Control, and the records in community health organizations and hospitals.

Critical Thinking Questions

1. From clinical practice, identify two examples that illustrate how epidemiologic knowledge can assist clinical decision-making.
2. During a health history, the following information is collected from Mr. X: age 50, height 5 ft. 10 in., weight 240 pounds, BP 190/90, cholesterol level of 240 mg/dl, 40-pack years of smoking, father died at age 45, cause myocardial infarction.

   For what disease processes is Mr. X at risk?

   Identify appropriate intervention to develop with Mr. X to modify his risk?

   Explain how epidemiologic knowledge influenced your responses to the above questions.
3. Of Community C's population, 20% is 65 years of age or older. Based on this limited information identify two preventive health programs for Community C.

REFERENCES

Aiken L: Assuring the delivery of quality patient care, *State of the Science Invitational Conference: nursing resources and the delivery of patient care,* NIH Publication No. 89-3008: 3-10, Washington, DC, 1988, US Department of Health and Human Services, Public Health Service.

Alfaro R: *Application of nursing process: a step-by-step guide,* Philadelphia, 1986, JB Lippincott.

American Nurses' Association: *Nursing: a social policy statement,* Kansas City, MO, 1980, The Association.

Carpenito LJ: *Nursing diagnosis, application to clinical practice,* Philadelphia, 1989, JB Lippincott.

Cohen IB: Florence Nightingale, *Sci Am, 250,* (3):128-137, 1984.

Cope Z: *Florence Nightingale and the doctors,* Philadelphia, 1958, JB Lippincott, pp 98-107.

Davis W: The many paths of a healer. In Smolan R, Moffit P, Naythons M: *The power to heal, ancient arts and modern medicine,* New York, 1990, Prentice Hall, pp 11-26.

Graunt J: *Natural and political observations made upon the bills of mortality: London, 1662,* Baltimore, 1939, Johns Hopkins Press.

Hennekens CH, Buring JE: *Epidemiology in medicine,* Boston, 1987, Little, Brown.

Hood GH: Epidemiology. In Jarvis LL: *Community health nursing: keeping the public healthy,* Philadelphia, 1985, FA Davis, pp 59-70.

Hippocrates: On airs, waters, and places, translated and republished in *Med Classics* 3:19-42, 1938.

Humphreys NA: *Vital Statistics: A memorial volume of selections from the reports and writings of William Farr, 1807-1883,* London, 1885, Sanitary Institute of Great Britain.

Last JM: *A dictionary of epidemiology,* New York, 1988, Oxford University Press.

Lilienfeld AM: *Foundations of epidemiology,* ed 2, New York, 1980, Oxford University Press.

Mausner JS, Kramer S: *Epidemiology—an introductory text,* ed 2, Philadelphia, 1985, WB Saunders.

Snow J: *On the mode of communication of cholera,* London, 1855, Churchill. Reproduced in *Snow on cholera,* New York, 1965, Hafner.

2

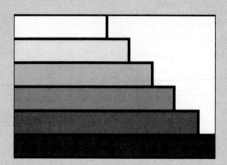

Epidemiology and Health Promotion

Objectives

1. Define the spectrum of health in terms of the individual.
2. Explain the relationship between the spectrum of health and the epidemiologic process.
3. Trace the conceptualization of health as it has evolved during the twentieth century.
4. Discuss the potential of nurse-initiated health promotion activities to reduce individual risk factors for illness.
5. Analyze the interaction of host, agent, and environment in epidemiologic models.
6. Relate the natural history of disease to the three levels of prevention.

Key Terms

- agents
  - biologic
  - chemical
  - nutrient
  - physical
  - psychologic
- environmental factors
  - biologic, physical, social
- epidemiologic triad
- health promotion
- host factors
- primary prevention
- risk factors
- secondary prevention
- spectrum of health
- tertiary prevention

The *spectrum of health* encompasses many diverse levels or phases of the human condition, extending from optimal wellness through illness and/or disability to death. The health spectrum for any individual, family, or group is never static but changes continuously as we grow and develop while interacting with our environments. The science of epidemiology describes, explains, and predicts the patterns of wellness and illness that constitute the phases of the spectrum of health. Epidemiologic studies also provide information about factors that influence the development of these patterns of health. Such information is vital for nurses in their efforts to facilitate health promotion, disease prevention, and the maintenance of optimal health and function.

CONCEPTS OF HEALTH

The way that health is defined and perceived has direct bearing on the health behaviors all of us pursue and the health services and programs that health care providers make available (see Fig. 2-1). For example, the long-held definition of health as the absence of disease has led health to be perceived only in negative terms of nondisease. In other words, health needs have been identified in terms of the pathologic changes of disease; individuals take health actions only in response to signs and symptoms of disease; and health policies and services are disease-oriented. Use of this definition has failed to emphasize health-promotion and disease-prevention services in the United States and in other nations. Thus a limited definition of health has adversely affected the health status of many population groups worldwide.

In an early effort to expand the concept of health, the World Health Organization in 1946 promulgated a definition of health as "a state of complete physical, mental, and social well-being and not merely the absence of disease or

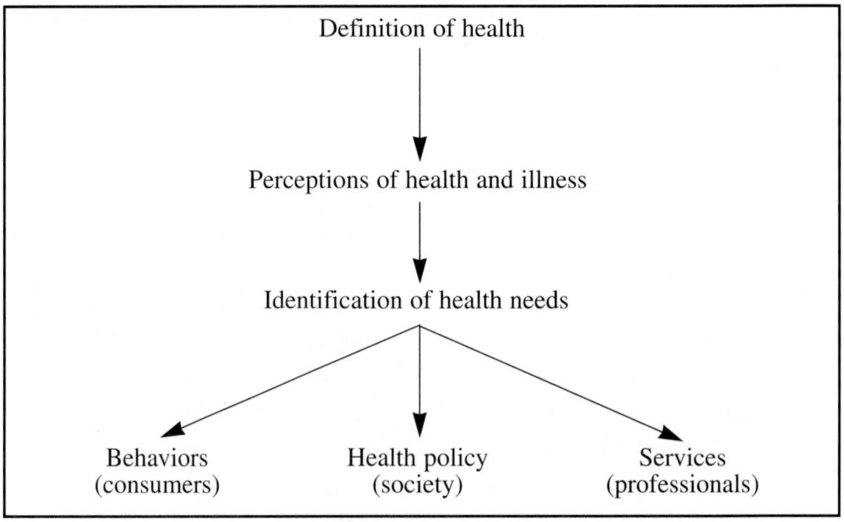

Fig. 2-1 The influence of definitions of health on health care.

infirmity" (World Health Organization, 1958). While this definition has been criticized as an ideal never capable of being accomplished, it did attempt to define health in terms of what it is instead of what it is not. In addition, it forced policy makers, health-care providers, and consumers to think of health holistically and consider issues having to do with the quality of life as part of health concerns. This definition remains a classic on which many additional definitions have been built.

Another broad concept of health that has been used extensively in nursing is Dunn's model of high-level wellness (Dunn, 1980). Rejecting the dichotomous view of health and illness prevalent in the medical model, Dunn proposed that wellness be envisioned on a continuum ranging from death to peak wellness. Wellness comprises four components—physical, psychologic, social, and spiritual. All aspects of wellness are influenced by the environment are represented by a continuum, ranging from very unfavorable to very favorable environments (Fig. 2-2). Dunn sees both the personal and the environmental continua as constantly changing and thus open to interventions that promote higher levels of wellness. The ultimate goal in Dunn's model is high-level wellness that is defined as ". . . an integrated method of functioning, which is oriented toward maximizing the potential of which the individual is capable within the environment where he is functioning." Dunn has also described high-level wellness for communities (Dunn, 1977). Nursing practice based on this concept views health in terms of maximal well-being individualized according to the client's potential. Health

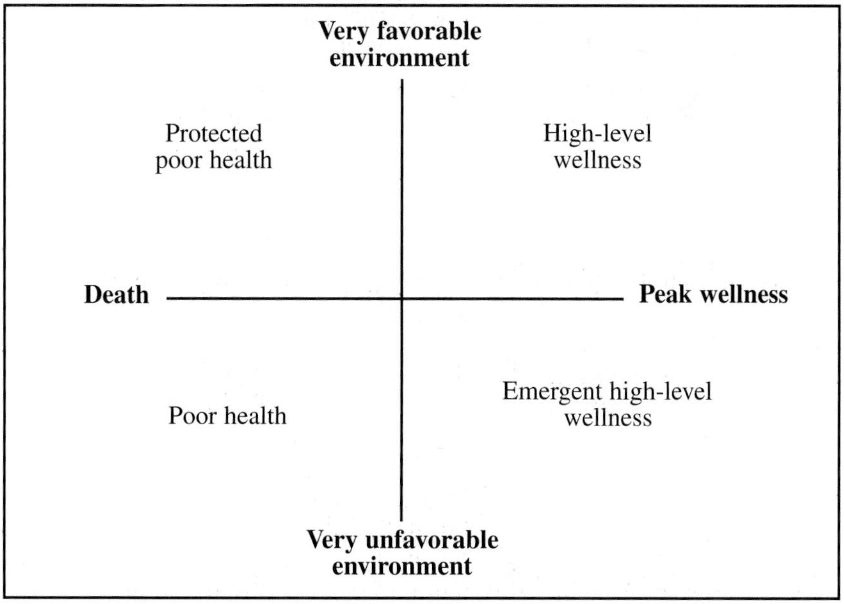

Fig. 2-2 Levels of wellness. (From Dunn HL: High level wellness for man and society, *AJPH* 49:788, 1959.)

needs are assessed holistically, including a focus on the environment, to identify factors that need to be supported or changed to reach higher levels of wellness. Health behaviors and programs or services include actions that improve the quality of life physically, psychologically, socially, and spiritually. The goal of health policy is no longer merely the eradication of disease but the achievement of high-level wellness for individuals, families, and communities.

In the years following these early efforts to define health beyond the mere absence of disease, countless definitions of health have appeared in the literature of many disciplines. Smith (1981) has provided a useful typology for categorizing the numerous definitions of health found in the literature (Table 2-1). Application of the steps outlined in Fig. 2-1 to each of the models of health described by Smith will demonstrate how different concepts of health can lead to very divergent ideas about health actions, services, and policies. This is especially problematic when nurses, clients, other health care professionals, and policy makers do not share similar definitions of health.

DETERMINANTS OF HEALTH STATUS

Vast amounts of information about the factors that influence various levels of wellness have been provided by epidemiologic, clinical, and laboratory studies. We know that some factors are necessary to promote or maintain health. For example, adequate amounts of vitamins A, C, and D are essential for healthy growth and mineralization of bone. We know too that some factors can produce disease or other health problems. For example, constant exposure to high levels of noise in the workplace can eventually cause deafness for most unprotected workers. This knowledge from epidemiology provides the basis for nurses to identify which of the factors influencing their clients will promote or maintain their health and which will contribute to the development of deviations from health.

Health promotion

Positive *health promotion* has been defined by the World Health Organization as " . . . the process of enabling people to increase control over and improve their own health" (Noack, 1987). Measures built on the Eudaimonistic Model of health exemplify this approach to health promotion. Although disease prevention may result from these efforts, the protection from disease is not the primary objective. Rather, vigorous well-being and self-actualization are the goals. Pender (1987) notes that it is important to differentiate between the goals of health protection and health promotion, because the motivation to pursue each is different. Fear of disease and its consequences often provides the motivation to take health-protective actions. However, motivation to engage in health-promotion behaviors depends on the desire for self-actualization and improving the quality of one's life. Pender has identified 10 parameters of life-style and health habits that provide a comprehensive basis for nursing assessments and interventions in positive health-promotion efforts. These assessment parameters are competence in self-care, nutritional practices, physical or recreational activity, sleep patterns, stress management, self-actualization, sense of purpose, relationships with others, environmental control, and use of the health care system (Pender, 1987).

Table 2-1 Smith's models of health

Clinical model

The health extreme of this model is the absence of signs or symptoms of disease or disability as identified by medical science. Conversely, conspicuous presence of these signs or symptoms is a model indicator of the illness extreme.

Role-performance model

In this model, the health extreme of the continuum constitutes performance of social roles with maximal expected output; the illness extreme is failure in performance of one's role. (It is assumed that the relevant role is the one in which the person earns or otherwise receives income.)

Adaptive model

Under the conditions of this model, the health extreme of the continuum is that in which the organism maintains flexible adaptation to the environment and interacts with the environment with maximal advantage. Conversely, alienation of the organism from the environment and failure of self-corrective responses are model indicators of the illness extreme.

Eudaimonistic model

Health is the condition of realization or actualization of one's unique potential. The health extreme of the continuum is seen as exuberant well-being, and the illness extreme is seen as enervation and languishing debility.

Adapted from Smith JA: The idea of health: a philosophical inquiry, *ANS* 3(3):44-46, 1981.

Risk factors

Factors that increase the probability that disease will develop are called *risk factors.* They are identified by epidemiologists who compare incidence rates (see Chapter 3) for a particular health problem among population groups characterized by varying levels of the factors of interest. When higher levels of the relevant factors are associated with higher incidence rates of the health problem, the factors are considered risk factors. For example, it has been found that there is a higher incidence of low birth weight babies born to women who smoke compared with women who do not smoke. Therefore maternal smoking has been identified as a risk factor in low birth weight babies.

The presence of risk factors does not necessarily predict that disease will always result, nor does their absence guarantee that disease will not occur. Rather, the knowledge of risk factors can identify individuals and groups who have a high probability of developing a particular disease or health problem. We designate these individuals or groups as being "at risk" in terms of that health problem. In instances where a number of risk factors are known, as in the case of cardiovascular disease, very comprehensive risk-appraisal instruments have been developed to collect data about health history and life-style. These data are reviewed for the presence of risk factors and factors that contribute to health maintenance. Statistical procedures are used to compute the extent of risk for the individual and project the likelihood of disease development within certain time frames. Risk-appraisal instruments also use statistical procedures to demonstrate how the individual's risk status could be changed by alterations in life-style, such as weight reduction and smoking cessation.

EPIDEMIOLOGIC MODELS

Epidemiologic triad model

The factors that influence health status come from sources both intrinsic and extrinsic to the client. One approach to examining these sources is provided by the *epidemiologic triad model* (Fig. 2-3).

Originally developed to examine the causative factors in infectious diseases, this approach has been applied to the examination of many other health problems. This model is based on the belief that health status is determined by the interaction of characteristics of the host, agent, and environment and not by any single factor. The host is the client whose health status concerns us. The agent is an element or force that under proper conditions can initiate or perpetuate a health problem. Environment refers to the context within which the agent and host interact. Some nursing texts have substituted a Venn diagram (Fig. 2-4) for the classic triangle to emphasize the interrelationships among host, agent, and environment.

Host factors, sometimes called intrinsic factors, include both variable and immutable factors. Age, race, and genetic makeup are examples of the latter. Life-style, exercise level, nutrition, health knowledge, and motivation for achieving optimal wellness are examples of host factors that are open to change.

Agents can be classified into five types (Clark, 1992). *Physical,* such as heat and trauma; *chemical,* including pollutants, medications, and drugs; *nutrient,* including absence and excess, such as some vitamins, proteins, and carbohydrates; *psychologic,* including stress, social isolation, and social support; and *biologic,* such as bacteria, viruses, and arthropods. The examples for each type are not comprehensive and are meant to be illustrative only.

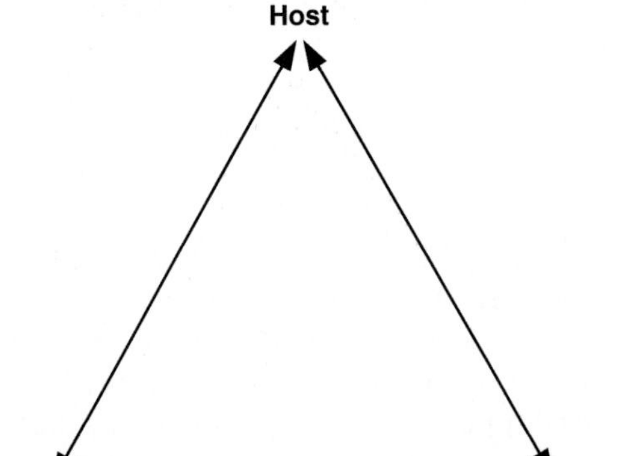

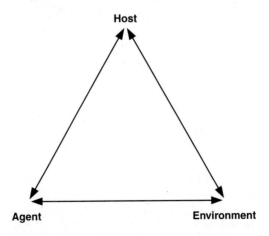

Fig. 2-3 The epidemiologic triangle.

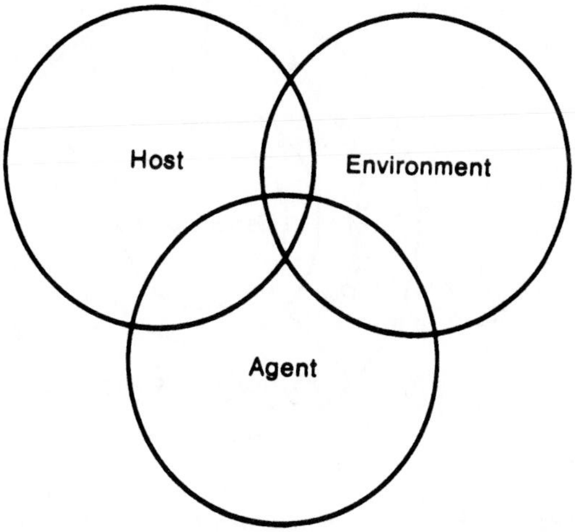

Fig. 2-4 The epidemiologic model. (From Turner JG, Chavigny KH: *Community health nursing: an epidemiologic perspective through the nursing process*, Philadelphia, 1988, JB Lippincott, p 54.)

Environmental factors are frequently divided into three categories—biologic, social, and physical aspects of the environment. The *biologic* environment is composed of plants and animals needed for food and includes pathogenic microorganisms, vectors of infectious agents, and reservoirs of infection. The *physical* environment comprises heat, light, air, atmospheric pressure, radiation, and water to name a few. Washington (1985) has identified a number of forces that should be considered in examining the *social* environment. They include cultural, technologic, educational, political, demographic, sociologic (class structure and mobility), economic, and legal forces.

The use of this model in the epidemiologic analysis of any health problem mandates that the characteristics of the host, agent(s), and environment and their interactions be examined. Nursing interventions to prevent disease or maintain health attempt to change the character of any of these three components or alter the nature of their interactions.

Some modifications of the epidemiologic triad have appeared in the literature in recent years. For example, Mausner and Kramer (1985) argue that many diseases with which epidemiologists are concerned have no discernible agents. When there are agents, they are addressed as parts of the environment. To this end, they offer a model conceptualized as a wheel, where the host is represented as a circle with a genetic core and is surrounded by a larger, segmented circle representing the biologic, psychologic, and social environments (Fig. 2-5). Despite the modifications, the interactions between host and environment (with or without agents) remain major determinants of health status in all epidemiologic models.

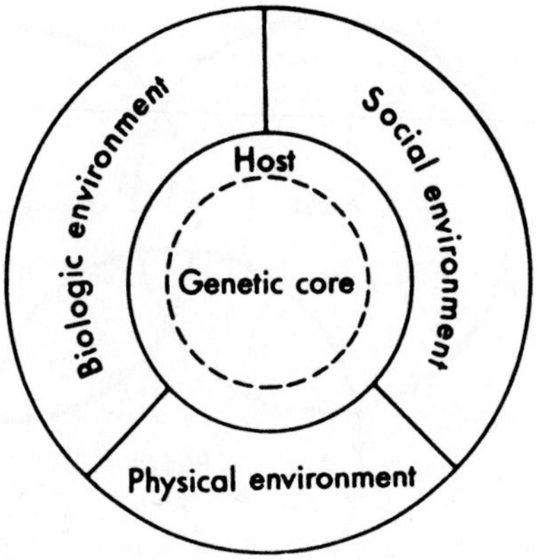

Fig. 2-5 The wheel model of human-environmental interactions. (From Mausner J, Kramer S: *Epidemiology—an introductory text*, Philadelphia, 1985, WB Saunders, p 36.)

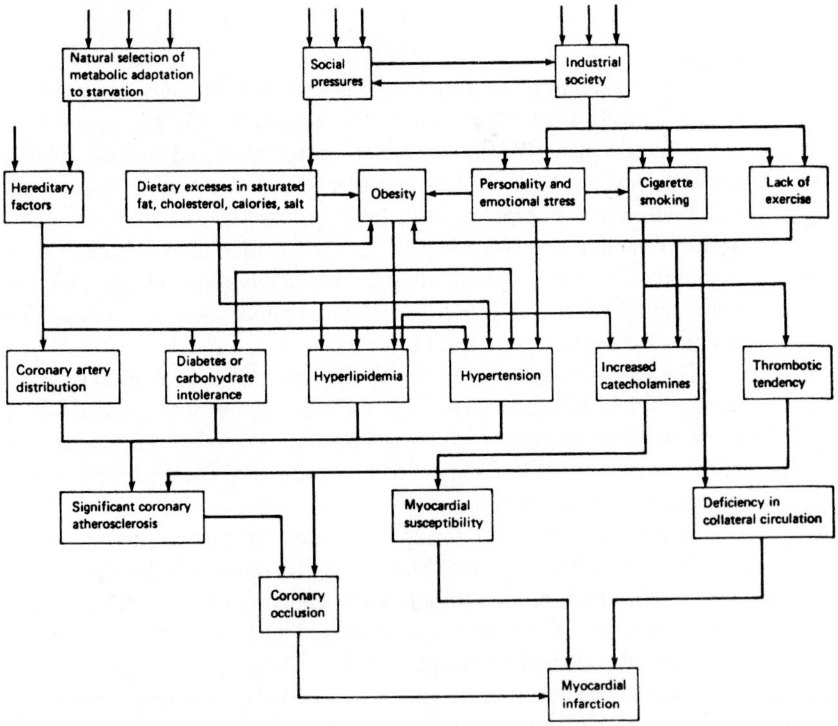

Fig. 2-6 The web of causation for myocardial infarction. (From Friedman GE: *Primer of epidemiology*, ed 3, New York, 1987, McGraw-Hill, p 4.)

Web of causation

An epidemiologic model that strongly emphasizes the concept of multiple causation was first published by MacMahon and Pugh (1970) (Fig. 2-6). In this model, all possible antecedent factors that could influence the development or prevention of a particular health problem are identified. Each factor is perceived as a link in multiple chains of causation that are interrelated in the very complex configuration of a web. This approach helps to identify direct and indirect factors that can be changed to produce higher levels of health. Fig. 2-6 illustrates a web of causation for myocardial infarction.

Natural history of disease

Leavell and Clark (1958), two public health physicians who championed the cause of preventive medicine in clinical and public health practice, have emphasized that prevention is required at every phase of the disease process. To explain their approach, they diagrammed their concept of the course of any disease process as it affects humans, which they called the natural history of disease (Fig. 2-7).

The course of any disease is divided into two phases—the prepathogenesis period and the period of pathogenesis. During the prepathogenesis period, there are factors within individuals and their various environments that have the capability of predisposing them toward health problems or actually precipitating disease. In many instances, these factors may exist indefinitely without producing the stimulus necessary for a health problem to occur. However, when conditions are favorable, the initial interactions between agents, host, and environmental factors that produce disease will take place in the prepathogenic period. Prodromal stage and incubation period are terms also applied to the latter stage of the prepathogenic phase.

Once the host begins to respond to the disease stimulus with biophysical, psychologic, or social changes, the period of pathogenesis begins. It is manifested by signs and symptoms that are clinically diagnosed and lasts until the condition is terminated by time or treatment. Termination may include recovery, disability, defect, or death.

For each of the stages of the disease process, Leavell and Clark have identified types of interventions and goals perceived as levels of prevention. *Primary prevention* should occur during the prepathogenesis period, when the goal is to prevent the incidence of disease. Early in the prepathogenesis period, health-promotion interventions are used to strengthen the general health of the host, thus increasing overall resistance to disease. An example of such an intervention is ensuring an adequate balance between work and leisure. Environmental improvements that ensure general good health, such as adequate handling of toxic waste, are also part of primary prevention. In the latter part of the prepathogenesis period, the potentially pathogenic agent(s), host, and environmental factors are present, but they have not yet interacted to produce disease. Specific protection measures or risk-reduction efforts are used to alter these factors, and their ability to

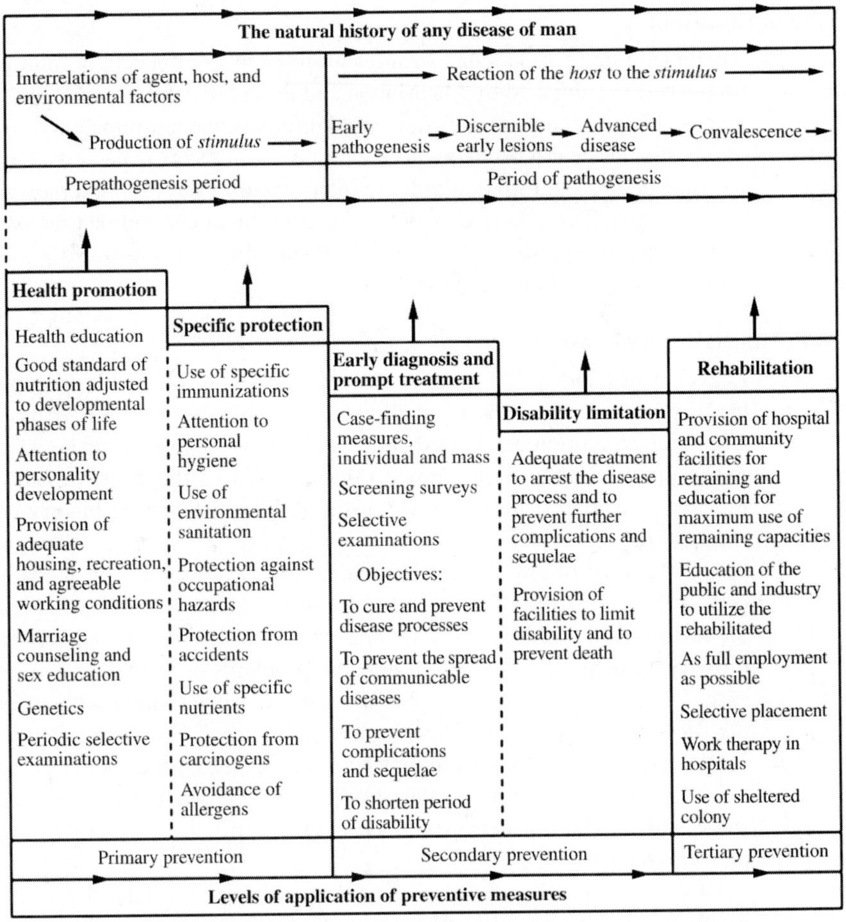

Fig. 2-7 Levels of application of preventive measures in the natural history of disease. (From Leavell HF, Clark EG: *Preventive medicine for the doctor in his community: an epidemiologic approach,* New York, 1965, McGraw-Hill, p 21.)

interact before health problems can occur. Efforts to reduce stress in the workplace and lower blood-cholesterol levels are examples of risk-reduction measures.

Secondary prevention occurs during the period of pathogenesis. The goals of secondary prevention include limiting the spread and severity of the disease and preventing complications and sequelae. Early diagnosis, when the initial changes occur within the host, and prompt treatment are the keystones of early secondary prevention. For example, early diagnosis of cervical cancer through periodic Pap smears leading to prompt treatment has been credited with reducing the severity of the disease for women worldwide. In addition to periodic examinations like mammography, colonoscopy, and Pap smears, the processes of individual case-finding and screening programs have been successful in achieving secondary prevention for many health problems. When the course of the disease advances, because early diagnosis and treatment were impossible or ineffective, secondary preventive measures are used to prevent death, shorten the course of the disease when possible, and limit adverse sequelae that may result from it. Nurses in intensive care units practice secondary prevention when they turn and position unconscious patients on a scheduled basis, perform range-of-motion exercises, and keep their patients hydrated and relatively free of pain.

Tertiary prevention is employed after irreversible changes have resulted from the disease process. The goal at this stage is to limit unnecessary disability and return the individual to a useful place in society by maximizing his or her remaining capacities. Interventions help the individual to adapt to or transcend disabilities, help the family and significant others adapt to the individual's changed abilities, and promote environmental adaptations that enhance his or her abilities. Although not addressed in Leavell and Clark's diagram, nurses also practice tertiary prevention when they assist dying patients to achieve a dignified and peaceful end to life.

SUMMARY

The spectrum of health for each individual is a dynamic process ranging from optimal wellness through illness and disability to death. Present concepts of health emphasize this continuum along with the individualistic nature of health. In defining health, it is also necessary to include psychologic and spiritual components along with physical needs. Epidemiology describes, explains, and predicts the wellness and illness patterns within the spectrum of health.

Enabling people to control and improve their states of health is the process of health promotion. Individual life-styles and health habits are strong determinants of health and disease. Characteristics that increase the probability that disease will develop are called risk factors. Health-promotion activities, such as smoking-cessation or weight-reduction programs, have been shown to reduce the risk of illness.

The basic epidemiologic model used in studying the distribution and determinants of states of health involves interaction of the host, agent, and environment. Host factors include immutable factors, such as age, sex, race and genetic makeup, and variable factors, such as life-style, nutrition, and motivation. Agents include physical, chemical, nutrient, psychologic and biologic stressors. Environmental factors can be biologic, physical, and social. Modifications of this model include the wheel (Mausner and Kramer, 1985) and the web of causation (MacMahon and Pugh, 1970).

The natural history of disease includes all aspects of the cycle of disease in humans. Leavell and Clark (1958) perceive the prepathogenesis and pathogenesis periods to be three levels of prevention. The goal of primary prevention is to prevent disease by increasing the general health and resistance of the host. Secondary prevention goals include limiting the spread and severity of the disease through early diagnosis and treatment. Tertiary prevention goals limit unnecessary disabilities, maximizing the individual's capacity to contribute to society.

Critical Thinking Questions

1. Compare and contrast the epidemiologic triad model with the web of causation model.
2. From nursing practice, give an example in which the concept of "at risk" has been used in care of an individual; an aggregate.
3. Discuss the concept of health as it has evolved over the twentieth century.
4. Using Leavell and Clark's levels of prevention, trace the natural history of osteoporosis. Identify at least one specific preventive activity for each phase of the disease process.

REFERENCES

Clark MJ: *Nursing in the community,* Norwalk, 1992, Appleton & Lange.

Dunn HL: Points of attack for raising the level of wellness, *J Natl Med Assoc,* 49:223-235, 1977.

Dunn HL: *High level of wellness,* Throrofare, NJ, 1980, Charles B Slack.

Friedman GD: *Primer of epidemiology,* ed 3, New York, 1987, McGraw-Hill.

Leavell HR, Clark EG: *Preventive medicine for the doctor in his community,* ed 3, New York, 1958, McGraw-Hill.

MacMahon B, Pugh TF: *Epidemiology principles and methods,* Boston, 1970, Little, Brown.

Mausner JS, Kramer S: *Epidemiology—an introductory text,* ed 2, Philadelphia, 1985, WB Saunders.

Noack H: Concepts of health and health promotion. In Abelin T, editor: *Measurement in health promotion and protection,* Copenhagen, 1987, World Health Organization.

Pender NJ: *Health promotion nursing practice,* ed 2, Norwalk, CT, 1987, Appleton & Lange.

Smith NJ: The idea of health: a philosophical enquiry, *ANS,* 3(3):43-50, 1981.

Turner JG, Chavigny KH: *Community health nursing: an epidemiologic perspective through the nursing process,* Philadelphia, 1988, JB Lippincott.

Washington WM: An interactive model for wellness: a systems approach, *Fam Community Health,* 7(4):44-52, 1985.

World Health Organization. *The first ten years of the World Health Organization,* New York, 1958, The Organization.

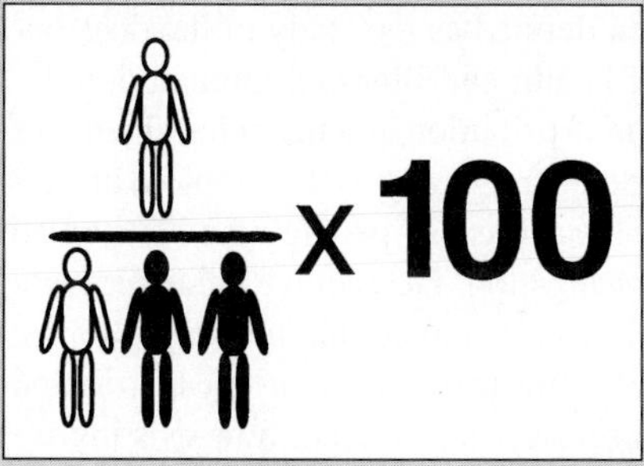

3

Descriptive Epidemiology
Using Rates

Objectives

1. Describe the primary method of measuring the existence of disease in a population during a given time period.
2. Explain the formula and rules for calculation of a rate.
3. Differentiate between crude, specific, and adjusted rates.
4. Identify the differences between the use of incidence and prevalence rates.
5. Contrast incidence density with incidence rates.
6. Define relative risk ratio.
7. Using examples, interpret the relevance of the use of rates in nursing practice.

Key Terms

adjusted rate
attack rate
attributable risk
crude rate
denominator
direct method
incidence density
incidence rate
indirect method
infection rate
morbidity rate
mortality rate
numerator
period prevalence
point prevalence
population at risk
prevalence rate
proportion
proportional mortality ratio
rate
ratio
relative risk ratio
risk factor
specific rates

The discipline of epidemiology has been defined as the study of the distribution and the determinants of states of health and illness in human populations. The first steps in investigating both the distribution and the determinants of states of health are to describe the magnitude or frequency of the problem or outcome, and determine the characteristics of the groups of people who have or do not have the problem or outcome under investigation. Descriptive epidemiologic techniques can tell us what people are likely to develop certain health problems; what diseases, disabilities, or needs they have; how these problems are distributed within the community; what kind of health services are needed; how existing resources are used; and who provides the services they need.

Using the information about the frequency and distribution of various states of health, nurses and other health-care professionals can identify the characteristics of groups of people in the community or within institutions who are most likely to develop health problems. These groups are considered to be *populations at risk*. Populations at risk can then be studied to determine the specific *risk factors* that increase the probability of developing the health problem. Knowledge about the population at risk and risk factors can be used to set priorities within the institution or community for the development, expansion, or change of programs that target specific health problems. Strategies to meet emerging health needs can then be implemented. Plans can be made to use established health resources more effectively, and the effectiveness of the measures used to control or prevent spe-

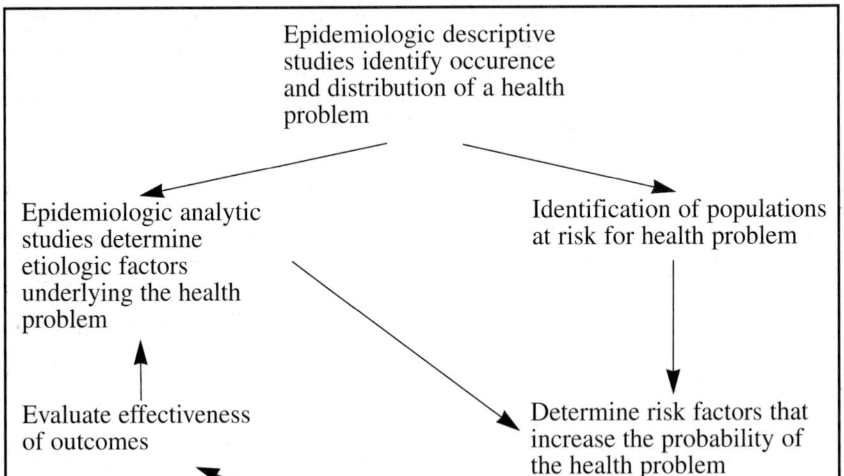

Fig. 3-1 Use of epidemiologic techniques to generate new knowledge about a health problem and to plan control and prevention strategies.

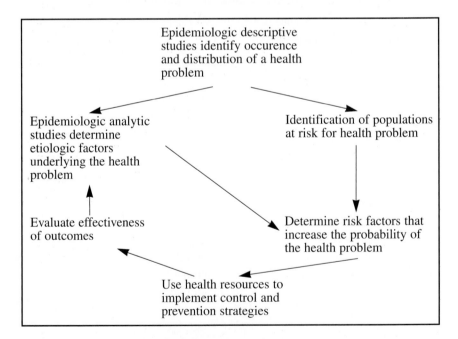

cific problems can be evaluated. Also, descriptive information provides clues to the cause of health problems that can be studied using analytic epidemiologic techniques. This process of using epidemiologic techniques to generate a knowledge base about a specific health problem and plan for its control and prevention is outlined in Fig. 3-1.

Perhaps the most successful example of this process has been the epidemiologic study of cardiovascular disease, the leading cause of death in the United States. The knowledge gained from the study of populations at risk and predisposing risk factors has been the foundation for primary, secondary, and tertiary prevention strategies. A national focus on health-promotion activities, such as good eating habits and exercise, has contributed to the decrease in occurrence of cardiovascular disease (primary prevention). Programs for reduction of high-risk behaviors, such as smoking-cessation clinics, have been instituted in communities throughout the country (secondary prevention). Treatment for those with cardiovascular disease includes rehabilitation programs with a primary focus on increasing cardiovascular health (tertiary prevention).

Although Fig. 3-1 is focused on a specific health problem, it should be emphasized that this process also can be used to study states of wellness. For example, studies of the factors that are associated with healthy, community-dwelling, elderly people over the age of 85 can lead to the implementation and evaluation of strategies to enhance wellness in the elderly population.

THE CONCEPT OF RATES

The ability to quantify the occurrence of a health problem or any other state of health is an essential prerequisite for any epidemiologic investigation. The most basic measure of frequency is to count the number of affected individuals. While this information is important to health planners as they plan control and prevention strategies, it may result in misleading impressions and has limited use in epidemiology. The number of people in the population who could have acquired the health problem and the time period during which the health problems occurred should also be taken into consideration.

For example, compare 17 cases of acquired immunodeficiency syndrome (AIDS) diagnosed during 1 year in Brown County, population 114,000, with 156 cases of AIDS diagnosed during 1 year in Orrin County, population 1,268,000. If only the frequency count is examined, Orrin County has the greatest number of persons with AIDS, and therefore it would appear that Orrin County has the greater community problem. However, it is not appropriate to compare the raw numbers alone. Obviously, more cases would be expected in a more populated county.

Ratios, proportions, and rates are used in epidemiology to provide a more valid description of the frequency of health problems. A *ratio* is a fraction that represents the relationship between two numbers. It is the value obtained by dividing one quantity by another quantity; the numerator is not included in the denominator. For instance, the number of male patients on a medical unit could be contrasted with the number of female patients on the same unit using a ratio.

A *proportion* is a type of ratio that includes the quantity in the numerator as a part of the denominator. It is the relationship of a part to the whole. Dividing the number of male babies in a nursery by the total number of both male and female babies results in a proportion. The *proportional mortality ratio* is an epidemiologic statistic where the number of deaths from a specific cause are divided by the total number of deaths in the same time period.

The *rate* is the primary measurement used to describe the occurrence of a health problem. A rate is defined as a measure of the quantity of a health-related event or health problem in a specific population within a given period of time. It is a proportion that includes the factor of time. Therefore rates are the best indicators of the risk or probability that a disease, condition, or event will occur (Last, 1988; Mausner and Kramer, 1985).

A rate consists of a *numerator* and a *denominator*. The numerator is composed of the number of health-related conditions or events of interest that occurred within a designated period of time. The denominator is the population at risk during the same period of time. Therefore the numerator is a portion of the denominator. If the time period is long, often the population at risk is estimated at midperiod, such as midyear. The construction of rates is a basic tool in health care calculations, making it possible to compare events that occur at different times, in different places, and with different people.

When examining the frequency of AIDS in Brown and Orrin counties in the example presented earlier, the calculation of rates would allow a more valid comparison to be made between the two counties with different populations. In a similar way, the calculation of rates makes it possible to compare such events as the number of postoperative pneumonia cases on one hospital unit with another during the same time period or the types of functional disabilities of residents in one nursing home with another during the same time frame.

CALCULATION OF RATES

There are some general rules that apply to the calculation of rates. These rules should be carefully considered in the construction of any type of rate.

1. The numerator should include all of the events that are being measured, such as the number of people diagnosed with AIDS, cases of pneumonia, or various types of functional disabilities. This means that there must be adequate information available about the population to determine that the condition or event either has or has not occurred to each member of the population at risk in the denominator.
2. The denominator must be valid. Everyone included in the denominator must be at risk for the event in the numerator. Alternatively stated, the events in the numerator must have occurred to the population in the denominator. For example, it would be inappropriate to include males in the denominator when calculating a rate for ovarian cancer because no males are at risk for the illness. Ideally, the denominator should not include those who already have the disease, condition, or problem, nor should it include those who are not susceptible. In calculating a rate for a large population, this type of correction may not be made since it would not signif-

Table 3-1 Example of calculation of rates

Brown County	Orrin County
AIDS rate = $\frac{17}{114{,}000} \times 100{,}000$	AIDS rate = $\frac{156}{1{,}268{,}000} \times 100{,}000$
AIDS rate = 0.0001491 × 100,000	AIDS rate = 0.000123 × 100,000
AIDS rate = 14.9 cases per 100,000 people	AIDS rate = 12.3 cases per 100,000 people

icantly alter the statistical outcome. However, in calculating specific rates for smaller populations, such as the rate for postoperative pneumonia in a surgical intensive care unit, corrections to the denominator should be made.

3. A specific period of time for the observations must be clearly indicated. This can range from a single point in time to several years, depending on the type of rate that is being calculated.
4. Since a rate is a fraction or a proportion, it is necessary to multiply by a base, which is usually a multiple of 10. This procedure removes the decimal points and makes the comparison of rates easier to interpret. Any base multiple of 10 may be chosen that results in a rate above the value of one. The rate should be a reasonable size not a fraction. For large populations, 100,000 is often used. For smaller populations, 100 is often used, and the rate can then be expressed as a percent. The formula for calculation of a rate is:

$$\text{Rate} = \frac{\text{Number of conditions or events occurring in a period of time}}{\text{Population at risk during the same period of time}} \times \text{Base multiple of 10}$$

Using the example of the number of AIDS cases diagnosed in Brown and Orrin counties, rates can be calculated as illustrated in Table 3-1. The comparison of rates shows that Brown County actually had a higher rate of AIDS (14.9 per 100,000 people) during the year than did Orrin County (12.3 per 100,000 people), even though Brown County had fewer cases than Orrin County. A base multiplier of 10,000 would result in a rate of approximately 1.5 cases per 10,000 people for Brown County and 1.2 cases per 10,000 people for Orrin County. A more accurate figure for the denominator in this example would be the midyear population of both Brown and Orrin counties. If the midyear population is not known, an estimated midyear population can be calculated by averaging the population statistics at the beginning and end of the year.

CRUDE, SPECIFIC, AND ADJUSTED RATES

Crude rates or general rates measure the experience of the entire population in a designated geographic area in regard to the condition being investigated. Since crude rates include the total population, subgroups of the population that may have significant differences in the risk of developing the condition may be obscured. For instance, the formula for a crude birth rate has the midyear population as its denominator. Since births can only occur to females who are of childbearing age, the total population may not be an ideal denominator. However, crude rates require a minimum of information and are commonly calculated as summary rates.

Specific rates refer to population subgroups. These more detailed rates are frequently used for understanding the distribution of various health-related conditions by age, sex, race, and other demographic characteristics. Specific rates are discussed on page 59, and examples can be found on page 42. *Adjusted rates* have been standardized, removing the effect of differences in the composition of the population. Rates are often adjusted for age thereby removing age as a factor in the interpretation of the rate. An example of adjusted rates can be found on page 45.

INCIDENCE RATES

The number of new cases of AIDS that were diagnosed during 1 year in Brown and Orrin counties in relation to each county's population is called an *incidence rate* or occurrence rate. Incidence or occurrence rates measure the probability that people without a certain condition will develop the condition over a period of time, often a year. It measures the pace at which new illnesses, such as AIDS, occur in a previously disease-free group of people. When this information is known, the factors that affect the development of the illness can be investigated. The formula for an incidence rate is a variation of the general formula for a rate:

$$\text{Incidence rate} = \frac{\text{Number of } \textit{new} \text{ conditions or events occurring in a period of time}}{\text{Population at risk during the same period of time (often midyear)}} \times \text{Base multiple of 10}$$

The general rules that apply to rates apply to incidence rates. Also, crude, specific, and adjusted incidence rates can be calculated. The numerators and denominators must be well-defined and valid; knowledge of the health status of the population must be available; and the period of observation must be stated. In addition, determination of the date of onset is required for studies of incidence. For acute conditions, this can be quickly established. For other conditions, such as cancer, depression, or other chronic conditions, it may be difficult to determine a specific time of onset. In these instances an event that can be verified, such as the date of diagnosis, is chosen as the time of onset.

Also, when specifying the numerator of an incidence rate, sometimes more than one event can occur to the same person within the chosen time period. For example, this frequently occurs when monthly rates of nosocomial infections are calculated in acute care facilities. Two different types of incidence rates can be calculated. The first rate results in the probability that a person will develop a nosocomial infection during the month. This is an *attack rate,* representing the onset of illness in an exposed population. The formula is:

Table 3-2 Incidence rates and ratios that provide indices of community health

General mortality rates		
Crude mortality rate	$\frac{\text{Number of deaths occurring during 1 year}}{\text{Midyear population}}$	× 100,000
Cause-specific mortality rate	$\frac{\text{Number of deaths from a stated cause during 1 year}}{\text{Midyear population}}$	× 100,000
Case-fatality rate	$\frac{\text{Number of deaths from a specific disease}}{\text{Number of cases of the same disease}}$	× 100
Proportional mortality ratio	$\frac{\text{Number of deaths from a specific cause within a given time period}}{\text{Total deaths in the same time period}}$	× 100
Age-specific mortality rate	$\frac{\text{Number of persons in a specific age group dying during 1 year}}{\text{Midyear population of the specific age group}}$	× 100,000
Maternal and infant indices		
Crude birth rate	$\frac{\text{Number of live births during 1 year}}{\text{Midyear population}}$	× 1000
General fertility rate	$\frac{\text{Number of live births during 1 year}}{\text{Number of females aged 15-44 at midyear}}$	× 1000
Maternal mortality rate	$\frac{\text{Number of deaths from puerperal causes during 1 year}}{\text{Number of live births during same year}}$	× 100,000
Infant mortality rate	$\frac{\text{Number of deaths of children under 1 year of age during 1 year}}{\text{Number of live births during same year}}$	× 1000
Perinatal mortality rate	$\frac{\text{Number of fetal deaths plus infant deaths under 7 days of age during 1 year}}{\text{Number of live births plus fetal deaths during the same year}}$	× 1000
Neonatal mortality rate	$\frac{\text{Number of deaths of children under 28 days of age during 1 year}}{\text{Number of live births during the same year}}$	× 1000
Fetal mortality rate	$\frac{\text{Number of fetal deaths during 1 year}}{\text{Number of live births plus fetal deaths during the same year}}$	× 1000

$$\frac{\text{Number of people developing a nosocomial infection in a period of time}}{\text{Number of people hospitalized during the same period of time}} \times \text{Base multiple of 10}$$

The second rate indicates the probability of the event, a nosocomial infection, developing during the month. This is an *infection rate.* The formula is:

$$\frac{\text{Number of nosocomial infections that occurred in a period of time}}{\text{Number of people hospitalized during the same period of time}} \times \text{Base multiple of 10}$$

When the number of persons and the number of events are different, the composition of the numerator should be clearly defined as one of the other. Normally it is assumed that the numerator of an incidence rate refers to people. Some common examples of the calculation of incident rates that provide indices of the health of a population are found in Table 3-2.

The incidence of violence is a significant health problem that was investigated by a nurse specialist associated with the Philadelphia Department of Public Health and the Philadelphia Injury Prevention Program (Wishner and others, 1991). In this study, all interpersonal, violence-related injuries (IVRI) in a 97.2% African-American community were assessed for 1 year by an active emergency room surveillance system. There were occasions when the IVRI involved more than one type of violence. In this case, the investigators chose one classification that best described the sequence that lead to a physical injury. By doing so, the investigators calculated attack rates rather than event rates. The violence-specific rates are shown in Table 3-3. Age- and sex-specific rates are illustrated in Fig. 3-2. In this study, firearm-related injuries had the highest case-fatality rate (CFR) with a sex-specific CFR of 26.5% for males and 16.7% for females. Data such as these pro-

Table 3-3 Total number of interpersonal, violence-related injuries by type of violence

Type of violence	No. of events	Rate per 1000 population
Abuse	63	3.28*
Rape	7	0.10
Stabbing	296	4.35
Firearms	74	1.09
Other assaults	1518	22.29
Total	1958	28.71

*Rate per 1000 population 0-18 years of age.

From Wishner AR and others: Interpersonal, violence-related injuries in an African-American community in Philadelphia, *Am J Pub Health* 81(11): 1471-1476, 1991.

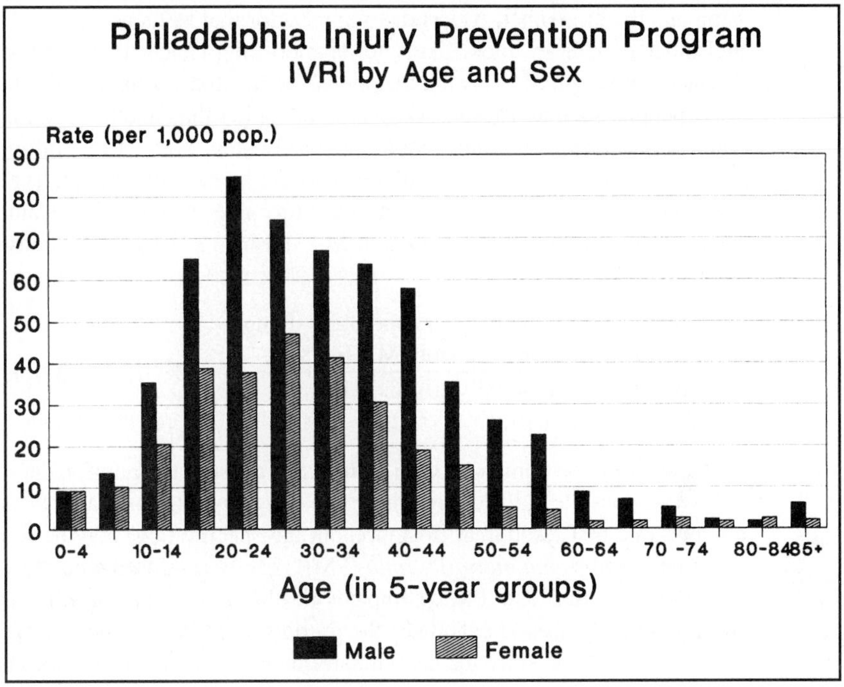

Fig. 3-2 Interpersonal violence-related injuries by age and sex, Philadelphia Injury Prevention Program. (From Wishner and others: Interpersonal violence-related injuries in an African-American community in Philadelphia, *Am J Pub Health,* 81(11):1471-1476, 1991.)

vide dramatic evidence of the extent of violence in the neighborhoods of our large cities. The investigators urge that these data be used to develop new efforts to control and prevent these injuries.

Mortality rates

Mortality rates or death rates are common incidence rates that are calculated for public health purposes. Crude mortality rates indicate the probability of death from any cause among the entire population in a designated geographic area. Cause-specific (disease-specific) mortality rates are crude rates that indicate the probability of death from a specific cause among the entire population in a designated geographic area. For instance, a crude mortality rate for cancer of the lung would include deaths from lung cancer among the population at risk regardless of sex, age, or other characteristics. Case-fatality rates refer to the proportion of people with a particular illness who die as a result of that illness (Table 3-2).

Since crude rates provide a very broad measure of the experience of a designated population, it is sometimes difficult to compare the rates from different populations with valid results. For example, death rates from lung cancer may vary between communities, but one community may have many more elderly inhabitants than the other. Age is the major factor that influences the risk of death, and older people are more likely to develop lung cancer than younger people. Therefore it would be expected that the crude rate for a community with more elderly people, such as Tucson, AZ, would be higher than another community with a higher proportion of young people, such as Boston, MA. Further information regarding subgroups of these populations would be helpful, and age-specific rates could be calculated. An age-specific mortality rate for lung cancer among those 65 years of age and older in Boston, MA during 1995 would be constructed as follows:

$$\frac{\text{Number of people 65 years and older dying from lung cancer in Boston, MA in 1995}}{\text{Number of people 65 years and older in Boston, MA in 1995}} \times \text{Base multiple of 10}$$

This rate could be compared with a similarly constructed rate for Tucson, AZ in 1995. It is possible that although the crude mortality rates indicated that there was a higher rate in Tucson than Boston, their age-specific rates may be similar.

The *proportional mortality ratio* (PMR) can be confused with the cause-specific mortality rate. The PMR compares deaths from a specific illness to deaths from all other causes; it calculates the proportion of deaths due to a specific disease. It is not a rate, since the denominator includes all deaths that are in the given time period. In contrast, the cause-specific mortality rate indicates the risk of death from a specific disease for a given living population. Both the PMR and cause-specific mortality rates should be calculated when death statistics are being examined for public health purposes. The formula for PMR is found in Table 3-2.

Adjusted rates

Although specific rates can provide helpful data for comparison purposes, there is often a need to remove the effects of differences in the composition of a population. This occurs when an investigator wishes to compare two or more groups, knowing that they differ in a characteristic that may influence the results. Since age is a significant factor in the development of health problems, age is the characteristic that often requires adjustment or standardization. *Adjusted rates* control for such differences.

There are two methods for removing the effect of a confounding variable such as age—a *direct method* and an *indirect method.* In the direct method, age-specific rates for each of the populations being compared are applied to a population with a known age distribution or the standard population. Choice of the standard population is an arbitrary one. It can be the population of a geographic area; often, it is the total population or a subgroup of the study being performed (Friedman, 1987).

Friedman (1987) uses an example of age-adjusted rates using the direct method in evaluating the association between parental-loss and back pain. Table 3-4 shows direct age adjustment by applying the age-specific rates of lower-back pain observed in the subgroup without parental loss to a standard population con-

Table 3-4 Example of direct age-adjustment: observed lower-back pain rates applied to standard population consisting of all study subjects

Age	Observed lower back pain rate	×	Total number in age subgroup of standard population	=	Number that would be observed in standard population
30-39	10%		200		20
40-49	20%		200		40
50-59	30%		200		60
		TOTAL	600		120
Age-adjusted rate = 120/600 = 20%					

From Friedman GD: *Primer of epidemiology,* ed 3, New York, 1987, McGraw-Hill, p 178.

sisting of all study subjects. The result is the number that would be observed or expected in each age category in the standard population. These numbers are then added, and the total is divided by the total standard population, yielding an age-adjusted rate of 20%.

The same process would be used to calculate an age-adjusted rate for the subgroup with parental loss. If the results were the same, the conclusion would be that parental loss was not related to lower-back pain. If the results were different an association between parental-loss and lower-back pain is possible. Although age-adjusted and other types of adjusted rates are artificial, they provide a valid way to compare two populations without the confounding variable (age) affecting the results. Age-adjustment is meaningful only as a comparison and should not be used if an accurate description of a population is desired rather than a comparison of populations.

In situations where age-specific rates for two or more groups cannot be calculated or are not known, the indirect method of adjustment may be calculated. Rather than apply the age-specific rates of the study population to the standard population with a known age structure, the age-specific rates of the standard population are applied to the subgroups of the study (Friedman, 1987). It is the reverse of the direct method. A more detailed description of the indirect method of rate adjustment can be found in Mausner and Kramer (1985).

An example of removing the effect of a confounding variable through adjustment of rates can be found in Fig. 3-3. *Haemophilus influenzae* (Hi) causes disease among persons in all age groups, and type b (Hib) is the most common cause of bacterial meningitis among children in the United States. Hib vaccines were introduced in 1988, resulting in a decreased incidence of invasive Hib infections. Hib disease among children under 5 years of age is targeted for elimination in the United States by 1996. Hib disease rates are generally higher for blacks than whites, probably reflecting differences in socioeconomic risk factors, such as overcrowding, for the disease. These socioeconomic characteristics could have accounted for the variance in incidence rates between the two groups. Therefore race-adjusted incidence rates per 100,000 children were calculated

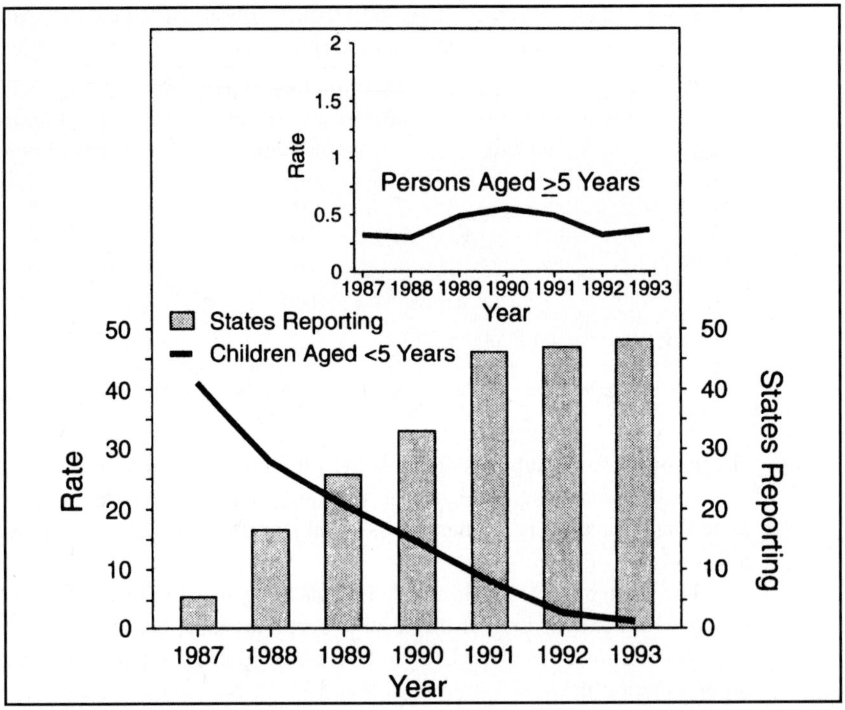

Fig. 3-3 Race-adjusted incidence rate* of *Haemophilus influenzae* (Hi) disease among children aged < 5 years, incidence rate† of Hi disease among persons aged ≥ 5 years, and number of states reporting Hi surveillance data—United States, National Notifiable Diseases Surveillance System, 1987-1993. (*Per 100,000 children age < 5 years. †Per 100,000 persons age ≥ 5 years.) (†From Centers for Disease Control: Progress toward elimination of *Haemophilus influenzae* type b disease among infants and children—United States, 1987-1993, *MMWR* 43(8):144-148, 1994.)

(Centers for Disease Control, 1994). Fig. 3-3 shows the marked decrease in incidence rates since introduction of the vaccine with the rates adjusted for the confounding variable of race. Another example of adjusted rates is shown on page 62.

Incidence density

When there are unequal periods of observations for study subjects, a person-time denominator may be used in the calculation of incidence rates. This technique provides a measure of *incidence density.* Individuals often enter a study period at different times and therefore contribute unequal periods of time to the population at risk. To identify the precise period of observation for each individual and weigh that period of observations properly in calculating rates, a person-time unit, such as person-day or person-year, can be constructed. A person-day reflects one person at risk for 1 day, and a person-year represents one person at risk for 1 year. Incidence density can be constructed as follows:

Table 3-5 Incidence rates for development of nosocomial pneumonia in the elderly

Setting	Number of cases	Number at risk	Patient or resident days	Crude incidence (%)	Incidence Density (per 1000 patient days)
Acute care	33	2249	19,102	1.5	1.75
Long-term care	27	366	37,064	7.4	0.73

From Harkness GA, Bentley DW, Roghmann K: Nosocomial pneumonia in the elderly, *Am J Med* 89:459, 1990.

$$\text{Incidence density} = \frac{\textit{New}\text{ cases occurring during a study period}}{\text{Person-time units accumulated by the study subjects during the study period}} \times \text{Base multiple of 10}$$

Harkness and others (1990) demonstrated the difference between the calculation of crude incidence rates and incidence density when studying the development of nosocomial pneumonia in both an acute care facility and a long-term care facility (Table 3-5). These incidence data illustrate the need to calculate and compare both crude incidence and incidence-density rates when comparing different settings. In this example, the incidence rate in long-term care was almost five times that of the acute care setting. However, when patient-days were included in the denominator, the acute care setting reflected two times the incidence density of the long-term care setting. More patients contributed shorter periods of time in the acute care setting, while there was relatively little turnover among residents in the long-term care setting.

Measures of incidence density can account for those persons who die, those who are lost to follow-up, or those who have acquired the illness and are therefore not at risk for the entire study period (Valanis, 1992). Normally, it is assumed that the risk of acquiring the illness is constant throughout the entire period of study.

Attributable risk

Attributable risk is the difference between the incidence rates in exposed and unexposed groups. It measures the risk of a disease or health-related event in an exposed group that is attributable to the exposure but not to other factors. In almost any health-related event, some risk occurs normally in a population without exposure. In calculating attributable risk, the risk of the event that would have occurred normally without exposure is subtracted from the risk of the event in the exposed group:

$$\text{Attributable risk} = \text{Incidence rate in the exposed} - \text{Incidence rate in the nonexposed}$$

Although normally focused on disease states, these calculations are also used to document benefit from exposure to therapeutic interventions.

To determine the proportion of the disease or health-related event among the exposed group that is attributable to the exposure, discounting those cases that would have occurred anyway, the attributable risk is often presented as a percentage. To calculate the attributable risk percentage, the attributable risk is divided by the incidence rate among the exposed:

$$\text{Attributable risk percent} = \frac{\text{Attributable risk}}{\text{Incidence rate exposed}} \times 100$$

Table 3-6 presents a hypothetical example of attributable risk calculation regarding the onset of pneumonia following aspiration. The risk of pneumonia attributable to aspiration is 21.47, resulting in an attributable risk percent of 84.2% as determined in Table 3-6.

Relative risk ratio

Incidence rates indicate the occurrence of a health-related event in a population in a given period of time. It is an indicator of the probability that people without a specified condition will develop the condition within a designated period of

Table 3-6 Attributable risk and relative risk ratio calculation in a hypothetical cohort of hospitalized patients

Aspiration	Pneumonia		Total
	Yes	No	
Yes	102	298	400
No	41	976	1017
Total	143	1538	1417

From Harkness GA, Bentley DW, Roghmann K: Nosocomial pneumonia in the elderly, *Am J Med* 89:459, 1990.

$$\text{Incidence rate in exposed} = \frac{102}{400} = 0.2550 \times 100 = 25.5$$

$$\text{Incidence rate in nonexposed} = \frac{41}{1017} = 0.0403 \times 100 = 4.03$$

$$\text{Attributable risk} = 25.5 - 4.03 = 21.47$$

$$\text{Attributable risk percent} = \frac{21.47}{25.5} \times 100 = 84.2\%$$

$$\text{Relative risk ratio} = \frac{25.5}{4.03} = 6.33$$

time. Therefore it is a measure of the risk of developing the condition. Incidence rates for different groups of people can be compared, particularly when examining the cause of the condition. Often incidence rates for groups exposed to a certain factor (risk factor) are compared with the incidence rates for those not exposed. This procedure results in a *relative risk ratio.* It is a ratio of the incidence rate in the exposed group and the incidence rate in the nonexposed group:

$$\text{Relative risk ratio} = \frac{\text{Incidence rate in the exposed}}{\text{Incidence rate in the nonexposed}}$$

A relative risk of 1.0 indicates that the risk is equal for both groups. A relative risk greater than 1.0 indicates that the risk is greater in the exposed group. For example, the relative risk of 6.33 in Table 3-6 indicates that pneumonia is 6.33 times more common in the group that was exposed to aspiration than those who were not exposed. A relative risk less than 1.0 indicates that there is less risk in the exposed group and that the factor may possibly protect against the condition under study. Although this finding is not very common, it may signify that further study is warranted. Statistical tests, such as the calculation of the chi-square statistic, are used to determine whether the relative-risk ratios are greater than (or less than) those that would be expected by chance. In this way, the statistical significance of the findings can be established.

PREVALENCE RATES

The *prevalence rate* measures the number of people in a given population who have a specific (existing) condition at a given point in time. Prevalence rates are often used to measure the total burden of a condition or illness that exists in a community. Both incidence rates and prevalence rates are measures of *morbidity,* which has been defined as a departure from a state of physiologic or psychologic well-being. With knowledge of the prevalence of morbidity within a population, nurses and other health-care professionals can plan for services to meet the needs of the community.

$$\text{Prevalence rate} = \frac{\begin{array}{l}\text{Number of \textit{existing} conditions or}\\ \text{events occurring in a period of time}\end{array}}{\begin{array}{l}\text{Population at risk during the same}\\ \text{period of time}\end{array}} \times \text{Base multiple of 10}$$

The general rules for constructing rates apply to the calculation of prevalence rates. Crude, specific, and adjusted prevalence rates can be calculated. The numerator and denominator must be clearly defined and valid, the health status of the population should be known, and the period of observation should be stated. Also, person-time denominators may be used as they are in incidence rates. Knowledge of the time of onset, which is so important in the calculation of incidence rates, is not required. In addition, the numerators in prevalence rates include both "old" and "new" cases, and the denominators in prevalence rates include the entire population (Mausner and Kramer, 1985).

There are two types of prevalence rates, period prevalence and point prevalence. *Period prevalence* indicates the existence of a condition during a period or an interval of time, and a midyear or average population may be used in the denominator. *Point prevalence* refers to the existence of a condition at a specific point in time. It provides a picture of an existing situation for a group of people. If period or point prevalence is not stated, point prevalence is inferred. Point prevalence does not have to be expressed in calendar time; it can refer to an event that happens to different people at different times. For instance, it could refer to the first postoperative day or a specific day of attendance at a screening clinic.

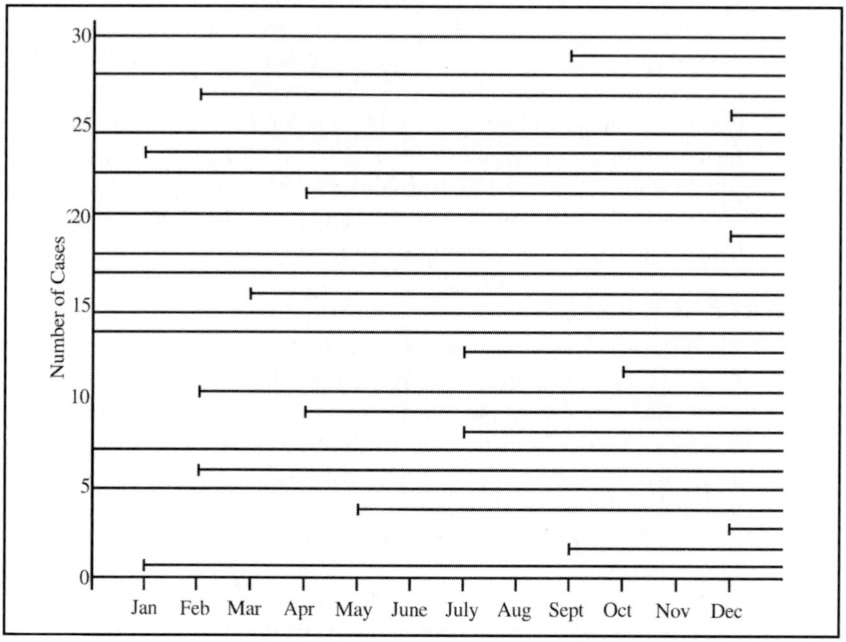

Fig. 3-4 Incidence and prevalence of AIDS in Brown County, population 114,000 during 1 year.

$$\text{Incidence rate, July} = \frac{2}{114{,}000} = 0.0000175 = \frac{1.75}{100{,}000} \text{ people}$$

$$\text{Prevalence rate, July} = \frac{24}{114{,}000} = 0.000211 = \frac{21.1}{100{,}000} \text{ people}$$

$$\text{Incidence rate, 1 year} = \frac{17}{114{,}000} = 0.000149 = \frac{14.9}{100{,}000} \text{ people}$$

$$\text{Prevalence rate, January} = \frac{15}{114{,}000} = 0.000132 = \frac{13.2}{100{,}000} \text{ people}$$

$$\text{Prevalence rate, December} = \frac{30}{114{,}000} = 0.000263 = \frac{26.3}{100{,}000} \text{ people}$$

Prevalence is influenced by two factors—the number of people who have developed the condition in the past and the duration of their illness. The longer the duration of a condition, the higher the prevalence rate will be in the community. This is best illustrated with chronic diseases. Even if the incidence rate is low, the prevalence rate may be high in the community. For instance, there are many more existing cases of cancer in a community than are indicated by examining the number of new cases. Fig. 3-4 is an example of the difference between incidence and prevalence. A person with AIDS may live for several years following diagnosis. In this hypothetical data from Brown County, the annual incidence rate of new cases is 14.9 per 100,000 people. In contrast, the prevalence rate at the end of the year was 26.3 per 100,000 people, reflecting the extended duration of the illness.

Nurses can use prevalence rates to gather information about many clinical situations. One example is a study of jaundice in healthy breast-fed infants during the first month of life (Brown and others, 1993). Using a noninvasive, transcutaneous bilirubinometer, jaundice levels were assessed on the second day of hospitalization, and at home on alternate days until the bilirubin level was below 10 mg/dl. Fig. 3-5 shows the prevalence of jaundice from day 2 through day 21. One of the difficulties for practitioners is the determination whether the jaundice is related to reduced milk intake, a finding that has been demonstrated in several studies. Since mothers and infants are often discharged within 12 to 48 hours after birth, the nursing staff have only a limited time to provide breast-feeding information. It is important that plans of care for the breast-feeding mother and infant include interventions that help promote adequate milk volume and appropriate feeding techniques. Given the prevalence patterns found in this study, it may be possible to screen infants just prior to discharge. The mothers of those infants demonstrating significant jaundice could be provided with further information about assessment of the jaundice, adequacy of the feedings, and recording the infants' output. A routine follow-up visit could be scheduled during the first post-discharge week (Brown and others, 1993).

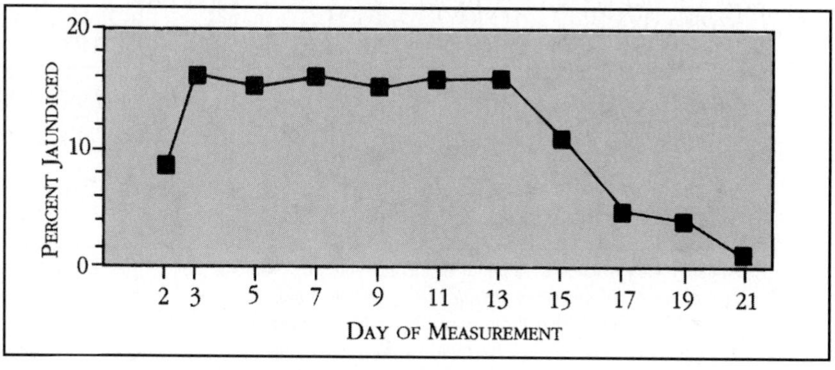

Fig. 3-5 Frequence of jaundice from day 2 through day 21: infants jaundiced at day 13 (n = 16). (From Brown LP and others: Incidence and pattern of jaundice in healthy breast-fed infants during the first month of life, *Nurs Res* 42(2):106-109, 1993.)

Prevalence statistics are important in identifying public health problems that exist in a community. They are particularly useful in determining the necessity for facilities, programs, and staff to meet the needs of a community. With alcohol and drug problems among the foremost health problems of our times, there has been an increased interest in identifying these problems in the populations served by health and social-service agencies. Table 3-7 identifies the prevalence and relative risk of problem drinking, illicit drug use, and multiple drug use in a variety of settings (Weisner and Schmidt, 1993). This table shows that all agency-based populations, with the exception of primary health-care patients on some measures, had a significantly elevated risk of alcohol and substance use problems when compared to the general public. The criminal justice subjects were 4.9 times more at risk for problem drinking than the general population. Mental-health subjects were 2.3 times more likely to be illicit drug-users, and 21 times more likely to be multiple drug-users. These differences could not be explained by age, sex, or ethnicity, since all samples were adjusted (standardized) according to the distributions of the general population.

Data such as these have multiple implications for targeted interventions. For example, those settings that have a larger number of individuals with alcohol and drug problems, such as the criminal justice, welfare, and mental health settings, should be targeted for screening and intervention efforts. Settings with a lower frequency and severity of substance abuse may prove optimal for education, prevention, and early intervention efforts.

In 1984, the Behavioral Risk Factor Surveillance System (BRFSS) was established to collect, analyze, and interpret state-specific data that could be used to

Table 3-7 Prevalence* and relative risk† of problem drinking, illicit drug use, and multiple drug use, by percentages.

	General population n=3069 (%)	**Primary health n=394 (% RR)**	**Welfare n=621 (% RR)**	**Criminal justice n=1147 (% RR)**	**Mental health n=406 (% RR)**
Problem drinker‡	11	15 (1.4)	24 (2.2)	54 (4.9)	26 (2.4)
Illicit drug§ user	27	41 (1.5)	58 (2.1)	59 (2.2)	61 (2.3)
Multiple drug§ user	1	7 (7.0)	21 (12.0)	12 (12.0)	21 (21.0)

Adapted from Weisner C, Schmidt L: Alcohol and drug problems among diverse health and social service populations, *Am J Pub Health* 83(6):824-829, 1993.

* Results are standardized to age, sex, and ethnicity distributions in the general population. The general population was the base for relative-risk calculations.

† The ratio of the prevalence of each indicator in each agency-based sample to the prevalence in the general population is in parentheses.

‡ All differences are significant at $p < 0.007$ with the exception of primary health.

§ All differences are significant at $p < 0.007$.

Table 3-8 Annual estimated prevalences of smoking* and overweight† among blacks—Michigan, Behavioral Risk Factor Surveillance System, 1987-1991‡

	Smoking		Overweight	
Year	**%**	**(95% CI§)**	**%**	**(95% CI)**
1987	34.8	(±7.0)	24.4	(±6.3)
1988	19.9	(±6.8)	32.5	(±8.0)
1989	34.5	(±6.7)	39.3	(±6.8)
1990	29.4	(±6.1)	29.5	(±5.7)
1991	31.5	(±6.1)	36.5	(±6.9)

Centers for Disease Control: Behavioral risk factor surveillance system—Michigan, 1987-1991, *MMWR* 42(36): 692-695, 1993.

* Defined as current cigarette smoking by a person who has ever smoked 100 cigarettes.

† Defined as body mass index ≥85%.

‡Annual sample sizes ranged from 130 to 290 persons aged ≥18 years.

§ Confidence interval.

plan, implement, and monitor public health programs. Through a random sampling process, the BRFSS gathers data about seven life-style variables: leisure-time physical activity, sedentary life-style, smoking, overweight, binge drinking, drinking and driving, and safety-belt nonuse (Centers for Disease Control, 1991). States have found this information very helpful in supporting their control and prevention activities. Periodically, portions of these data are published. For example, Table 3-8 presents the annual estimated prevalence of smoking and overweight among blacks in Michigan. The reduction of excess deaths in at-risk minority populations is a primary goal of the Michigan Department of Public Health. These data indicated that blacks should be targeted for health education programs about cardiovascular disease (Centers for Disease Control, 1993).

SUMMARY

In investigating the occurrence and distribution of health problems, the first steps are to describe the magnitude of the problem and to describe the characteristics of the people who have or do not have the problem. The primary measurement used to describe either the existence of a problem or the occurrence of a problem is the rate. Rates are ratios or proportions that measure the quantity of a health-related event in a specific population within a given period of time. The general rules that apply to the calculation of rates include: (1) a numerator that includes all of the events that are being measured; (2) a denominator that includes everyone at risk for the event in the numerator; (3) a specific time period of observation; and (4) adequate information about the population to determine that the event either has or has not occurred to each member of the population.

Incidence rates indicate the relationship between the number of new conditions or events occurring in a time period and the population at risk during the same time period. The determination of the date of onset is required for studies of incidence. Mortality rates or death rates are common incidence rates that provide indices of the health of a community. Incidence density calculations use a person-time denominator and are used when individuals in a study period contribute unequal periods of time to the population at risk. A relative-risk ratio is a ratio of an incidence rate in a group exposed to some factor and an incidence rate in an unexposed group. A relative-risk ratio greater than 1.0 indicates that the risk is greater in the exposed group.

Prevalence rates measure the number of people in a given population who have an existing condition at a given point in time. It is influenced by the number of people who have developed the condition in the past and the duration of their illness. The longer the duration of a condition, the higher the prevalence rate will be in the community. Therefore prevalence rates are very helpful for nurses in determining how problems are distributed within the community and in establishing programs to meet the needs of the community.

Critical Thinking Questions

1. It is determined from a report that City A has 50 new cases of an infectious disease and City B has 150 new cases. What conclusion can be made concerning the incidence of the disease in the two populations? Explain the rationale for your response.
2. Compare crude rates with specific rates. Which provides the most detailed information?
3. In Fantasy City between January 1 and December 31, 1993, 35 new cases of tuberculosis were diagnosed. There were a total of 300 cases on the list of active cases on December 31, 1993. The population of Fantasy City was 400,000. Due to tuberculosis, 20 deaths have been recorded during this 1 year period.

   What is the incidence rate per 100,000 population for tuberculosis during 1993?

   What is the prevalence rate of tuberculosis per 100,000 on December 31, 1993?

   What is the cause-specific death rate per 100,000 for tuberculosis?
4. Define attack rate, infection rate.

REFERENCES

Brown LP and others: Incidence and pattern of jaundice in healthy breast-fed infants during the first month of life, *Nurs Res,* 42(2):106-109, 1993.

Centers for Disease Control and Prevention: Progress toward elimination of *Haemophilus influenzae* type b disease among infants and children—United States, 1987-1993, *MMWR* 43(8):144-148, 1994.

Centers for Disease Control and Prevention: Behavioral risk factor surveillance system—Michigan, 1987-1991, *MMWR* 42(36):692-695, 1993.

Friedman GD: *Primer of epidemiology,* ed 3, New York, 1987, McGraw-Hill.
Harkness GA, Bentley DW, Roghmann K: Risk factors for nosocomial pneumonia in the elderly, *Am J Med* 89(4):457-463, 1990.
Hennekens CH, Buring JE: *Epidemiology in medicine,* Boston, 1987, Little, Brown.
Last JM: *A dictionary of epidemiology,* New York, 1988, Oxford University Press.
Mausner JS, Kramer S: *Epidemiology—an introductory text,* ed 2, Philadelphia, 1985, WB Saunders.
Siegel PZ and others: Behavioral risk factor surveillance, 1986-1990, *MMWR* 40(SS-4):1-7, 1991.
Valanis B: *Epidemiology in nursing and health care,* Norwalk, CT, 1992, Appleton & Lange.
Weisner C, Schmidt L: Alcohol and drug problems among diverse health and social service populations, *Am J Pub Health* 83(6):824-829, 1993.
Wishner AR and others: Interpersonal violence-related injuries in an African-American community in Philadelphia, *Am J Pub Health* 81(11):1471-1476, 1991.

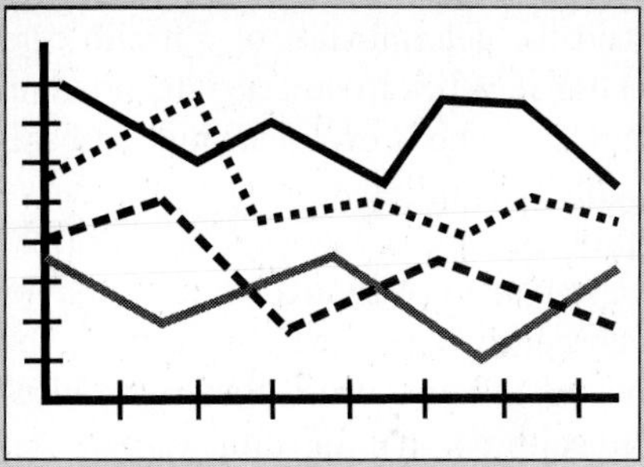

4

Descriptive Epidemiology
Person, Place, and Time

Objectives

1. Describe three ways that descriptive information about person, place, and time can be analyzed to help explain the occurrence of a health care problem.
2. Explain four ways that individuals differ in regard to person.
3. Identify the reasons why specific rates should be calculated when describing a problem.
4. Explain the value of describing a health care problem in terms of place.
5. Differentiate between short-term, periodic, and long-term fluctuations in time in relation to the development of a health care problem.
6. Present the rationale for conducting epidemiologic descriptive research studies in nursing.

Key Terms

age-specific rate
case reports
correlation coefficient
correlational studies
demography
epidemic curve
epidemiologic descriptive studies
long-term change
periodic change
short-term change

When investigating the distribution and the determinants of a health care problem, one of the first steps is to use statistics to describe the problem in terms of person, place, and time. This indicates who is experiencing the health problem (person), where it is occurring (place), and when it appears (time). Describing the characteristics of a health problem in this way provides information about the distribution of the problem, a step that is essential in the search for possible solutions. This information can subsequently be used to investigate the determinants of the health problem or how the problem occurs. Success in identifying the reasons for the occurrence of a health problem in certain groups depends on the accurate collection of this descriptive data.

There are three ways of examining descriptive information that can be helpful in developing plausible hypotheses that explain the occurrence of the health care problem. The first method is to look for **differences** in frequency of characteristics or events between various groups. The second method is to look for areas of **agreement**. A single factor may be a common finding in the study of several similar health problems, or several factors may be common to a specific health problem. The third method is to look for **variations** in the data. For instance, the frequency of a risk factor may vary with the frequency of the problem. Rates are usually used in this process, but it is often helpful to plot the numbers of conditions or events (numerators) on graphs or charts to examine the distribution of the health care problem.

PERSON

Within any general population, whether it consists of members of a neighborhood, the clients in a community clinic, or the patients in an institution, there are differences among the individuals. These differences are (1) genetic, such as race and sex; (2) biologic, such as age and nutritional state; (3) behavioral, such as religion and habits; and (4) socioeconomic, such as marital state, level of education, and characteristics of residence. Because of these variations, incidence and prevalence rates should be calculated according to these specific characteristics. This information indicates who is experiencing the health problem. Statistics of this type gathered to describe populations are referred to as demographic data. *Demography* is the study of the size, distribution, and characteristics of human population groups.

Examining individual case data

In investigating outbreaks of health problems, it is very helpful to list first the characteristics of each case, including the events surrounding the outbreak. Usually outbreak investigations begin before the end of the outbreak and before rates can be calculated. Table 4-1 lists the characteristics of four people who developed a postoperative group A *Streptococcus* wound infection (Paul, Genese, and Spitalny, 1990). Characteristics of person, place, and time of the outbreak are presented. The first three patients had an onset of infection within 24 hours of surgery, indicating that a potential source of the organism was the operating room.

Table 4-1 Case characteristics of a postoperative group A beta-hemolytic *Streptococcus* outbreak with the pathogen traced to a member of a health-care worker's household

Characteristic	Case no. 1	Case no. 2	Case no. 3	Case no. 4
Sex	Male	Male	Female	Female
Age (years)	42	52	44	72
OR*	OP†	IP #11‡	IP #11‡	IP #5
Procedure	Hernia	Thyroid lobectomy and isthmusectomy	Thyroid lobectomy and parathyroid excision	Exploratory laparotomy
Procedure duration§	85 min	150 min	190 min	255 min
Anesthesia	Local	General	General	General
Perioperative antibiotics	None	None	None	Yes
Onset	POD 1 ǁ	POD 1	POD 1	POD 16
Reoperations	2	2	2	0
ICU admission	Yes	No	Yes	Yes

From Paul SM, Genese C, Spitalny K: Postoperative group A beta-hemolytic *Streptococcus* outbreak with the pathogen traced to a member of a health-care worker's household, *Infect Control Hosp Epidemiol* 11(12):643-646, 1990.

* Operating room

† Outpatient

‡ Inpatient

§ Median 170 min.

ǁ Postoperative day

Further study determined that the only common human contact for these three patients was an anesthesiologist who had a positive culture for group A *Streptococcus.* The fourth patient had surgery during the same time frame as the others but developed signs and symptoms of the infection 16 days postoperatively. She was elderly and was the only one to receive perioperative antibiotics. Although she was not directly exposed to the anesthesiologist, she was in the operative suite at the same time as the other patients. This kind of descriptive case-listing gives clues to the investigator as to possible determinants or the origin of the problem. It serves as a guideline for further data collection.

Examining specific rates

There are two characteristics that are considered routine descriptors of a person: age and sex. Age is the most important characteristic to address when describing the person. Most illnesses vary in both frequency and severity by age, therefore morbidity and mortality rates for almost all health problems vary by age. Age can also be related to variations in time, place, and other characteristics of the person as indicated in the example that follows. Therefore age-specific incidence and prevalence rates should be calculated when describing a problem. *Age-specific rates* are figured using the number of conditions or events in a given age group in

Table 4-2 Age-specific rates for falls per 10,000 patient days

	Service					
	Neuro/psych department			Other clinical departments		
Age group	**Falls**	**Patient days**	**Rate/10,000**	**Falls**	**Patient days**	**Rate/10,000**
10-19	10	3984	25	16	7711	21
20-29	34	9256	37	35	26,092	13
30-39	17	9139	19	38	31,838	12
40-49	35	7647	46	51	26,322	19
50-59	46	8793	52	80	39,206	21
60-69	58	9132	64	144	49,042	29
70-79	80	7349	109	144	34,242	42
80 +	21	1404	150	51	10,711	50
TOTALS	**301***	**56,704†**	**53**	**562***	**225,164†**	**25**
Age-Adjusted Rate			**58.4**			**24.6**

Rohde JM, Myers AH, Vlahov D: Variation in risk for falls by clinical department: implications for prevention, *Infect Control Hosp Epidemiol* 11(10):521-524, 1990.

* Total falls were 874: 11 without age recorded were excluded from numerator.

† Total patient days were 282,713: 620 patient days for those with age missing variables were excluded from denominator.

the numerator and the population at risk in the given age group in the denominator (see Chapter 3).

An example of the use of age-specific rates is found in a study of the risk of falls in a 1000-bed, acute care hospital during a 1 year period. Table 4-2 shows age-specific incidence rates for falls per 10,000 patient days (Rohde, Myers, and Vlahov, 1990). The overall rate of falls on all hospital services was 31 out of 10,000 patient days. When falls were examined by service the highest rates were found in the neuroscience and psychiatric department, where 53 falls out of 10,000 patient days occurred. Age-specific rates indicated that the rate of falls increased steadily for all services after the age of 40. The rate for those 80 years of age and older was the highest, reaching 150 falls per 10,000 patient days in the neuroscience and psychiatric departments and 50 falls per 10,000 patient days in other clinical departments.

It is clear that the risk of falls was positively associated with increasing age in this study. Also, the age-specific rates for falls were consistently higher at all ages on the neuroscience and psychiatric services than on the other clinical services. This comparison of rates between services indicates that the increased fall rate on the neuroscience and psychiatric services was independent of age. Other factors, such as neurologic deficits and medications, were contributing to this increased overall risk, suggesting that this is an area for further study. This descriptive information about the distribution of falls is very helpful for nurses and other health professionals in developing individual fall assessment protocols and fall prevention programs for patients. It appears that falls are not random events, and that specific age groups and services should be targeted for prevention programs.

Another example of the use of age-specific rates can be found in a study of the prevalence of chronic bronchitis among the Hispanic population in the United States. Table 4-3 contrasts age-specific prevalence rates by sex and Hispanic subgroup (Bang, Bergen, and Carroll 1990). The information was based on the Hispanic Health and Nutrition Examination Survey (HHANES) conducted by the National Center for Health Statistics, 1982-1984. The HHANES data show higher rates in the 55 to 74 age group with the highest rates among Puerto Rican women between the ages of 35 and 74. The total prevalence rates indicate a higher prevalence of chronic bronchitis among Puerto Ricans. This kind of information identifies specific groups to target for further study. This information can also be used by health care practitioners in planning primary intervention programs for preventing health problems such as bronchitis.

Specific rates can also be developed for other characteristics. *Sex* is the second most important characteristic of the person. The incidence rates and death rates from various conditions often vary by sex. For instance, cancer of the lung has historically been associated with males, but this condition has rapidly increased in women. It is now estimated to be the leading cause of cancer deaths in women as well as men (American Cancer Society, 1993). Ethnicity, socioeco-

Table 4-3 Age-specific prevalence (%) of chronic bronchitis among Hispanic subgroups

	Males/age (years)			**Females/age (years)**			
	12-34	**35-54**	**55-74**	**12-34**	**35-54**	**55-74**	**Total†**
Mexican Americans							
Number	1578	624	336	1688	798	416	5440
Prevalence	0.9	1.5	3.6	0.9	2.5	3.1	1.7
95% CI	0.7, 1.1	0.4, 2.7	1.8, 5.4	0, 1.8	1.4, 3.7	0.8, 5.4	1.3, 2.1
Cuban Americans							
Number	256	221	162	268	260	217	1384
Prevalence	*	3.5	2.3	1.5	2.7	1.8	1.7
95% CI	*	0.3, 6.7	0, 5.3	0, 3.3	0.2, 5.2	0, 4.8	0.9, 2.5
Puerto Ricans							
Number	552	229	135	701	389	201	2207
Prevalence	1.1	2.0	2.5	2.7	5.0	4.9	2.9
95% CI	0.2, 2.0	0, 4.1	0, 7.3	1.3, 4.1	2.5, 7.5	1.9, 7.9	2.2, 3.6

Bang KM, Gergen PJ, Carroll M: Prevalence of chronic bronchitis among US Hispanics from the Hispanic Health and Nutrition Examination Survey, 1982-84, *Am J Public Health,* 80(12):1495-1497, 1990.

CI: Confidence interval.

* No reported chronic bronchitis.

† Age-adjusted prevalence.

nomic factors, religion, marital status, family relationships, occupation, educational level, habits, residence, and many factors can be characteristics of a person that may be of value to investigate when describing a certain condition or event.

An example of the use of several other descriptors of person is found in Table 4-4. Data from a southwest Hispanic sample of the HHANES survey were studied to determine the use of a curandero, a folk-medicine practitioner, by Mexican Americans (Higginbotham, Trevino, and Ray 1990). Examination of the specific rates (presented as percents) in Table 4-4 indicates that the users of curanderos were slightly more likely to be male, less-educated, and born outside the United States. It is interesting to note that being interviewed in Spanish was found to be highly predictive of curandero use. The investigators proposed that Mexican Americans may be reluctant to discuss the use of curanderos with English-speaking interviewers who are not familiar with the culture. Other demographic characteristics of this population of users and nonusers of curanderismo, such as age, marital status, and family size, were not found to vary significantly. This suggests that direct care-givers should strengthen their efforts to deal with the linguistic and cultural differences in establishing relationships with clients, planning care, and evaluating the results.

Examining age-adjusted rates

A third study using the HHANES data looked at behavior patterns of cigarette smoking among Hispanics in the United States. Fig. 4-1 illustrates age-adjusted prevalence rates of current smoking among the same three Hispanic groups (Haynes and others, 1990). Age-adjustment controls for variation in age when comparing two or more populations; in other words, age is removed as comparison factor (see Chapter 3). With the exception of Puerto Ricans, men were almost twice as likely to smoke as women. Among women, Puerto-Rican women had the highest rates of smoking.

The information obtained from the descriptions of the characteristics of Hispanics with chronic bronchitis and the descriptions of smoking patterns of Hispanics can be very helpful to nurses and other health professionals in community health settings who work with these populations. Smoking-prevention programs and smoking-cessation programs could target specific groups, such as Puerto-Rican women between the ages of 35 and 74. Puerto-Rican women in these age groups have the highest rates of bronchitis (Table 4-3), and Puerto-Rican women have the highest rate of smoking among the three groups when age is removed as a factor (Figure 4-1). Smoking-prevention and cessation programs could help reduce their risk of chronic bronchitis and the resulting complications.

PLACE

Differences in occurrence of diseases, conditions, or events by place are often helpful in determining health needs, planning prevention or control measures, and allocating resources. Examination of the characteristics of place determines where the rates of the disease or health problem are the highest or the lowest. Natural boundaries are considered along with political boundaries and environmental characteristics when appropriate.

Table 4-4 Demographic characteristics of reported Mexican-American users and nonusers of curanderismo

(N)	% Users (148)	% Non-Users (3475)
Gender		
Male	58.1	50.0
Female	41.9	50.0
Ages (years)		
18-44	64.2	65.2
45-64	31.1	29.2
65-74	4.7	5.6
Marital status		
Married: spouse in household	67.1	66.3
Married: spouse not in household	3.3	1.9
Widowed	5.4	3.5
Divorced	5.3	5.5
Separated	3.3	3.9
Never married	15.6	19.0
Education		
0-8 years	46.6	36.6
9-11 years	15.4	20.0
12+ years	37.9	43.5
Nativity		
United States	52.0	61.0
Other	48.0	39.0
Acculturation		
1.0-1.9	48.4	33.9
2.0-2.9	17.6	21.1
3.0-3.9	31.1	38.5
4.0-4.9	2.9	6.4
Language of interview		
English	48.6	61.3
Spanish	51.4	38.7
Family size (persons)		
1 or 2	22.2	19.6
3 or 4	39.6	40.5
5 or 6	25.3	27.6
7 or more	12.9	12.4
Size of place (population)		
500,000 or more	27.9	24.2
100,000-499,999	14.4	15.0
25,000-99,999	28.2	27.5
200-24,999	21.7	24.1
Not in a place	7.9	9.2

Higginbotham JC, Trevino FM, Ray LA: Utilization of curanderos by Mexican Americans: prevalence and predictors, *Am J Public Health,* 80(suppl):32-35, 1990.

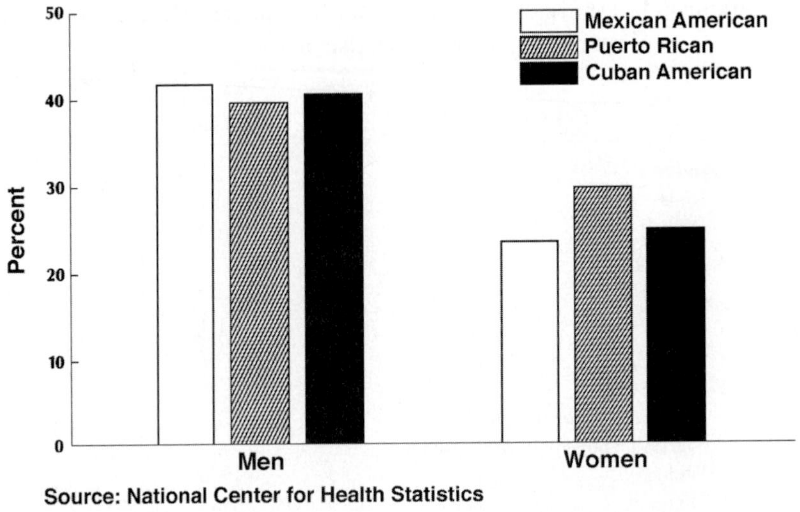

Fig. 4-1 Age-adjusted prevalence rates of current smoking among three Hispanic groups in the HHANES, by sex. (From Haynes SG and others: Patterns of cigarette smoking among Hispanics in the United States: results from HHANES 1982-84, *Am J Public Health* 80(suppl):47-53, 1990.)

Variations in incidence and prevalence rates can be examined worldwide, by continents, nations, states, counties, cities, census tract, city blocks, or any other geographic area. Differences in urban and rural sectors or between smaller localities may be helpful in investigating specific health needs of a community. Place of occurrence is almost always examined with investigations of outbreaks of illness, both in the community and within institutions. The variation in rates can be computed between institutions, units in a single institution, or different groups within any health-care facility. This information shows where prevention and control measures and health resources should be concentrated to decrease incidence and prevalence of the problem.

The Centers for Disease Control and Prevention in Atlanta, GA monitors the health problems of the United States population on a continual basis (see Chapter 9). Many of their reports depict specific illness or events by state. The human immunodeficiency virus/acquired immunodeficiency syndrome (HIV/AIDS) epidemic has been followed closely. Fig. 4-2 illustrates the rate of reported AIDS cases by sex and place of residence (CDC, 1991). The wide diversity in geographic distribution is evident. The health care systems in the states and territories with high rates have already been severely challenged. As HIV infection spreads in the heterosexual population and in women, the ability of these systems to provide preventive and therapeutic services will be further stressed.

A unique example of the description of place characteristics is presented in Fig. 4-3. Following an outbreak of surgical-wound infections by *Penicillium*

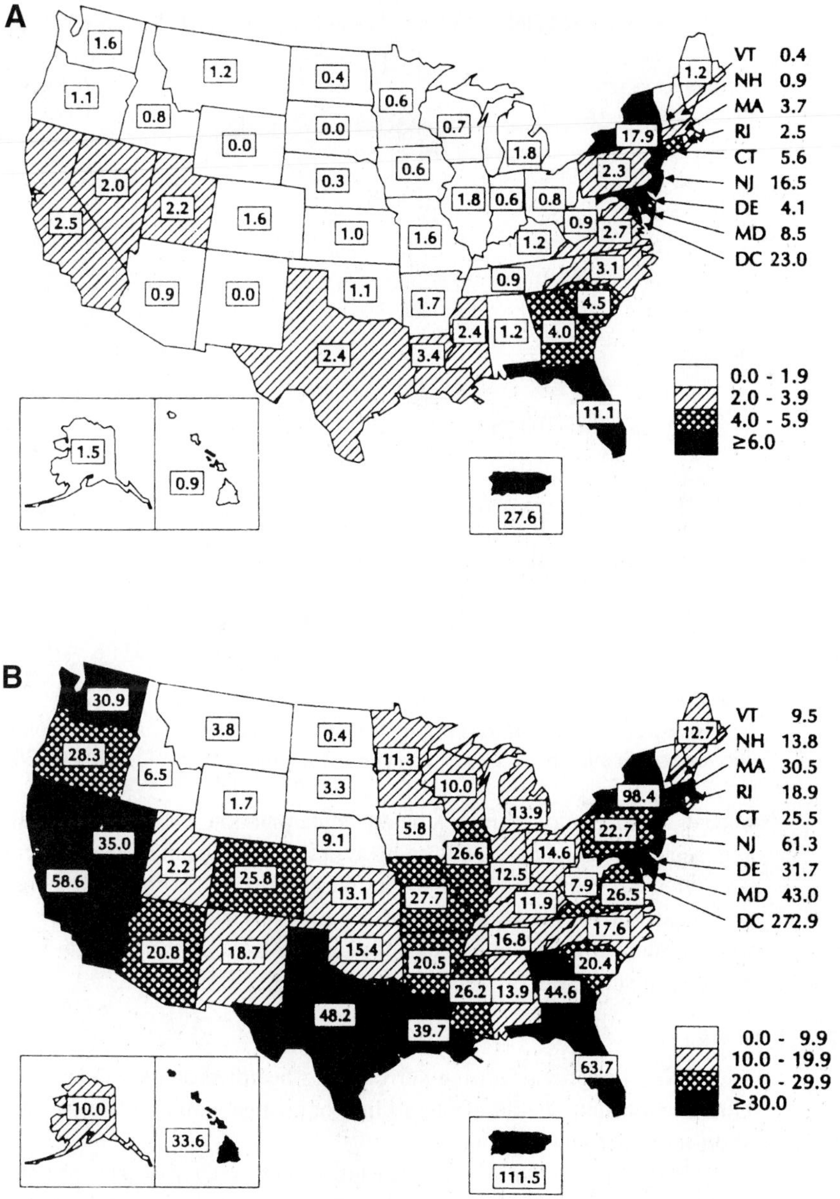

Fig. 4-2 Rate of reported AIDS cases per 100,000 population among adolescents and adults, by sex (**A,** women; **B,** men) and state of residence, United States, 1990. (From Centers for Disease Control: The HIV/AIDS epidemic: the first 10 years, *MMWR,* 40(22):357-363, 1991.)

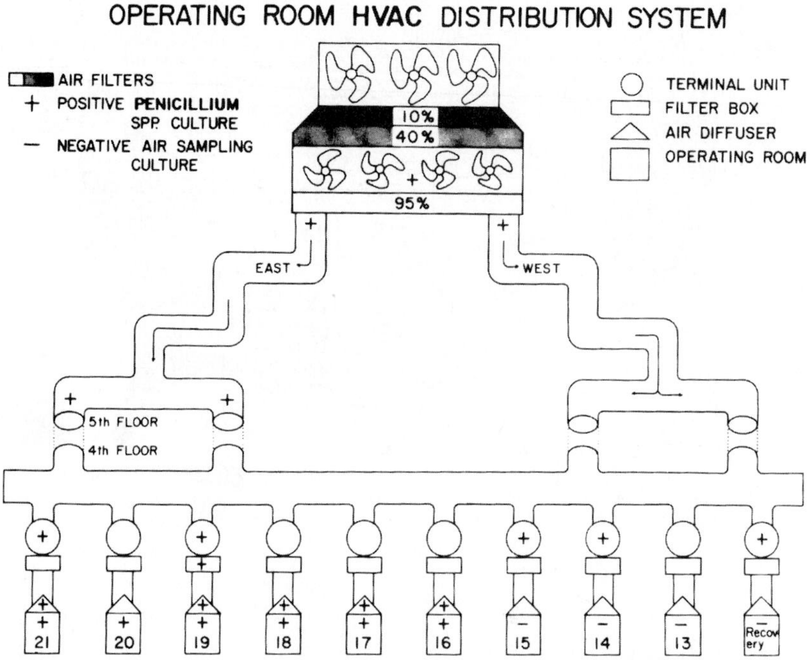

Fig. 4-3 Contamination of operating room air by *Penicillium.* (From Fox BC and others: Heavy contamination of operating room air by *Penicillium* species: identification of the source and attempts at decontamination, *Am J Infect Control,* 18(5):300-306, 1990.)

species, a filamentous fungi, a heavy contamination was discovered in the heating, ventilation, and air-conditioning system of the hospital operating rooms (Fox and others, 1990). The air-distribution system to 10 operating rooms is diagrammed, and the contamination of five rooms is shown. Corrective measures included filter replacement and use of an aerosolized chlorine solution to decontaminate the ventilation system.

TIME

Describing variations in time surrounding health problems indicates *when* the condition occurs. The three major kinds of change with time are considered to be short-term, periodic, or long-term.

Short-term fluctuations are measured in hours, days, weeks, or months. They are commonly found in epidemics of infectious disease. Fig. 4-4 presents the *epidemic curve* of an outbreak of measles in Chicago in 1989, by age and week of the rash onset. At the time of the report, the epidemic was continuing. During this epidemic, 2232 confirmed cases of measles were reported in a 6 month period with a rate of 74 cases per 100,000 population, a rate that was 10 times higher than the overall U.S. incidence rate for that year. Nearly 75% of the reported patients were unvaccinated, indicating a continuing need for immunization clinics for preschool children. Outbreaks like these have stimulated a nationwide drive to increase the percentage of children who are immunized to childhood diseases.

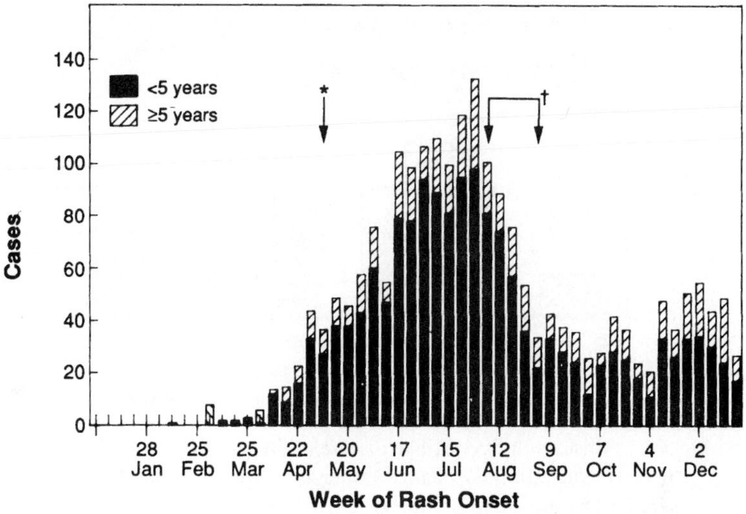

Fig. 4-4 Patients with confirmed measles, by age and by week of rash onset—Chicago, February 14 through December 31, 1989. (* On May 5, the minimum age for vaccination was lowered citywide to 12 months. † On July 31, the minimum age for vaccination was lowered to 6 months in communities with high attack rates. Additional outbreak-control activities during July 31 through September 1 included intensified surveillance; publicity; audits of school vaccination records; vaccination clinics; and door-to-door vaccination in housing projects.) (From Centers for Disease Control: Update: measles outbreak, *MMWR* 39(10):317-319, 1990.)

Outbreaks, such as the epidemic of influenza-like disease that occurred in hospitalized patients in West Virginia (Fig. 4-5), can be defined in terms of time (CDC, 1980). Diagramming variables, such as the date of onset and location, provides indications as to the mode of transmission and spread of the organism. Once the influenza B virus infection appeared in one patient on the unit, several more cases followed in succession, indicating the possibility of person-to-person transmission between patients. It is known that the transfer of virus-containing respiratory secretions from an infected person to a susceptible person occurs through small-particle aerosols dispersed through sneezing, coughing, and talking (Betts and Douglas, 1990). More information regarding epidemic curves, transmission of infectious disease, and investigation of epidemics is found in Chapter 7.

Periodic changes may be seasonal or cyclic. For instance, respiratory diseases are more common in winter and spring, and infectious hepatitis often increases in incidence every 7 to 9 years. *Long-term changes* extend over decades and reflect gradual changes. Changes in trends of the mortality of various cancers can be seen when examined over many years (Fig. 4-6). Most cancer death rates have either decreased or stabilized with the exception of lung cancer, which has risen dramatically (American Cancer Society, 1991). In contrast, statistics from the American Heart Association (1993) indicate that age-adjusted death rates for major cardiovascular diseases have steadily decreased in recent years (Fig. 4-7).

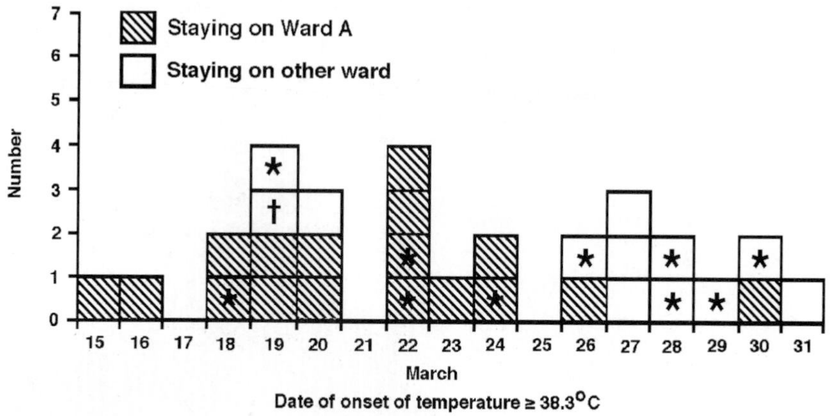

Fig. 4-5 Cases of influenza-like disease (* influenza B virus isolated; † respiratory syncytial virus isolated) in hospitalized patients in West Virginia, March 15-31, 1980. (From Centers for Disease Control: *MMWR* 29:26, 1980.)

Knowledge of periodic and long-term changes are helpful in evaluating disease-prevention programs and planning for future allocation of resources.

EPIDEMIOLOGIC DESCRIPTIVE STUDIES

Epidemiologic descriptive studies are designed to acquire more information about the occurrence of states of health, such as characteristics of person, place, and time. These studies provide a picture of the events as they naturally occur. Therefore this type of data is very helpful for nurses involved in health planning or administration in both community and institutional settings. Knowledge of the groups of people that are the most, or least susceptible to a health problem can help in decisions to implement programs for prevention or control of health problems and to allocate resources.

Descriptive studies are very useful in describing the characteristics of disease occurrence and generating hypotheses for further study. They are the first studies to be done in investigating the determinants of a health problem. A substantial base of descriptive data is necessary to build the rationale for an experimental or intervention study. *Epidemiologic descriptive studies* include the description of an epidemiologic problem, case reports, and correlational studies.

Description of an epidemiologic problem

When specific studies are conducted that examine the morbidity rates, mortality rates, or other characteristics of one or more health problems in a population, it is considered a description of an epidemiologic problem. Descriptive statistics are used, such as a presentation of specific rates broken down by person, place, and time. However, no sample is selected from the population to study, and no inferential statistical analysis is done that compares groups for statistically significant results. For example, Table 4-2 is a descriptive study of the problem of falls in the

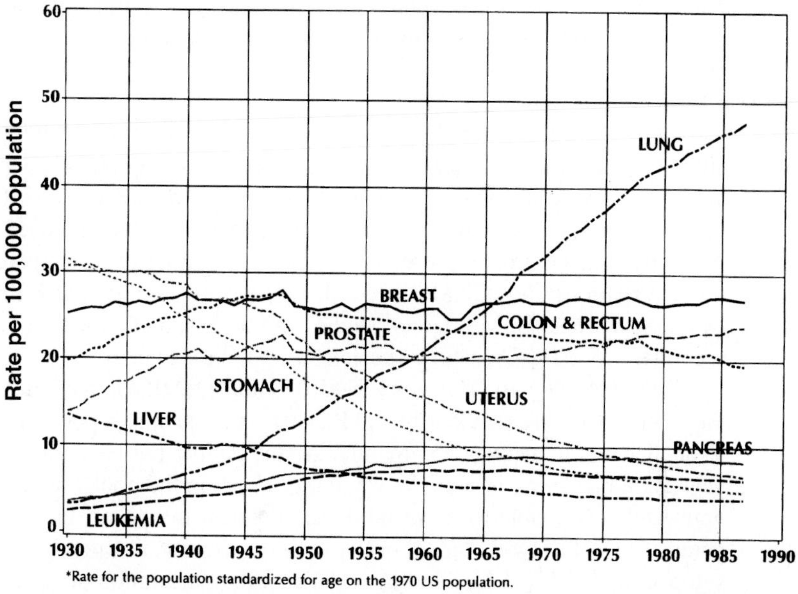

Fig. 4-6 Cancer death rates by site, United States, 1930-1987. (Rate for the population standardized for age on the 1970 U.S. population.) (Sources of data: National Center for Health Statistics and Bureau of the Census, United States. Note: Rates are for both sexes combined except breast and uterus [female population only] and prostate [male population only].) (From American Cancer Society: Cancer facts and figures—1991, Atlanta, GA 1991, The Society.)

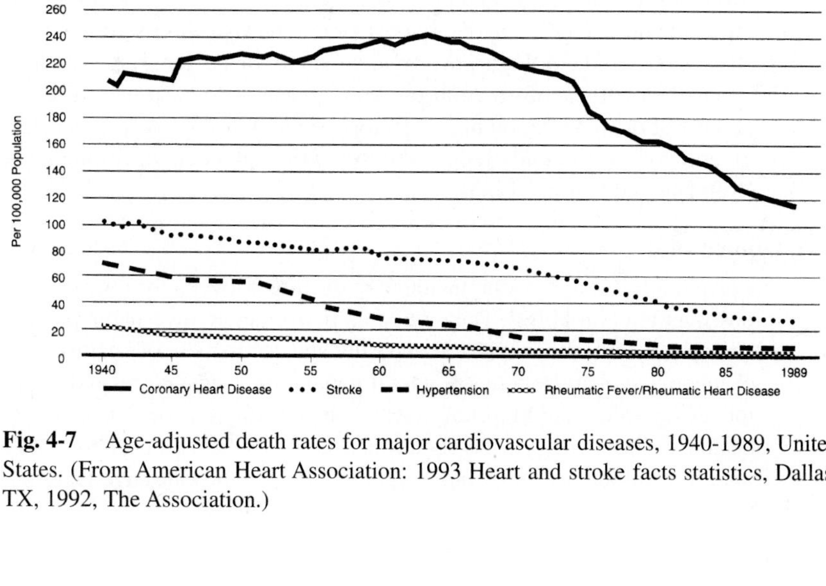

Fig. 4-7 Age-adjusted death rates for major cardiovascular diseases, 1940-1989, United States. (From American Heart Association: 1993 Heart and stroke facts statistics, Dallas, TX, 1992, The Association.)

clinical departments of an acute care hospital. Fig. 4-3 illustrates a descriptive study of the source of operating room air contamination.

Case reports

Case reports like those in Table 4-1 examine the experience of individuals. The study of unusual occurrences of single individuals or a group of people with the same condition can lead to the identification of new disorders. Knowledge of the circumstances surrounding the unusual occurrence can then be used to develop prevention and control measures. Case reports or a series of case reports are based on the experience of individuals and therefore cannot be used to establish statistical associations. However, case studies can be invaluable for forming hypotheses. Case reports can raise the question but not answer it.

The *Morbidity and Mortality Weekly Report (MMWR),* published weekly by the Centers for Disease Control and Prevention frequently reports unusual events as an alert to the medical community and the public. For example, in 1991, a 3-year-old girl playing in a public wading pool sat on the pool's uncapped suction drain and was unable to move until the attendant turned off the pool's suction pump. The girl's rectal mucosa prolapsed from the negative pressure, and she developed peritonitis. A laparotomy revealed a long laceration of the rectosigmoid colon that required a sigmoid colostomy. Along with documentation of the event, safety measures to prevent childhood injuries from pool suction drains were published (CDC, 1992).

Perhaps the best example of the usefulness of case reports is illustrated by the events surrounding the initial recognition of the syndrome that was later identified as AIDS. Between October 1980 and May 1981, five cases of *Pneumocystis carinii* pneumonia were reported in young homosexual men who had been previously healthy (CDC, 1981a). This type of pneumonia had previously occurred only in immunosuppressed elderly people, such as cancer patients. This report was quickly followed by another unusual report of Kaposi's sarcoma in young homosexual men (CDC, 1981b). Kaposi's sarcoma also was usually seen only in the elderly. An epidemiologic investigative surveillance program was immediately initiated to gather information on what appeared to be a new disease, and the process of documentation of risk factors began. Within 4 years a substantial body of epidemiologic knowledge about AIDS had been developed (Peterman, Drotman, and Curran, 1985).

Correlational studies

Correlational studies examine the relationships between the characteristics under investigation (variables). They are often performed to investigate possible associations between various types of exposure and adverse use of health outcomes. For example, the characteristics of a total population can be correlated with such factors as mortality and morbidity rates from specific diseases or patterns of use of health services within a specified time frame. The results of these studies can be used to formulate assumptions (hypotheses) as to the causative factors involved.

The measure of association in correlational studies is the *correlation coefficient, r.* It measures the extent to which changes in the characteristic (exposure) are related to an increase or decrease in adverse health outcomes. The value of r can vary from +1 (direct relationship) to -1 (inverse relationship); 0 indicates no relationship. Although correlational studies often can be performed quickly and at relatively low cost, there are limitations to their interpretation. It can be incorrectly reasoned that if two variables are related, one must cause the other to occur. Causality cannot be established by correlation techniques; many other intervening variables may be present. For example, lower socioeconomic status is associated with tuberculosis, but it is not a causative relationship. Nevertheless, this information is valuable. Knowledge of this relationship can help public health officials to target specific groups for prevention and control of tuberculosis.

SUMMARY

One of the first steps in the epidemiologic investigation of the distribution and the determinants of a health care problem is to describe the problem statistically in terms of person, place, and time. This information provides us with the who, where, and when characteristics of the problem. These data can subsequently be used to examine the reasons why and how the problem occurs. This is done by examining the data for differences, areas of agreement, and variations in frequency of the characteristics between groups.

Differences in individuals can be genetic, biologic, behavioral, and socioeconomic. Individual case data can be listed as a first step in the investigation. However, the calculation of specific rates will provide the most valid information regarding the problem. Age-specific incidence and prevalence rates are frequently calculated when describing a problem. Age-adjusted rates can be calculated when two or more groups are to be compared. When this is done age is standardized for the groups to be compared and is removed as a factor for comparison.

Differences in the occurrence of health problems by place are helpful in determining need, planning for prevention and control, and allocating resources. Incidence and prevalence rates are used to compare groups by geographic location. These geographic areas are diverse, ranging from international comparisons to examining differences between groups of people in a single institution.

Variations in time can be short-term, found in outbreaks of infectious diseases, periodic, such as seasonal or cyclic, and long-term, such as the changes in trends of mortality over time. Evaluating these trends over time give evidence of the effectiveness of health-promotion and disease-prevention programs and are useful in planning for future use of resources.

Epidemiologic descriptive research studies are designed to acquire more information about the occurrence of states of health, providing a picture of events as they naturally occur. Epidemiologic descriptive studies include the description of an epidemiologic problem, case reports, and correlational studies. They are useful in describing characteristics of disease occurrence, identifying relationships between characteristics, and generating assumptions as to origin of the problem.

Critical Thinking Questions

1. Identify three methods for examining descriptive information that are helpful in developing a hypothesis explaining the occurrence of a health-care problem.
2. List at least four characteristics of individuals that may be of value when describing a health condition or event.
3. A recent report from the Connecticut State Health Department included a map indicating the distribution and number of rabid animals for each of the 167 towns in the state during the time period of January 1, 1993 to October 31, 1993. What type of information about the occurrence of rabies does this report include? How might this information be used to control rabies?
4. Occurrence of health events may be short-term, periodic, or long-term. Give an example of each. How does knowledge of change in the occurrence of health events over time contribute to evaluation of disease-prevention programs?

REFERENCES

American Cancer Society: *Cancer facts and figures—1991,* Atlanta, 1991, The Society.

American Cancer Society: *Cancer facts and figures—1993,* Atlanta, 1993, The Society.

American Heart Association: *1993 Heart and stroke facts statistics,* Dallas, TX, 1992, The Association.

Bang KM, Gergen PJ, Carroll M: Prevalence of chronic bronchitis among US Hispanics from the Hispanic Health and Nutrition Examination Survey, 1982-84, *Am J Public Health* 80(12):1495-1497.

Betts RF, Douglas RG: Influenza virus. In Mandell GL, Douglas RG, Bennett JE: *Principles and practice of infectious diseases,* ed 3, New York, 1990, Churchill Livingstone.

Centers for Disease Control: Influenza B in a hospital—West Virginia *MMWR* 29(26), 1980.

Centers for Disease Control: *Pneumocystis* pneumonia—Los Angeles, *MMWR* 30:250, 1981a.

Centers for Disease Control: Kaposi's sarcoma and *Pneumocystis* pneumonia among homosexual men—New York City and California, *MMWR* 30:305, 1981b.

Centers for Disease Control: Update: measles outbreak, *MMWR* 39(10):317-319, 1990.

Centers for Disease Control: The HIV/AIDS epidemic: the first 10 years, *MMWR* 40(22), 357-363+, 1991.

Centers for Disease Control: Suction-drain injury in a public wading pool—North Carolina, 1991, *MMWR* 41(19):333-335, 1992.

Fox BC and others: Heavy contamination of operating room air by *Penicillium* species: identification of the source and attempts at decontamination, *Am J Infect Control* 18(5):300-306, 1990.

Haynes SG and others: Patterns of cigarette smoking among Hispanics in the United States: results from HHANES 1982-84, *Am J Public Health* 80(Supp), 47-53, 1990.

Hennekens CH, Buring JE: *Epidemiology in medicine,* Boston, 1987, Little, Brown.

Higginbotham JC, Trevino FM, Ray LA: Utilization of curanderos by Mexican Americans: prevalence and predictors, *Am J Public Health* 80(Supp): 32-35, 1990.

Mausner JS, Kramer S: *Epidemiology—an introductory text,* ed 2, Philadelphia, 1985, WB Saunders.

Peterman TA, Drotman DP, Curran JW: Epidemiology of the acquired immunodeficiency syndrome (AIDS), *Epidemiol Rev* 7(1), 1985.

Paul SM, Genese C, Spitalny K: Postoperative Group A beta-hemolytic *Streptococcus* outbreak with the pathogen traced to a member of a health care worker's household, *Infect Control Hosp Epidemiol* 11(12):643-646, 1990.

Rohde HM, Myers AH, Vlahov D: Variation in risk for falls by clinical department: implications for prevention, *Infect Control Hosp Epidemiol* 11(10):521-524, 1990.

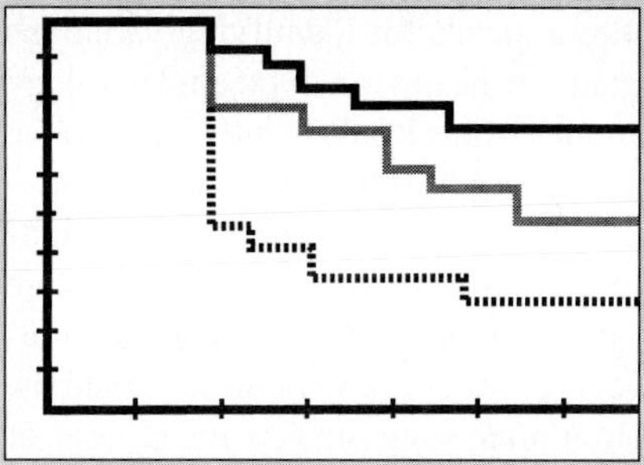

5

Analytic Epidemiology
Cross-sectional, Case-control, and Cohort Studies

OBJECTIVES

1. Explain the meaning of statistical associations and the role of chance.
2. Compare cross-sectional, case-control, and cohort study designs in terms of exposure and outcome variables.
3. Discuss the use of epidemiologic study designs in answering questions associated with nursing care.
4. Describe how confounding variables can affect the validity of an epidemiologic study.
5. Explain potential bias in epidemiologic study designs.
6. Identify the differences in time frame involved in cross-sectional, case-control, and cohort studies.
7. Contrast the similarities and differences between cohort and historical cohort studies.
8. Assess the importance of choosing representative control groups in case-control and cohort studies.
9. Define relative risk and odds ratio in terms of exposure and outcomes.

KEY TERMS

association bias
case-control study
cohort studies
confidence intervals
cross-sectional study
epidemiologic analytic study
historical cohort study
hypothesis
logistic regression
longitudinal study
odds ratio
P-value
prospective study
retrospective study
statistical significance
Type I error
Type II error
variables
- confounding
- dependent
- independent

While descriptive epidemiology provides a means for identifying variations in the distribution or occurrence of states of health, analytic epidemiology focuses on identifying the determinants of states of health. When the descriptive data are analyzed, the variations in the occurrence of health conditions often suggest tentative explanations or hypotheses. Hypotheses are testable propositions that attempt to explain *why* the variations occur. Analytic research processes are then used to test these hypotheses, either accepting or rejecting them, in an attempt to find the reasons or determinants that are associated with these variations. This is a cyclic process, since new information often suggests new hypotheses or the need for further descriptive studies (Fig 5-1).

STATISTICAL ASSOCIATIONS

Finding a statistical association between an exposure and an outcome means that when the exposure varies the outcome changes. There is a statistical dependence between the two variables. In epidemiology, it usually means that the state of health of people who have had a specific exposure is different from those people without the exposure. Exposures and states of health are broadly defined. Exposures can include any factors internal to the individual or external in the environment. States of health or health outcomes can be positive, such as health states or behaviors, or negative, such as disease or disability.

Both epidemiologic research and nursing research are usually conducted among people in a community or institutional setting. Control over many outside factors (confounding variables) that are not being studied but could affect the study results is not possible. As a result, statistical associations may have alternative explanations. While the association hopefully is a valid association, it might also be due to chance, bias, or the effect of confounding variables (Hennekens and Buring, 1987).

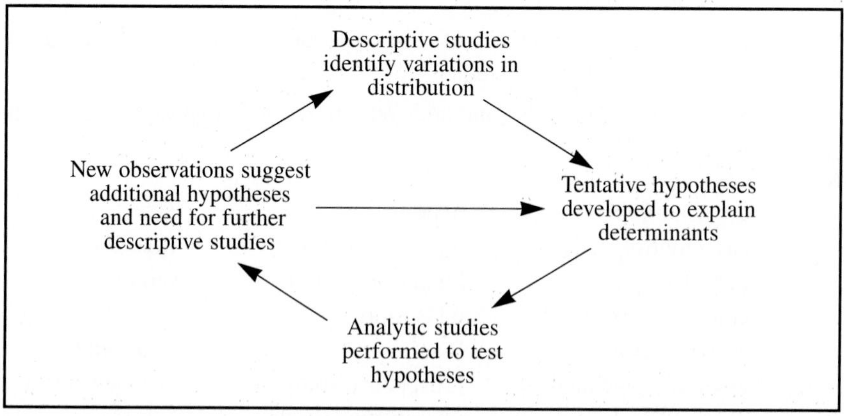

Fig. 5-1 The epidemiologic study cycle. (Adapted from Mausner JS, Kramer S: *Epidemiology—an introductory text,* Philadelphia, 1985, WB Saunders, p 155.)

Chance

An association due to chance occurs as a result of the sampling process. It is assumed in most studies that information about an entire population can be obtained by studying a sample of that population. However, if two samples of people are randomly selected from a population, it is unlikely that they would be identical. The variation between the two samples is due to chance. Therefore selecting any sample may result in a sample that is not representative of the entire population due to chance. There are sampling techniques that reduce this possibility. A sampling text will explore these in detail. In general, larger sample sizes will produce less variability, and the results will be more reliable.

A test of statistical significance, such as a t-test or chi-square test, measures variability due to chance in analytic and intervention studies. The result is calculation of a *P-value,* the probability that the obtained results occur from chance alone. It is generally accepted that a P-value less than or equal to 0.05 is considered *statistically significant.* This figure is interpreted to mean that there is no more than a 5% probability that the observed result would be due only to chance.

Bias

An association between variables may also be due to bias or error. *Association bias* is any factor that produces a distortion in the results of a study. Usually this means that information was collected differently for the study groups involved. For example, the criteria for enrolling subjects into a study may vary (case detection or selection bias). Information may be obtained using unstructured methods resulting in differences between the groups to be compared (observation bias), or investigators may interpret information inconsistently (observer or interviewer bias). Subjects may also remember events differently (recall bias). Biases such as these make the data collected incomparable. Any statistical analysis, even if it resulted in a p-value equal to or less than 0.05, would not be valid if flaws existed in the study design.

Confounding variables

Along with study bias, the presence of additional *variables* can result in the observation of differences between study groups when they really do not exist (*Type I error*) or no differences between study groups when they do exist (*Type II error*). Methods for the control of *confounding variables,* either in the study design or in the analysis of data, have been developed and should be considered prior to initiating any study.

The primary objective of *epidemiologic analytic studies* is to produce valid results where the study has measured and examined what it was supposed to measure; chance, bias, and confounding variables have been excluded. There are four types of studies frequently used in epidemiologic analytic investigations: (1) cross-sectional (prevalence) studies, (2) case-control (retrospective) studies, (3) cohort (prospective, longitudinal) and historical cohort studies, and (4) intervention (experimental) studies. Intervention studies are discussed in Chapter 6. A comparison of these study designs is found in Fig. 5-2.

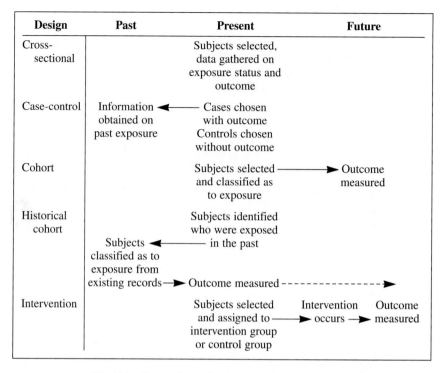

Design	Past	Present	Future
Cross-sectional		Subjects selected, data gathered on exposure status and outcome	
Case-control	Information obtained on past exposure ←	Cases chosen with outcome Controls chosen without outcome	
Cohort		Subjects selected and classified as to exposure →	Outcome measured
Historical cohort	Subjects classified as to exposure from existing records ← →	Subjects identified who were exposed in the past; Outcome measured - - - →	
Intervention		Subjects selected and assigned to intervention group or control group →	Intervention occurs → Outcome measured

Fig. 5-2 Comparison of epidemiologic study designs.

CROSS-SECTIONAL STUDIES

Cross-sectional studies are surveys that produce prevalence data and can be classified as either descriptive studies or analytic studies. In a traditional cross-sectional study, a sample is chosen from a population and information is gathered about the variables of interest at a given point in time. Sometimes, a cross-sectional study will be designed to gather data from two or more groups of people who have different characteristics or who have had different exposures in the past. Comparisons can then be made between the groups. In either case, information about both risk factors (exposure) and health outcomes (either positive or negative) are ascertained during the same period of time. As a result, relationships or associations can be identified, but it is usually not possible to determine whether the risk factor (exposure) preceded or resulted from the health problem (outcome). In other words, it cannot be clearly established which came first, the risk factor or the outcome. An exception is when the exposure variables do not alter over time, such as an inherited predisposition to an illness.

The content of cross-sectional studies varies widely and can include information on personal background, health status, environmental data, behavior characteristics, knowledge, opinions, attitudes, values, and motives. A specific time period is designated, such as a calendar year, a month, or a week, during which data are collected. Alternatively, a fixed point in a course of events can be identified that varies in time for each individual person. Examples of the latter would include a survey of nursing history and physical assessment findings on the day of admission to a clinic or a study of status of patients on their first postoperative day. Information is gathered on the day of the event, the admission day or first postoperative day, but the real time varies from patient to patient. Therefore cross-sectional surveys provide a glimpse of the health status of a sample of the population at a specific time and place (Fig. 5-2).

Cross-sectional survey information may be obtained in a variety of ways, through examination of records, observation of behavior, personal and telephone interviews, and written questionnaires. The more precise the sampling and data-gathering techniques are, the less bias is introduced into the study. Observational techniques and interview forms should be carefully designed, and training sessions for interviewers are essential. Following data collection, the information is analyzed descriptively and the relationships between the variables are examined.

Cross-sectional studies can cover a range of topics and serve many purposes. Usually, they are easy to put into operation, are flexible and economical, and produce results in a reasonable length of time. Some studies have been criticized for being too superficial, and others may demand much personnel time and financial resources. A summary of the features of cross-sectional studies is found in the box below.

The National Health Survey consists of a series of on-going cross-sectional prevalence surveys of the U.S. population. The survey was established in 1956, is administered by the National Center for Health Statistics, and is conducted by the Bureau of the Census. It is the only nationwide source of data for the prevalence of acute and chronic illnesses, disabilities, functional problems, health needs, and

FEATURES OF CROSS-SECTIONAL STUDIES

Purpose

Describe health states
Explore data for tentative hypotheses to explain determinants of health states

Design

Both exposure and outcome variables are ascertained at the same point in time

Data collection techniques

Documentary sources
Observation
Personal and telephone interviews
Written questionnaires

Advantages

Flexibility
Broadness
Uncomplicated
Economical
Rapid results
Large sample possible

Disadvantages

Cannot infer cause and effect
Relatively superficial
Can demand significant resources

use of resources as they exist in the population. The Health Interview Survey collects data through random personal household interviews, and the Health and Nutrition Examination Survey gathers information about physical examinations and laboratory tests. Statistics generated from these studies can be used to document the magnitude of specific health problems and provide a comparison for the findings of studies that have used samples from smaller or more local populations. Also, the data are available on computer tapes for research studies by other investigators. An example is a study of the prevalence, severity, and impact of childhood chronic illness using data from the 1988 National Health Interview Study (Newacheck and Taylor, 1992). This study demonstrated that chronic illnesses have highly variable impacts on the activities of children and their use of health care resources.

Another example of the use of national data is a study of risk factors for suicide attempts among Navajo adolescents, using the 1988 Navajo Adolescent Health Survey, a subset of the Indian Health Service Adolescent Health Survey (Grossman, Milligan, and Deyo, 1991). The study was conducted by two physicians and a nurse working collaboratively. One question in the survey was used as the outcome variable: "Have you ever tried to kill yourself?" In a sample of 7241 adolescents, students who reported a past suicide attempt were compared to those with no such report on a number of risk-factor variables.

Table 5-1 presents the nine significant risk factors for lifetime prevalence of suicide attempts that were obtained in the study. The researchers chose to calcu-

Table 5-1 Crude and adjusted odds ratio of risk factors for suicide attempts in Navajo adolescents

	Odds ratios		
Category/risk factor	**Crude**	**Adjusted**	**95%CI**
Physical child abuse	4.0	1.9	1.5-2.4
Sexual child abuse	3.4	1.5	1.2-1.9
Female gender	1.8	1.7	1.4-2.0
Family history of suicide attempt/ completion	3.9	2.3	1.6-3.2
Friend history of suicide attempt	5.0	2.8	2.3-3.4
Perception of poor health	4.4	2.2	1.3-3.8
History of mental/behavior problems requiring professional help	3.7	3.2	2.2-4.5
Extreme alienation from family and community	5.0	3.2	2.1-4.4
Weekly use of hard liquor	4.2	2.7	1.9-3.9

Adapted from Grossman DC, Milligan BC, Deyo RA: Risk factors for suicide attempts among Navajo adolescents, *Am J Pub Health* 81(7):871, 1991.

late the *odds ratio* (OR), an estimate of relative risk (see page 49). The crude odds ratios that estimate relative risk are presented in column one. Odds ratios that have been adjusted to remove age as a factor in the logistic regression analysis are found in column two. The difference in odds ratios between these two columns represents the effect of age as a confounder. For example, those having a friend with a history of a suicide attempt were 5 times more likely to have had a suicide attempt themselves on the crude estimate of relative risk but were only 2.8 times more likely to have had a suicide attempt themselves when age was removed as a factor. The two strongest associations were a history of a mental, behavioral, or emotional problem requiring professional help (OR = 3.2) and extreme alienation from family and community (OR = 3.2). The weekly consumption of hard liquor was also significantly associated with suicide attempts. The correlation between liquor use and suicide attempts is illustrated in Fig. 5-3.

The prevalence of self-reported suicide attempts among Navajo students is high. However, the risk factors found for Native American youth are similar to those that have been reported for the general population. Although this cross-sectional study design found a number of important risk factors that will be helpful in designing preventive programs, it was not able to establish the temporal relationships between the risk factors and the suicide attempts. It is important that preventive strategies focus on those risk factors that can be modified. Therefore the authors suggest that carefully designed, population-based, case-control studies be conducted to further explore the determinants of suicidal behavior in native populations.

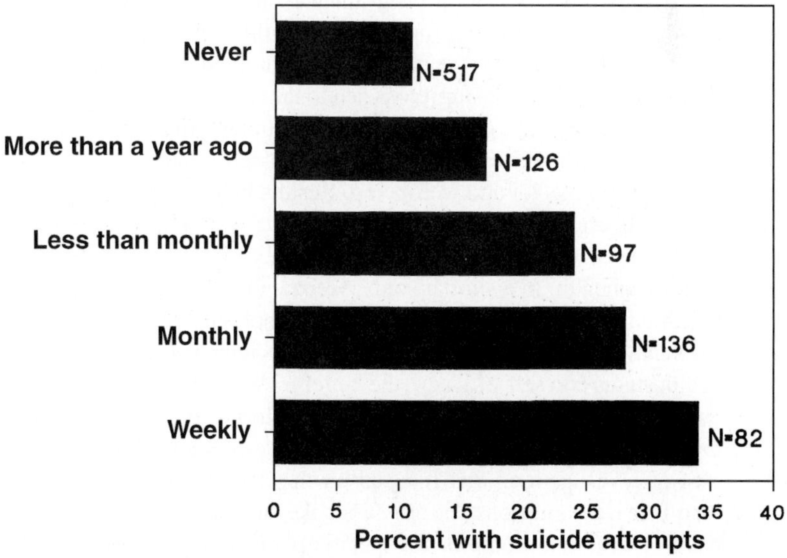

Fig. 5-3 Correlation between alcohol use and suicide attempts in Navajo adolescents. From Grossman DC, Milligan BC, and Deyo RA: Risk factors for suicide attempts among Navajo adolescents, *Am J Pub Health* 81(7): 871, 1991.

Many nurse researchers have used cross-sectional survey techniques on a smaller scale to obtain data that will assist in the health promotion of various population groups. For example, a nursing study of home apnea monitoring and disruption in family life used cross-sectional survey techniques (Ahmann, Wulff, and Meny, 1992). The association between apnea and sudden infant death syndrome (SIDS) has lead to the use of home apnea monitors for preventive and diagnostic purposes. This study investigated possible detrimental effects from home apnea monitors on family life. Of those families of infants considered at high risk for SIDS, 93 had home apnea monitoring and were compared with 86 families with infants not requiring home apnea monitoring. The families of infants at high risk for SIDS were participants in one of two monitoring programs that provided support and follow-up. The comparison families were identified from birth or nursery record and therefore were more representative of the general population. They were matched to the home apnea monitoring families on infant age, race, sex, and mother's marital status. The matching process ensured that the infants in both samples were of the same age, race, and sex and that their mothers were of the same marital status. Therefore these characteristics were removed as variables in the study design.

The survey techniques used in this study involved telephone interviews and questionnaires that measured 12 family life variables. The comparison of family life variables between the two groups indicated that the home apnea monitoring mothers were at an increased risk of poor health. However, the absence of other significant differences between the case and comparison families indicated that adequate resources for families in supportive monitoring programs have enabled them to cope well with the stresses of home monitoring. This study indicated that the support and follow-up program was achieving satisfactory results, but a health-promotion program for mothers should be considered.

A number of nurse researchers have examined factors associated with health-promotion behaviors using cross-sectional study designs. Duffy (1988) studied 262 midlife women, gathering data on demographic variables, health locus of control (belief that health outcomes can be self-controlled), self-esteem, and an assessment of health and well-being. Results indicated that women with high levels of self-esteem, who are health-conscious and believed that they could affect their own health outcomes, were most likely to take an active responsibility for their own health. In a similar study, Weitzel (1989) examined the relationship between demographic variables, several psychologic variables, and health-promoting behaviors in blue-collar workers. Results indicated that people's perception of health status and self-efficacy (the belief in one's ability to successfully complete an action), were most strongly related to health-promoting behaviors. Both of these studies support Pender's (1987) health-promotion model. They are examples of investigations that focused on the determinants of healthy states rather than disease conditions. Information like this is helpful for nurses in targeting health-promotion programs for specific population groups.

An example of a cross-sectional study that provided data for nurses involved in long-term health care planning was performed by Pfeffer and others (1987).

They studied the prevalence of Alzheimer's disease in a retirement community. The data suggested that Alzheimer's disease is more prevalent than previously suspected; current observed rates underestimated the actual community prevalence. It was recommended that added attention be given to this phenomenon in social and health care planning and in the assessment of future research priorities.

CASE-CONTROL STUDIES

Case-control studies involve the investigation of two groups of people, one group that has a specific health problem (cases) and another group that does not have the health problem (controls), who are similar in all other characteristics. The sample for these studies is chosen on the occurrence (cases) or absence (controls) of the health problem being studied. Therefore the outcome variable, or dependent variable, has already occurred. Data collection goes back in time to look for factors related to exposure, and the cases and controls are examined for differences (Fig. 5-2). The investigators are looking for exposure factors that are associated with the development of the condition, but not associated with those without the condition. This type of study is often called a *retrospective study,* since the design looks backward from outcome to possible exposure or causative factors.

Case-control studies evolved during the time that major public health concerns were shifting from acute to chronic diseases in developed countries (Cole, 1979). Chronic diseases often develop slowly and have long latency periods during which the condition is present but not apparent. This study design allows investigators to identify groups of affected and unaffected people and to look backward to identify exposure factors, rather than wait years for the condition to develop. This design is also excellent for studying rare diseases or events. A very large number of people would have to be followed for a significant length of time to adequately study the development of a rare condition. Also, if the information is available, many exposure factors can be studied in the affected and unaffected groups. Case-control studies are relatively inexpensive to perform, and results can be obtained quickly. A summary of the features of case-control studies is found in the box on page 84.

Case-control studies are usually the first to be performed when determining whether a specific characteristic—personal or environmental—is related to the onset of a health problem. They are exploratory in nature, attempting to determine whether there is any significant evidence that the *hypothesis* or tentative explanation is correct. Most studies that assess risk factors associated with a specific illness or a social problem are case-control studies.

The first evidence of the relationship between smoking and cancer was documented by a case-control study (Doll and Hill, 1950). This classic study obtained information on smoking history and other health-related variables from a large sample of people with lung cancer. These cases were compared with controls that were selected from hospitalized patients who did not have a malignancy. They found that their hypothesis was valid; a significant association between smoking and lung cancer was demonstrated. Following the identification of an unusual syndrome in 1981 that was later defined as acquired immunodeficiency

FEATURES OF CASE-CONTROL STUDIES

Purpose

Determine if two groups, one with and one without the condition under study, differ in proportion of exposure to specific factors

Design

Select sample of "cases" that have the condition (dependent variable) to be studied
Select sample of "controls" that do not have the condition to be studied
Trace past experience to determine relevant exposure (independent) variables
Compare cases and controls

Selection of cases and controls

Define criteria for selection of cases
Choose controls that resemble cases closely except for presence of condition under study
When there is evidence that two conditions are related, the use of one as a control for the other is contraindicated

Advantages

First step in hypothesis testing
Inexpensive
Relatively small samples can be used
Good design for studying rare conditions, chronic diseases, and long-term effects of exposure
Results obtained quickly
Can examine multiple exposure factors for a single health condition

Disadvantages

Information about past exposure or past events may not be available
Selection of appropriate control groups may be difficult
Incidence or risk can only be estimated
The temporal association between exposure and outcome may be difficult to determine
Potential selection, recall, observation, and recall bias

syndrome (AIDS), descriptive studies provided tentative hypotheses or clues as to possible cause. Subsequently, case-control studies found that specific exposure factors, such as male homosexuality and intravenous drug abuse, were associated with the development of AIDS. These data contributed to the identification of the human immunodeficiency virus (HIV) as the causative agent (Peterman, Drotman, and Curran, 1985).

Case-control studies often are performed when investigating an outbreak. Agents from the Centers for Disease Control frequently use case-control studies in investigating unusual outbreaks of illness throughout the United States. Nurses and physicians have also used this study design in investigating outbreaks, particularly in hospitals or institutions where infection control programs are in place. An example is the investigation of an outbreak of *Staphylococcus aureus* sternal wound infections in patients undergoing coronary artery bypass graft (CABG) surgery (McLeod and others, 1991). When contrasting the data from the cases and controls, the two statistically significant predisposing factors for sternal wound infections after CABG procedures were found to be increased operative time and increased time between administration of preoperative antimicrobials to the incision time. Consequently, the authors identified control measures for epidemics of this type and made a number of recommendations to prevent such occurrences.

Due to the fact that both the exposure factors and the outcome have already occurred in case-control studies, there is potential for study bias either in selection of the cases and controls or in obtaining information about exposure. Information about past exposure or events may not be available or may be incomplete. Very careful consideration must be given to the criteria for case selection and the choice of a control group. If personal interviews are used, people may not recall events appropriately. Also, the temporal association between exposure factors and outcome may be difficult to establish—did exposure truly precede the outcome? All of these factors must be considered when initiating a case-control study. However, well-designed case-control studies, conducted carefully, can provide valuable information about the relationships between exposure factors and outcomes.

Selection of cases

The criteria for cases must be precisely defined. A basic assumption is that the cases are representative of the people who have the condition under study. The definitions must be such that it is absolutely clear whether a person meets the criteria for inclusion as a case or not. In some studies, especially those that involve specific diseases, it is helpful to classify cases as definite, probable, or possible. If enough information is available, these categories can be analyzed separately.

Once the definitions have been clearly designated, people can be identified who have the condition during a specific period of time. It is best if cases represent incidence (new cases) rather than prevalence (new and existing cases) of the condition under study. Prevalence includes duration as well as development of the condition, and therefore the study findings may be more difficult to interpret.

Selection of controls

The selection of controls is one of the most crucial steps in constructing a case-control study. The control subjects should be comparable to the cases. They should represent the population of people (without the condition under study) who would have been included as cases had they developed the condition. However, they may not be representative of the general population of people without the condition. Any exclusions or restrictions applied to selection of the cases should be applied to the controls and vice versa (Hennekens and Buring, 1987). Without careful attention to details, study biases occur that can result in invalid conclusions.

Often, controls are chosen from the same institution or community agency from which cases are selected. These are usually people who are hospitalized or have been admitted into a caseload of a community agency for reasons other than the condition under study. There are several advantages to this source of controls. They can be easily identified and records are available. They may be more willing to participate in the study, more health-conscious, and therefore less prone to problems with recall of events. These factors reduce bias and make the study cost-effective.

The primary difficulty is that these controls also have a health problem. The people who are cases developed their condition while members of a community population. Control groups from institutions or other facilities may not be representative of the exposure in the community. For instance, research has indicated that hospitalized people are more likely to smoke cigarettes and use oral contraceptives than those not hospitalized (West, Schuman, and Lyon, 1984). If controls are chosen from the same institution or agency as the cases, it is best to select controls with a wide variety of other conditions than the one under study. When there is definite evidence that two conditions have similar causative factors, then the use of one as a control for the other is contraindicated. If the causative factors for the illness in the controls are very similar to those of the cases, true positive associations between exposure factors and the cases may be minimized in the study results.

Comparison groups may also be chosen from the general population, or from special community groups, depending on the objectives of the study. Occasionally, more than one control group is chosen often from a hospital or community setting. When the sample size of cases is limited or cost factors are problematic, more than one control also can be chosen for each case. As the number of controls increase, the statistical power of the study to detect a difference between the two groups also increases. A matching procedure is sometimes used to control for confounding variables prior to data collection. Controls are matched to cases on characteristics like age, sex, race, and length of stay in the institution. This procedure eliminates the matched factors as variables in the study since they are the same for both cases and controls. Matching can be difficult to achieve, expensive, and time-consuming. Several alternative statistical techniques for the control of confounding variables in the analysis are available.

Analysis of case-control data

The cases in a case-control study are chosen because they have the outcome or the health status that is being investigated, and the controls that are chosen do not. As a result, it is not possible to calculate the rate of development of the outcome; calculation of incidence or prevalence rates and relative risk ratios would not be valid (see Chapter 3). However, the analysis of case-control data compares the frequency of the risk factor or exposure between the cases and the controls. This usually is done by estimating the relative risk.

The relative risk is the ratio of the incidence rate in the exposed group and the incidence rate in the nonexposed group. The estimate of relative risk is performed by calculation of the odds ratio or the ratio of the odds of exposure among the cases to the ratio of the odds of exposure among controls. It indicates the level of increased risk associated with previous exposure. The odds ratio is interpreted in the same way as the relative-risk ratio. An odds ratio of 1.0 indicates that the risk is equal for both groups, an odds ratio greater than 1.0 indicates that the risk is greater in the exposed group, and an odds ratio less than 1.0 indicates that the risk is less in the exposed group. The mathematic basis for the odds ratio being a stable and unbiased estimate of the relative risk in case-control studies has been well-established (Cornfield, 1951; Miettinen, 1976).

An example of the calculation of an odds ratio is presented in Table 5-2. The formula for an odds ratio (OR) is:

$$OR = \frac{a/c}{b/d} = \frac{ad}{bc}$$

where

a = Yes (case), Yes (factor present)
b = No (control), Yes (factor present)
c = Yes (case), No (factor absent)
d = No (control), No (factor absent)

More simply stated, the formula becomes:

$$OR = \frac{\text{YesYes} \times \text{NoNo}}{\text{NoYes} \times \text{YesNo}}$$

In this hypothetical data, patients who aspirated were 3.8 times more likely to develop pneumonia than those who did not aspirate. Odds ratios are often accompanied by calculation of a *confidence interval* (CI). Confidence intervals measure the range in which the true magnitude of the effect lies within the population. Further analysis of case-control data can be performed by chi-square tests for individual risk factors and by multivariate analysis through logistic regression. In a matched study, a different method of calculating the relative risk is required and the unit of analysis becomes the matched pair (Mausner and Kramer, 1985).

A case-control study that examined the risk factors for nosocomial pneumonia in the elderly provides a good example of the design and analysis of case-control studies (Harkness, Bentley, and Roghmann, 1990). The research was undertaken simultaneously in an acute care setting and a long-term care setting. The study was initiated to gather more information about those characteristics of pa-

Table 5-2 Calculation of an odds ratio using hypothetical data

Risk factor	Cases with pneumonia	Controls without pneumonia	Total
Aspiration			
Present	(a) 42	(b) 16	58
Absent	(c) 58	(d) 84	142
Total	100	100	200

$$OR = \frac{ad}{bc} = \frac{\text{YesYes} \times \text{NoNo}}{\text{NoYes} \times \text{YesNo}} = \frac{(42)\,(84)}{(58)\,(16)} = \frac{3528}{928} = 3.8$$

tients that contribute to increased risk of pneumonia. With this knowledge, patients at high risk can be identified and assessed, and preventive measures taken.

In both settings, cases of nosocomial pneumonia were identified during an 18-week period through surveillance and follow-up of chest radiograph reports 3 days or more after admission. Precise criteria for identification of cases were established (see box below). All cases that were identified during the 3-month period were admitted into the study; therefore the incidence rate for that period of time could be calculated. (The incidence data from this study is presented on p. 90.) For each case, two matched control subjects were chosen who did not have any respiratory infection and did not develop pneumonia. Matching was performed to control for age, sex, hospital service or resident unit, and length of stay. Two control subjects were chosen for each case to maximize the statistical power of the study to differentiate the risk factors between the two groups, since a small sample size was anticipated. The use of hospitalized and institutionalized people for controls was very appropriate, since risk of a hospital-acquired infection was being investigated.

Data were collected through review of the medical record with verification of data obtained by patients, residents and medical and nursing personnel when necessary. The information about risk factors was abstracted retrospectively as soon as the subjects were entered into the study, primarily for the week prior to the onset of the pneumonia. This design helped minimize bias, since information was readily available.

The data from acute care and long-term care settings were analyzed separately. Each variable was analyzed separately as a potential risk factor for nosocomial pneumonia. An odds ratio and 95% confidence interval calculation was performed for the matched triplets. The association between the potential risk fac-

CRITERIA FOR DEFINITION OF NOSOCOMIAL PNEUMONIA CASES IN THE ELDERLY

1. A person 65 years and older
2. Hospitalized on a medical/surgical unit or residing in a skilled nursing facility or intermediate care facility for 3 or more days
3. New, radiographically confirmed findings consistent with pneumonia
4. Accompanied by one or more clinical signs and symptoms compatible with pneumonia occurring within the prior week:
   a. Fever greater than 37.8° C
   b. Productive or non-productive cough
   c. Purulent respiratory secretions
   d. Respiratory rate equal to or greater than 26 per minute

From Harkness GA, Bentley DW, Roghmann K: Risk factors for nosocomial pneumonia in the elderly, Am J Med 89(4):458, 1990.

tor and nosocomial pneumonia was evaluated for significance by a chi-square test, using the Yates correction. Table 5-3 summarizes the statistically significant risk factors that were identified in the study. Aspiration had the strongest association with the onset of pneumonia with an odds ratio of 17.0 in the acute care setting and 130.0 in the long-term care setting. These odds ratios are interpreted to mean that pneumonia was 17 times more common in patients who aspirated in the acute care setting and 130 times more common in patients who aspirated in the long-term care setting. Patients with difficulty handling oropharyngeal secretions were 5.8 times more likely to develop pneumonia in the acute care setting and 23 times more likely to develop pneumonia in the long-term care setting. The presence of a nasogastric tube also predisposed to the development of pneumonia in both settings.

A series of stepwise *logistic regressions* were performed to determine the best multivariate model for identifying patients who would be the most likely to develop pneumonia. The relatively small sample sizes in both settings required that only a few variables be entered into the logistic regression. Therefore only those factors that were considered to be valuable for assessing future risk of pneumonia were entered into regression procedures. For development of the model, variables were removed if the significance levels were greater than 0.1 (rather than 0.05). Table 5-4 indicates the significant predictors of pneumonia along with the new odds ratios calculated for the model. It is interesting to note that risk factors varied by setting, but difficulty with oropharyngeal secretions was a risk factor for patients in both settings.

COHORT STUDIES

In *cohort studies* a group or groups of people are classified according to their exposure to risk factors (*independent variables*) and followed forward in time to determine the onset of the states of health or illness (outcomes) being studied (*dependent variables*). A cohort is defined as a group of people who share a common experience within a defined time period (Mausner and Kramer, 1985). The groups are chosen based on the category of exposure; the outcome has not occurred. These studies are also called *prospective* or *longitudinal* studies, since they are often used to follow a group of people for a long period of time (see Fig. 5-2).

Cohort studies are often conducted after an hypothesis has been preliminarily tested by a case-control study. One cohort may be chosen, classified as to exposure, and followed forward to determine the outcome. The experience of people with varying levels of exposure are later compared according to the outcome. Alternatively, two or more cohorts may be selected based on the magnitude of the exposure; one of these cohorts may be a nonexposed group. The groups are followed forward in time to determine the outcome. A major consideration in any cohort study is the availability of accurate and complete information about exposure factors and the ability to determine accurately whether specific outcomes occur.

Data regarding exposure can be obtained from medical or employment records, interviews or questionnaires completed by the subjects enrolled in the study, examination of the subjects, or environmental assessments (Hennekens and

Table 5-3 Significant risk factors for nosocomial pneumonia in the elderly

Risk factor	Cases with risk factor (%)	Controls with risk factor (%)	Odds ratio (95% confidence interval)
Acute care	**n = 33**	**n = 66**	
State of health			
Neurologic disease	42.4	16.7	4.4* (1.4, 13.5)
Renal disease	18.2	4.5	10.0* (1.2, 80.4)
Deteriorating health	45.5	23.1	2.7* (1.1, 6.7)
Decreased consciousness	42.4	21.2	2.6* (1.01, 6.48)
Disorientation	48.5	24.2	3.0* (1.12, 8.03)
Dependent bathing	97.0	75.8	8.0* (1.52, 42.18)
Dependent bowel function	65.6	34.4	3.2* (1.32, 7.88)
Dependent feeding	74.2	40.9	4.8† (1.82, 12.8)
Predisposing events			
Aspiration	54.8	3.3	17.0‡ (5.53, 52.2)
Difficulty with oro-pharyngeal secretions	48.4	9.4	5.8† (2.26, 14.9)
Nasogastric tube	63.6	42.4	3.0* (1.01, 8.92)
Long-term care	**n = 27**	**n = 54**	
State of health			
Deteriorating health	48.1	5.6	24.0‡ (5.15, 111.18)
Malnourished	96.2	70.4	15.0* (1.72, 130.74)
Weight change	37.0	11.5	5.7* (1.5, 21.48)
Decreased consciousness	37.0	1.9	20.0‡ (4.15, 96.49)
Disorientation	55.6	20.4	10.5‡ (2.37, 46.58)
Dependent feeding	55.6	27.8	4.0* (1.28, 12.49)
Predisposing events			
Aspiration§	25.9	0.0	130.0‡ (5.83, 2897.50)
Difficulty with oro-pharyngeal secretions	44.4	3.7	23.0‡ (4.99, 106.07)
Suctioning§	18.5	0.0	80.0† (1.91, 3358.90)
Nasogastric tube§	18.5	0.0	120.0‡ (5.43, 2652.45)
Febrile upper respiratory infection	40.7	5.6	18.0‡ (3.24, 99.95)
Inhalation therapy§	22.2	0.0	120.0‡ (5.43, 2652.45)
Increased confusion	44.4	9.3	10.5‡ (2.61, 42.31)
Increased agitation§	77.8	0.0	120.0‡ (5.43, 2652.45)

From Harkness GA, Bentley DW, Roghmann K: Risk factors for nosocomial pneumonia in the elderly, *Am J Med* 89(4):460, 1990.

* $p = 0.05$.

† $p = 0.01$.

‡ $p = 0.001$.

§ 0.1 added to zero cells.

Table 5-4 Logistic regression models for nosocomial pneumonia in the elderly

Significant predictor	Coefficient	p Value	Odds ratio (confidence interval)
Acute care			
Difficulty with oropharyngeal secretions	2.13	0.0002	8.41 (2.75, 25.72)
Nasogastric tube	0.88	0.0707	2.41 (0.93, 6.23)
Long-term care			
Difficulty with oropharyngeal secretions	2.53	0.0123	12.55 (1.73, 90.89)
Deteriorating health	1.60	0.0872	4.95 (0.79, 30.88)
Unusual event	2.73	0.0001	15.33 (3.89, 60.46)

From Harkness GA, Bentley DW, Roghmann K: Risk factors for nosocomial pneumonia in the elderly, *Am J Med* 89(4):458, 1990.

Buring, 1987). Outcome information can be obtained in similar ways through medical records, periodic examinations, questionnaires, and observations. The goal is to obtain complete information about the state of health of each study subject that is comparable and unbiased.

Cohort studies have several advantages. This study design allows the magnitude of the risk for a condition to be determined for the populations who were or were not exposed to a specific factor. Therefore the relative-risk ratio can be calculated from incidence rates (see Chapter 3), and the data can be tested for statistical associations. The time sequence between exposure and outcome can be more clearly established than in other study designs, and the effects of rare exposures can be investigated. Multiple disease outcomes may be studied prospectively, and selection bias is minimized. However, prospective studies can be time-consuming, expensive, and subjects can be lost in the follow-up stages perhaps resulting in a study bias. The features of cohort studies are summarized in the box on p. 92.

The Framingham Heart Study is a classic example of a prospective, on-going, study of the health characteristics of a community. A cohort of 5209 men and women, representative of the total population, have been followed for 30 years with physical examinations every other year at the study clinic in Framingham, MA. Subjects were initially classified as to the presence or absence of specific exposure factors, such as blood pressure, blood cholesterol, activity, and smoking. The biennial examinations have assessed the onset of multiple conditions, ranging from coronary heart disease and related conditions, such as hypertension and congestive heart failure, to stroke, gout, gallbladder disease, and eye disorders. Medical journals periodically report findings, such as Dannenberg, Garrison, and

FEATURES OF COHORT STUDIES

Purpose

Determine if the incidence of the condition under study varies between the exposed and the nonexposed

Design

One sample or two samples may be chosen, one with and one without exposure
Subjects observed longitudinally for development of condition under study

Advantages

Incidence rates can be calculated directly
Time sequence between exposure and outcome can be more clearly established
Effects of rare exposures can be investigated
Selection bias is minimized
Multiple outcomes may be studied

Disadvantages

May extend over a long period of time, especially when studying chronic conditions or slowly developing disorders
Expensive
Bias from losses to follow-up may occur

Kannel (1988) in their article on the incidence of hypertension in the cohort. Much of the information about risk factors for coronary heart disease that underlies preventive programs was established by the Framingham Heart Study.

The Nurses Health Study is another large, well-known cohort study. More than 120,000 married female nurses, 30 to 55 years of age, who were licensed in one of eleven states, were enrolled in the study in 1976 (Belanger and others, 1978). An initial questionnaire assessed demographic characteristics, reproductive history, state of health, life-style, and other variables. Since 1976, the nurses have completed follow-up questionnaires every 2 years that focused on the development of cancer and cardiovascular diseases. The medical literature has reported the data periodically, looking at the relationship between these diseases and exposure factors, such as the use of oral contraceptives and hormones, amount of dietary fat, use of hair dyes, and family history of illness. This cohort is providing much needed information regarding women's health.

However, not all cohort studies are so large, comprehensive, and lengthy. Studies that use smaller samples or that are limited to one geographic area or institution are common in the medical and nursing literature. Nurses have used prospective designs in identifying factors that predispose to specific patient outcomes and observing the outcomes of therapeutic measures and nursing interventions. For example, Flynn, Norton, and Fisher (1987) assessed patients fed daily by way of enteral tube to describe feeding practices and document associated problems. Northouse and Swain (1987) studied the adjustment of patients and husbands to the initial impact of breast cancer by observing them approximately 3 days after surgery and again 30 days later. A prospective study of health care workers and visitors was undertaken by Pettinger and Nettleman (1991) to determine their compliance with isolation protocols.

Table 5-5 illustrates the risk factors for postoperative pneumonia found to be statistically significant in a cohort study of coronary artery bypass graft (CABG) patients (Harkness, 1994). Of CABG patients, 165 were assessed preoperatively by thoracic intensive care nurses and postoperatively on Day 1, Day 3, and Day 6. The data in Table 5-5 reflect significant risk factors found on postoperative Day 1, when the strongest associations between risk factors and pneumonia were found. A postoperative pneumonia risk scale based on these findings is being developed. It is anticipated that early identification of high-risk patients will enable preventive intervention protocols to be instituted immediately following surgical procedures.

Historical cohort studies

Occasionally, a group of people can be identified who were exposed to a risk factor at some time in the past. These people can be followed forward in time from

Table 5-5 Risk factors for postoperative pneumonia in CABG patients

	No pneumonia N = 144	Pneumonia N = 20	Odds ratio (95% CI)
Risk factor			
Altered respiratory status			
Impaired cough reflex	20.1	57.9	5.31 (1.77-16.17)†
Abnormal breath sounds	39.6	63.2	2.59 (0.88-7.80)*
Altered respiratory secretions	33.3	63.2	3.39 (1.15-10.29)*
Suction	21.5	68.4	7.90 (2.52-25.69)‡
Altered health status			
Re-exploratory surgery	1.4	26.3	27.12 (4.04-112.05)‡
Decreased mobility	7.6	42.1	8.79 (2.58-30.37)†
Decreased consciousness	7.6	42.1	8.79 (2.58-30.37)†
Increased severity of illness	4.9	31.6	9.79 (2.95-40.07)†

From Harkness GA: Risk of postoperative pneumonia following coronary artery bypass graft surgery, submitted for publication.

* = 0.05

† = 0.001

‡ = 0.0001

that point to determine whether a disease or condition develops. This type of study is called a *historical cohort study.* Both exposure and outcome are often known at the onset of the study. However, the study sample is chosen based on exposure and not outcome (see Fig. 5-2). Study subjects are followed from the past point in time to the present and sometimes into the future as well.

When rare exposures have occurred, such as those related to certain occupations or environments, historical cohort studies can shorten the length of time of the study if accurate and complete information on prior exposure is available. Investigators studying occupational exposures often use this study design, since a past cohort can be easily identified and industry records can be used to determine exposure. Classic epidemiologic studies linking asbestos exposure and lung cancer were historical cohort studies (Enterline, 1965; Selikoff and others, 1968). Although this study design has not been used often by nurses, there is a great potential for nurses in health maintenance organizations (HMOs) to use an historical cohort study design. A cohort of people entering the HMO at a specific time in the past could be followed forward to determine specific outcomes. Factors that contribute to wellness could be studied, as well as those factors that predispose to illness. Analysis of historical cohort studies parallels that of a cohort study, risk of developing specific outcomes can be calculated, and multiple outcomes can be studied. The features of historical cohort studies can be found in the box on page 95.

SUMMARY

Descriptive epidemiology examines variations in the distribution of states of health, while analytic epidemiology attempts to identify the determinants of states of health. Analytic epidemiologic research methods are used to test hypotheses generated from descriptive studies, looking for a statistical association between an exposure and an outcome. Statistical associations may be valid, true, or a result of chance, bias, or the effect of confounding variables.

There are four types of studies frequently used in epidemiologic analytic investigations: cross-sectional, case-control, cohort, and intervention studies. Cross-sectional studies are surveys that produce prevalence data and are conducted at one point in time. Information about exposure and outcome are obtained at the same time. Case-control studies choose cases that have experienced the outcome under investigation and choose controls that have not experienced the outcome. The investigators look back in time for factors related to exposure and the cases and controls are examined for differences. Cohort studies follow a group or groups of people who have been classified as to their exposure to risk factors forward in time to determine the outcome. Historical cohort studies are a type of cohort study that identifies the exposure of a group in the past and follows the group forward in time to assess the outcome. Nurse researchers have used these designs to identify populations at high risk so that control and prevention procedures can be instituted and to examine relationships between exposure and outcome variables that provide information for enhancing nursing practice.

FEATURES OF HISTORICAL COHORT STUDIES

Purpose

To determine whether the incidence of the condition under study varies between the exposed and nonexposed

Design

A previously exposed group of subjects is selected
Exposure status is identified on the basis of existing records at a specified point in time
A comparison group of unexposed subjects may be similarly identified
Groups followed forward and observed for onset of the outcome under study
The outcome may have been observed at the onset of the study

Advantages

Incidence of condition under study can be obtained
Shortens length of time of study, especially when chronic conditions or disorders with long incubation periods are studied
Less expensive
Multiple outcomes may be studied

Disadvantages

Accurate classification of exposure may not be available
Information may be incomplete or not comparable

CRITICAL THINKING QUESTIONS

1. Identify two purposes of cross-sectional studies.
2. Describe the design of a case-control study.
3. In an industry employing 10,000 people, 2500 were employed in areas where they were exposed to ionizing radiation; the remaining 7500 were not exposed. At the beginning of the study, all were free of disease. The entire population of 10,000 was followed for 10 years to determine whether exposure to radiation increased the risk of developing a particular disease.
   a. What type of study is the above example?
   b. List the advantages and disadvantage of this type of study.
4. In a particular study an association between exposure and the development of a health problem is reported. Besides being a valid association, what other explanations may account for the reported association?

REFERENCES

Ahmann E, Wulff L, Meny RG: Home apnea monitoring and disruptions in family life: a multidimensional controlled study, *Am J Pub Health* 82(5):719-722, 1992.

Belanger CF and others: The nurses' health study, *Am J Nurs* 78:1039, 1978.

Cole P: The evolving case-control study, *J Chronic Dis* 32:15, 1979.

Cornfield J: A method of estimating comparative rates from clinical data: applications to cancer of the lung, breast, and cervix, *J Natl Cancer Inst* 11:1269, 1951.

Dannenberg AL, Garrison RJ, Kannel WB: Incidence of hypertension in the Framingham study, *Am J Public Health* 78(6):676-679, 1988.

Doll R, Hill AB: Smoking and carcinoma of the lung: preliminary report, *BMJ* 2:739, 1950.

Duffy ME: Determinants of health promotion in midlife women, *Nurs Res* 37(6):358-362, 1988.

Enterline TE: Mortality among asbestos products workers in the United States, *Ann NY Acad Sci* 132:156, 1965.

Flynn KT, Norton LC, Fisher RL: Enteral tube feeding: indications, practices and outcomes, *Image: J Nurs Sch* 19(1):16-19, 1987.

Grossman DC, Milligan BC, Deyo RA: Risk factors for suicide attempts among Navajo adolescents, *Am J Pub Health* 81(7):870-874, 1991.

Harkness GA: *Risk of postoperative pneumonia following coronary artery bypass graft surgery*, submitted for publication.

Harkness GA, Bentley DW, Roghmann K: Risk factors for nosocomial pneumonia in the elderly, *Am J Med* 89(4):457-463, 1990.

Hennekens CH, Buring JE: *Epidemiology in medicine,* Boston, 1987, Little, Brown.

Mausner JS, Kramer S: *Epidemiology—an introductory text,* ed 2, Philadelphia, 1985, WB Saunders.

McLeod J and others: An outbreak of *Staphylococcus aureus* sternal wound infections in patients undergoing coronary artery bypass surgery, *Am J Infect Control* 19(2):92-97, 1991.

Miettinen OS: Estimability and estimation in case-referent studies, *Am J Epidemiol* 103:226, 1976.

Newacheck PW, Taylor WR: Childhood chronic illness: prevalence, severity, and impact, *Am J Public Health* 82(3):364-371, 1992.

Northouse LL, Swain MA: Adjustment of patients and husbands to the initial impact of breast cancer, *Nurs Res* 36(4):221-225, 1987.

Pender NJ: *Health promotion in nursing practice,* ed 2, Norwalk, CT, 1987, Appleton & Lange.

Peterman TA, Drotman DP, Curran JW: Epidemiology of the acquired immunodeficiency syndrome (AIDS), *Epidemiol Rev* 7:1, 1985.

Pettinger A, Nettleman MD: Epidemiology of isolation precautions, *Inf Control Hosp Epidemiol* 12(5):303-307, 1991.

Pfeffer RI and others: Prevalence of Alzheimer's disease in a retirement community, *Am J Epidemiol* 125(3):420-436, 1987.

Selikoff IJ and others: Asbestos exposure, smoking, and neoplasia, *JAMA* 204:106, 1968.

Weitzel MH: A test of the health-promotion model with blue-collar workers, *Nurs Res* 38(2):99-104, 1989.

West DW, Schuman KL, Lyon JL: Differences in risk estimations from a hospital and a population-based case-control study, *Int J Epidemiol* 13:235, 1984.

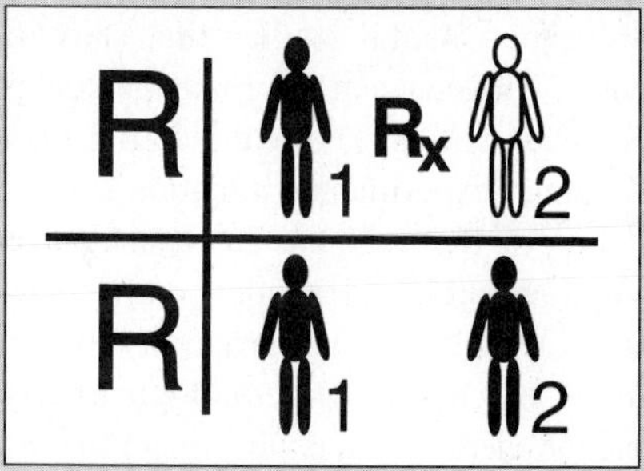

6

Analytic Epidemiology
Intervention Studies

Objectives

1. Define the characteristics of epidemiologic intervention studies.
2. Analyze intervention studies according to cause and effect criteria.
3. Critique intervention studies according to principles of sample selection.
4. Differentiate between therapeutic trials and preventive trials.
5. Apply common threats to internal validity to the design of epidemiologic intervention studies.
6. Explain the biases that can occur in the conduct of therapeutic and preventive trials, stating measures for reducing their occurrence.
7. Discuss factors affecting the external validity of intervention studies.
8. Outline the process of informed consent.

Key Terms

cause-and-effect
dose-response
double-blind study
experimental population
external validity
Hawthorne effect
indirect association
internal validity
multicausality
observation bias
placebo effect
power
preventive trial
quasi-experimental trial
random assignment
random selection
reference population
sampling error
therapeutic trial
Valsalva maneuver

Epidemiologic intervention studies are experimental studies that seek to determine a *cause-and-effect* relationship between exposure and outcome. Experimental studies have three primary characteristics: (1) manipulation of a variable, often a treatment variable, occurs (2) the experimental situation is controlled, and (3) randomization of subjects occurs so that each has an equal chance of being included in the study. In experimental research, independent and dependent variables are identified. Independent variables are qualities, properties, or activities that are manipulated or varied by the researcher. In epidemiologic experimental studies, or intervention studies, the characteristics of exposure are the independent variables that are manipulated by the investigator. The dependent variables are the responses, outcomes, or effects that the researcher wishes to explain or predict.

CAUSE-AND-EFFECT RELATIONSHIPS

The concept of causality is a controversial one. Some scholars believe that the concept of causality cannot be defended from either a metaphysical or an empirical basis, because cause can never be proven. Others, including epidemiologists, believe that the concept of causality is useful in science, despite the fact that causality can never be proven. In epidemiology, investigators are continually examining the relationships between exposure and outcome. They are looking for information about cause-and-effect relationships that can be used to prevent or control health problems and enhance positive states of health. The knowledge gained from epidemiologic investigations has contributed greatly to the improvement of health throughout the world. For example, epidemiologic investigations have provided information about risk factors for cardiovascular disease that are now the basis of many prevention programs. Epidemiologic data also contributed to the successful eradication of smallpox.

In establishing valid statistical associations between exposures and outcomes, it is necessary to eliminate chance, bias, and confounding variables as explanations for the study's findings (Hennekins and Buring, 1987). Valid statistical associations found in cross-sectional, case-control, and cohort studies imply that a relationship exists between exposure and outcomes. However, these study designs are such that a cause-and-effect relationship cannot be determined (see Chapter 5). It is important to understand that a valid statistical association in no way implies a cause-and-effect relationship.

For example, a significant statistical association found between lower socioeconomic status (exposure) and tuberculosis (outcome) could not be validly interpreted to mean that socioeconomic status caused tuberculosis. The lower socioeconomic status most likely would be related to other variables, such as crowding and poor sanitary conditions, that are more directly related to the transmission of the agent, *Mycobacterium tuberculosis.* The relationship between socioeconomic status and tuberculosis is an *indirect association.* The exposure and outcomes are associated because both are related to one or more common underlying conditions (Mausner and Kramer, 1985). Nevertheless, knowledge of this association is helpful to public health officials in planning prevention and control programs.

Similarly, an association between young nurses and medication errors in a hospital does not necessarily mean that being young is a causative factor for medicine errors. An increased rate of medication errors could be due to other variables, such as the fact that younger nurses more frequently work double shifts, and 90% of the medication errors are made on the nurse's second shift of the day. However, knowledge of this association is helpful in planning preventive strategies.

The first criteria for the establishment of causal associations were developed in the late nineteenth century. This followed the work of William Farr and John Snow and occurred after the relationship between bacteria and infectious processes had been identified. Koch's postulates put forth criteria for judging causality for one type of agent, microorganisms (Mausner and Kramer, 1985). These criteria have been modified and enhanced as knowledge of illness and wellness has expanded. A number of interrelated variables are almost always involved in the cause of a particular outcome. This is called *multicausality*. However, identifying cause-and-effect relationships between specific variables that comprise multicausality can explain a part of the process under investigation, leading to a greater understanding of phenomena (Burns and Grove, 1987).

Determination of a causal relationship is a dynamic, ongoing process. It can only be made in light of all the knowledge known at the time, and it should be continually re-evaluated as more information is accumulated. A causative association between two variables implies that when *x* variable occurs, there is a likelihood that *y* variable will occur. In epidemiology, there are specific criteria that assist in determining whether or not associations can be considered causal. Four primary criteria include (1) strength of the association, (2) time sequence, (3) consistency of the findings, and (4) biologic plausibility.

Strength of the association

Both descriptive and inferential statistical techniques are used when looking for relationships between specific exposures and outcomes. The stronger the statistical relationship between exposure and outcome, the less likely the results are due to confounding variables and the more likely the results represent a cause-and-effect relationship.

In epidemiology, strength of an association can be measured by the relative risk or an estimate of relative risk (see Chapter 3) that compares incidence rates in different groups. As the relative risk increases, the strength of association increases, and therefore the possibility of a causal association increases. For example, people who smoke heavily have a higher relative risk of developing lung cancer than those people who do not smoke heavily. This example also implies a *dose-response* relationship; the more people smoke the more likely they are to develop lung cancer. The likelihood of a causal relationship is strengthened if increasing levels of exposure to the risk factor result in a corresponding rise in occurrence of the outcome.

Time sequence

For a causal relationship to be considered, the exposure should precede the outcome for a period of time that is consistent with the biologic mechanisms involved. Sometimes this can be difficult to establish. When studying a condition, such as cancer, that has a long latency period, evidence that exposure preceded the initial cell abnormalities may be difficult to determine. Similarly, study factors that change over time make exposure difficult to determine. For example, life-style variables, such as smoking and eating habits, may change after the onset of the first symptoms of a disorder, such as cancer, making exposure difficult to document. Prospective studies, such as cohort or intervention studies, classify people as to exposure prior to the development of the outcome and therefore provide the most direct evidence that exposure precedes outcome.

Consistency of the findings

Consistency of the findings means that the results of one study are found to be similar to results in a variety of other studies. These other studies are usually conducted by different investigators using alternative study methodology with diverse populations at a different time and place. For example, the relationship between active smoking and increased risk of coronary heart disease has been found to be consistent in a number of studies over an extended period of time (Hennekens, Buring, and Mayrent, 1984). Alternatively, a lack of consistency between studies can be an indication that chance, bias, or confounding variables are affecting the study results. However, these inconsistencies can be preliminary cues to the development of new knowledge. Inconsistencies can generate ideas for further research that can lead to a better understanding of the state of health being investigated.

Biologic credibility

A stronger argument for a causal relationship between exposure and outcome can be made if the study findings are also plausible, according to current knowledge. For instance, aspiration is a risk factor for the development of pneumonia. There is a logical, known biologic mechanism that explains the reaction of lung tissue to gastric or oropharyngeal secretions that are aspirated into the lung. This knowledge produces the biologic credibility for the cause-and-effect relationship between aspiration and the development of pneumonia.

Biologic credibility depends on the current state of knowledge at the time. For example, Table 1-1 (see p. 6) demonstrates that John Snow identified water as the source of cholera in the 1853-1854 epidemic in London. However, bacteria had not yet been identified, and many of his critics believed that his findings were not credible. The state of knowledge at the time was inadequate to explain Dr. Snow's observations. Therefore it should be emphasized that the lack of biologic credibility does not necessarily mean that a relationship is not causal. It is also important to recognize that unusual or unexplained findings, along with inconsistencies, can sometimes be a clue to the unknown, and further study might result in an advancement of knowledge.

Of the four primary criteria for documentation of cause-and-effect relationships, strength of the association and time sequence are criteria that can be applied to each epidemiologic research study. These criteria can be used as a method of addressing the internal validity of each study (see the box on p. 107). Consistency of the findings and biologic plausibility criteria are not specific to individual research studies. These criteria depend on prior knowledge or prior research findings and should be considered when evaluating the external validity or ability of the study to generalize findings to other subjects or settings (Kleinbaum, Kupper, and Morgenstern, 1982).

EPIDEMIOLOGIC INTERVENTION STUDIES

True experiments that control all factors other than the one under investigation are rare when studying human populations. Many studies, although experimental in design, are not able to either randomize selection of subjects or exert the same degree of control of the study variables that would be found in true experimental studies. Manipulation of the independent variable occurs, but factors that may influence the manipulation of the independent variable may not be able to be controlled. When studying human responses to health problems in the person's environment, there are frequently factors that researchers are not able to manipulate or control. These studies are referred to as *quasi-experimental* studies. In epidemiology there are two types of intervention studies, *therapeutic trials* and *preventive trials.* Both can be experimental or quasi-experimental in design.

Therapeutic trials

Therapeutic trials attempt to determine the ability of interventions to decrease or prevent recurrence of symptoms and improve the outcomes for individuals with an actual or potential health problem. Therapeutic trials are also called clinical trials. Therapeutic trials are focused on concepts of secondary prevention (see Chapter 2). The treatment variable is the exposure (independent) variable that is manipulated by the investigator.

Many experimental or quasi-experimental studies performed by nurses meet the criteria for therapeutic trials. Most of these studies investigate the outcomes of nursing interventions. An example of such a study is the investigation of the effect of position (independent variable) on cardiovascular response (dependent variable) during the *Valsalva maneuver* (Metzger and Therrien, 1990). The Valsalva maneuver is defined as any forced expiratory effort against a closed airway. It occurs when any individual holds his breath and tightens muscles in a concerted, strenuous effort. For example, moving a heavy object, coughing, straining at stool, or changing position in bed can result in a Valsalva maneuver (Urdang and Swallow, 1983). Sudden cardiac death has been frequently associated with the Valsalva maneuver, which is accompanied by sudden intense changes in systolic blood pressure and heart rate.

Since many patients on bedrest have a history of cardiovascular disease, they are at increased risk for sudden cardiac death. It has been estimated that these patients may perform the Valsalva maneuver from 10 to 20 times an hour as they change position, cough, or strain at stool. Using this rationale, the investigators used an experimental design to determine the effect of body position on the variability and intensity of the cardiovascular responses to a Valsalva strain. Their results indicated that the most intense changes in systolic blood pressure during the Valsalva maneuver occurred when the person's head was elevated at a 30-degree angle and a 70-degree angle. The authors concluded that people with a history of cardiovascular disease, who were on bedrest, should be positioned with the head of the bed flat. This would reduce cardiovascular risks associated with the Valsalva maneuver. Since symptoms associated with the Valsalva maneuver decreased in a flat position and the outcome of sudden cardiac death could be potentially reduced, this study met the criteria for a therapeutic trial. However, further research is needed to validate these findings.

Therapeutic trials can also be conducted within the community. For example, a study of the use of telephone support for smoking cessation was provided to four smoker populations in Minnesota (Lando and others, 1992). Of the populations studied, 6777 smokers were randomly assigned either to an intervention group (4655 people) who received two 15-minute telephone calls from 1 to 3 weeks apart or to a nonintervention comparison group (2122 people). At a 6-month follow-up, the intervention group had a statistically significant validated quit rate, but these effects were not significant at 18 months. There are many extraneous factors that affected people and their smoking habits that could not be controlled in this study. However, the quasi-experimental design was such that these extraneous factors affected both the intervention group and the control group similarly. Therefore the study design produced some control over these extraneous factors. The authors concluded that the telephone intervention was moderately encouraging. However, more intensive telephone intervention and support may be needed to produce lasting changes in smoking prevalence (Lando and others, 1992).

Preventive trials

Preventive or prophylactic trials seek to reduce the risk of acquiring a specific health problem among a group of people who do not have that health problem at the onset of the study. Preventive trials focus on the concepts of primary prevention (see Chapter 2). The preventive strategies are the exposure (independent) variables that are manipulated by the researcher. Preventive trials also can be conducted among entire populations of healthy people. These studies are often referred to as community trials.

For example, a community-wide, smoking-prevention, quasi-experimental study was conducted as a part of the Minnesota Heart Health Program (MHHP). The MMHP was a population-wide, research and demonstration project designed to reduce cardiovascular disease. An intensive, school-based behavioral intervention for cigarette smoking was conducted with the class of 1989; it was initiated while the students were in the sixth grade. The intervention community was then compared with a matched comparison community. Throughout the follow-up period, smoking rates were significantly lower in the intervention community: 14.6% of the students were weekly smokers at the end of high school compared with 24.1% in the comparison community (Perry and others, 1992).

Issues regarding the design, implementation, and analysis of both therapeutic and preventive trials are similar. These include the selection of a sample, assignment of study groups, compliance with study protocols, and gathering and analyzing outcome data.

Selection of a sample

The *reference population,* or target population, is the entire group of people to whom the results of intervention studies are expected to apply. The reference population may be extensive, including all people. It also may be restricted to people with a specific combination of characteristics. The purpose and design of the study sets the parameters of the reference population. In general, the reference population represents the scope of the public health impact of the intervention under investigation (Hennekens and Buring, 1987).

The *experimental population* is the actual group of people that is being investigated. It is the group from which the sample is selected. This group of people should meet the sample selection criteria determined by the investigators and may be located in more than one site. Ideally, the sample of people chosen as subjects for the study should be randomly selected from the experimental population. *Random selection* of subjects will produce a study sample that is representative of the experimental population the majority of the time. This method assures that each individual in the experimental population has an equal opportunity to be selected for the sample. Random selection will usually result in a small *sampling error* or a minimal difference between the statistics generated from analyzing information from the sample and the true population parameters. Fig. 6-1 indicates the steps involved in the selection of participants in an intervention study.

Depending on the purpose of the research, the number of available subjects, and the number of people who refuse to participate, random selection may not be feasible. All those who meet the sample-selection criteria and who give their in-

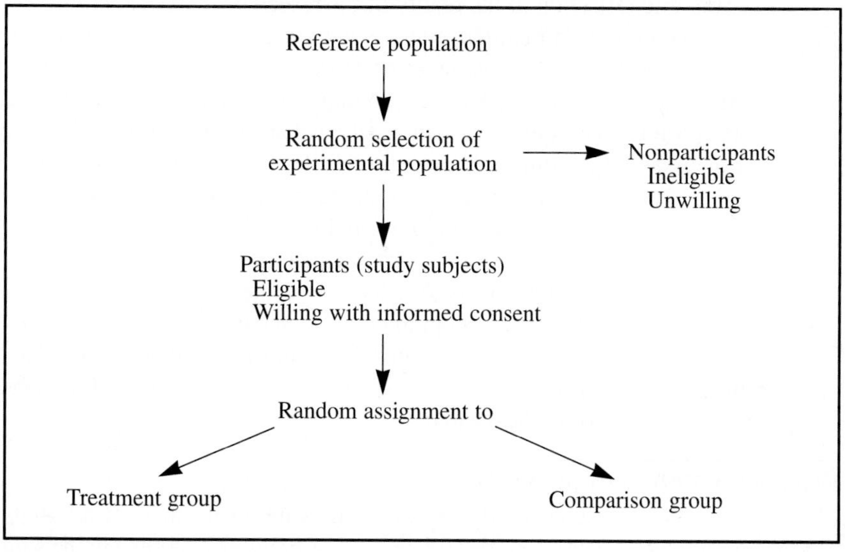

Fig. 6-1 Steps in the selection of participants in intervention studies.

formed consent may be admitted into the study and, subsequently, may be randomly assigned to either the intervention or the comparison group.

The final sample should be sufficiently large enough so that (1) a number of comparisons can be made and a number of outcomes studied; (2) small to moderate clinically important differences between the groups can be determined; and (3) accurate follow-up data can be obtained for the duration of the therapeutic trial. Many intervention studies have failed to find significant results because their sample size was inadequate. Without a large enough sample size, interventions may be interpreted as having no therapeutic effect. In reality, the small sample size may have failed to detect clinically important differences between the groups. True therapeutic effects could not be statistically determined; there was not adequate statistical *power* to detect the differences between groups. Sampling texts should be consulted for specific steps in probability sampling procedures and sample-size selection.

As the sample is being chosen, each study participant must give informed consent. The purpose of the therapeutic trial, the study protocols, and the risks and benefits from participation in the study should be presented clearly. Subjects must understand that they may or may not be allocated to the intervention group. They should also understand that they may not be informed of the intervention they receive until the end of the study (see p. 109).

Assignment of study groups

Once the participants have been recruited, they are assigned to the intervention group(s) or comparison group(s) by *random assignment.* Random assignment implies that each participant has the same chance of being placed in either group. Both random selection and random assignment help decrease study bias from selection procedures (selection bias) and reduce the threats to the *internal validity* or the true reflection of the reality of the research (see p. 107).

The process of randomization reduces threats to internal validity in intervention studies because any variations that occur, occur to both the intervention and the comparison groups. Any confounding or extraneous variables affecting the study should be equally distributed between the two groups. Therefore study groups should be comparable on all variables other than the interventions that are being evaluated. This is more likely to be true as the sample size increases.

Despite random selection and random assignment, it has been well documented that those who choose to participate in a study are often different from nonparticipants. Those who choose to give their informed consent have been found to have different demographic characteristics and different health beliefs. This can influence and lower morbidity and mortality rates (Hennekens and Buring, 1987). Therefore they are often not as representative of the experimental population as would be desired.

Compliance with study protocols

Intervention studies usually require significant involvement of the study subjects in following the procedures, treatments, or programs outlined in the study design.

It is important that the study participants comply as carefully as possible to these protocols. With a high degree of compliance with study protocols, the observed differences in outcomes between groups are more likely to reflect the true differences in the exposure variables being compared.

There are many reasons why subjects do not comply with study protocols. Compliance and noncompliance are directly related to the length and complexity of the study interventions. Sometimes participants cannot comply due to a change in their health status or the development of adverse reactions. Others may withdraw from the study after partial participation. Occasionally the subjects in the comparison group become aware of the alternative study protocols and change their own behavior. Similarly, research subjects sometimes change their behavior simply because they are subjects in a study and not because of the intervention. This is known as reactivity or the *Hawthorne effect* (page 108). Whatever the reason, noncompliance with study protocols will decrease the power of a study to detect a true effect of the intervention. Noncompliance makes the intervention and comparison groups more alike, and outcomes of the study can be affected. The characteristics of the participants and nonparticipants in a study should be statistically compared for differences.

Attempts to increase compliance have included frequent contact with participants through clinic visits or telephone calls and the use of incentives. Incentives have included such things as cash payments, long-term follow-up, or free, detailed information about the subjects health status. Some study designs include periodical measures of compliance. For example, pill counts for pharmaceutical trials have been conducted, and biochemical measurements have been used to verify drug levels or look for the presence of specific metabolites. These procedures can be expensive and of questionable reliability on a long-term basis. When interventions involve behavior modification, such as dietary change or exercise programs, self-report may be the only means of assessing compliance to study protocols. Regardless of the reason, those who do not comply should be followed for the duration of the study.

Gathering and analyzing outcome data

Baseline and outcome data are collected for all intervention and comparison groups. The primary objective is to collect equivalent and uniform information for all groups. Objective criteria should be developed to measure all outcomes. A bias may be introduced into the study if more information or more accurate data are collected for one group and not the other. This requires that the follow-up of study participants be as complete and detailed as possible for the duration of the study. As the time period of follow-up increases, the ability to gather complete, accurate, and comparable outcome data decreases.

When noncomparable information is obtained from different study groups, an *observation bias* may result. This can occur when either the researcher or the participant uses their knowledge of the study to influence the reporting of outcome data (experimenter/participant effect). For example, researchers collecting the data may unconsciously influence the results of a study if they know who is receiving the intervention protocol. They may look for a specific outcome more carefully in the intervention group.

The likelihood of observation bias is increased when the outcome variables are subjective in nature and thereby open to interpretation by either the researcher or the participant. For instance, outcome data involving laboratory tests are not likely to be biased. However, outcome data involving determination of levels of pain are more apt to be biased, either by the study subject or by the investigator who is observing the subject. Similarly, participants may respond differently if they know which intervention they are receiving.

One method for controlling observation bias is to conduct a *double-blind* study where neither the participants or the investigator know the status of the intervention until the study is complete. To accomplish this, both the intervention groups and the comparison groups should have very similar study protocols. This is often difficult to implement, and a *single-blind* or unblinded study is designed (Hennekens and Buring, 1987). In a single-blind study only the investigator knows the intervention that the subject is receiving. In an unblinded or open-intervention study, both investigator and participant know whether the participant is a member of the intervention group or the comparison group. In single-blind and unblinded studies, measures should be developed to reduce the possibility of observational bias.

Evaluation of outcome data can also be affected by the tendency for study subjects to report favorable responses to any intervention whether beneficial or not. This is called a *placebo effect* and is similar to the Hawthorne effect discussed earlier. The placebo effect is minimized if the study protocols are very similar for both the intervention group and the comparison group.

In the design of a therapeutic or preventive trial, consideration should be given to the possible necessity of modifying or completing the research earlier than anticipated. Data should be analyzed on an interim basis, while the trial is being conducted. For large, complicated trials, this is often done by a group that is not involved with the study. The possibility exists that the treatment or preventive strategies are so positive or negative that the study should be completed early to assure the health and welfare of the participants. For example, the Beta Blocker Heart Attack Trial was terminated 9 months before schedule due to the recommendation of an external monitoring group. There was a 26% decrease in the death rates of the experimental groups receiving a beta blocker but not in the comparison group that received a placebo (DeMets DL and others, 1984).

The first step in analyzing the data gathered during an intervention study is to compare the characteristics of the intervention group with the comparison group. Often, this is presented in table form when the results of the study are published. The primary objective in analysis of intervention studies is to compare the rate of the outcome variables in the intervention group with the corresponding rates in the comparison group. The techniques for analysis are similar to those for any epidemiologic analytic study.

Decisions regarding statistical techniques are based on the type of data collected and the research questions being investigated. There are always many issues to be addressed in this analysis. For example, should the analysis include those persons who were noncompliant with the study protocol? It is generally believed that once a person has been randomly assigned to a group, all data gathered about that person should be included in the analysis. This holds true even if the person has been noncompliant or lost-to-follow-up.

Threats to internal and external validity

The examination of internal and external validity is one way to evaluate the quality of a research study. Internal validity has been defined as the extent to which the effects found in the study are a true reflection of reality and not the result of the effects of confounding or extraneous variables (Burns and Grove, 1993). A summary of common threats to internal validity are found in the box below. These

COMMON THREATS TO INTERNAL VALIDITY

History

History refers to events external to the study that occur, while the study is being conducted. The response of subjects can be influenced, affecting the outcome (dependent) variables.

Maturation

Maturation refers to unplanned and often unrecognized processes affecting the subjects of study that are related to the passage of time. Events, such as physical growth, emotional maturity, knowledge development, and fatigue, can influence the findings of a study.

Testing

Testing refers to the effects of multiple measurements of the subject's responses. Gathering data at an earlier time may change the subjects responses at a later date.

Selection

Selection encompasses effects resulting from the choice of study subjects and the differences between study groups. This is more likely to occur when randomization is not performed. The subjects may not be representative of the target population, or the experimental and comparison groups may not be equivalent.

Instrumentation

Instrumentation reflects changes that occur in the tools used to measure variables during the course of the study. Inconsistent data collection occurs.

Mortality

Mortality refers to loss of subjects during the course of the study. Differences in the kinds of people who drop out of a study or differences in those who drop out of either the experimental or comparison group can influence the outcomes of the study.

factors can reduce the validity of a study and influence the results. These threats to internal validity are potential biases in any study, including cross-sectional, case-control, and cohort studies. A well-designed intervention study minimizes some of these biases, since the threat or bias applies to both the intervention group and the comparison group.

An objective of any research study is to generalize the findings to a larger group of people than the one that is being studied. If the results of a nursing intervention is found to be successful, other nurses will want to adopt the procedure in their setting with different patients. The degree to which this can be done with confidence is referred to as *external validity.* Some common threats to external validity are found in the box that follows. External validity is enhanced if there is

COMMON THREATS TO EXTERNAL VALIDITY

Reactivity

Reactivity refers to the subjects' responses to the phenomenon of being studied. Subjects may behave in a certain way because they know they are enrolled in a research study. This is commonly known as the Hawthorne effect.

Novelty

When a treatment or protocol is new, both researchers and participants may react with either skepticism or enthusiasm, affecting the outcome variables in the study.

Experimenter/participant effects

The researcher or participant may use their knowledge of the composition of the intervention or comparison groups to influence the reporting of outcome data. This results in noncomparable information being gathered from the different study groups.

Interaction of selection and intervention

Subjects who are willing to participate in a study, particularly one that requires an extensive time commitment, may not be representative of the target population. The characteristics of these subjects may affect the outcome of the intervention.

Interaction of setting and intervention

The characteristics of organizations that encourage the conduct of research studies in contrast to those that do not may influence the outcome data. Therefore the ability to generalize of the findings may be limited.

Interaction of history and intervention

The circumstances surrounding the conduct of a study (history) may influence the results obtained from the intervention and decrease the ability to generalize the findings.

consistency of findings with other studies. Depending on the purpose of the study, one type of validity may have to be compromised to improve the other.

Ethical considerations

Conducting research in an ethical manner is a fundamental priority in the development and implementation of any research study and involves three steps.

First, researchers should clearly delineate the benefits and risks of the study, considering the projected outcomes of the research. Benefits to participants can include access to an intervention that may not be available in other settings, knowledge that their information may be helpful to others, and increased attention from health professionals among others. Risks or costs to participants can include distress resulting from loss of privacy or time, self-disclosure, fear, financial costs, and possible physical discomfort or harmful side effects from therapeutic trials. All studies involve risk, although it may be missed in some study designs.

Second, researchers should obtain informed consent from subjects whenever appropriate. This includes a full disclosure of the benefits and risks of the study. The content of an informed consent document is outlined in the box below. Studies that abstract information from records of care or involve the completion of a questionnaire are often found to involve minimal risk and can be exempted from the informed consent process by institutional research review boards.

Third, researchers have an obligation to protect the human rights of study subjects. The fundamental principles of ethics should be upheld. A study should do no harm, maintain respect for human dignity, including the right to participate or not without prejudicial treatment, and be just. The latter includes the right of subjects to fair treatment and the right to privacy, including anonymity and confidentiality.

ELEMENTS OF INFORMED CONSENT

Description of the status of the subject as a participant
Statement of the purpose of the research
Description of the type of information that will be obtained
Time frame for data collection
Sponsorship of the research
Explanation of selection of research subjects
Description of data collection procedures
Description of benefits and risks
Assurance of privacy, anonymity, and confidentiality
Assurance of voluntary nature of participation
Assurance of option to withdraw at any time
Disclosure of alternative procedures or treatment that might exist
Name of contact person for further information

SUMMARY

Epidemiologic intervention studies seek to determine a cause-and-effect relationship between exposure and outcome. They are experimental studies that manipulate a variable, control for extraneous factors, and randomize the selection of subjects. Cause-and-effect relationships are determined by examination of (1) the strength of the association between the exposure and outcomes, (2) the time sequence involved, (3) the consistency of the findings, and (4) the biologic credibility of the relationship between exposure and outcomes.

Epidemiologic intervention studies may be experimental or quasi-experimental in nature and are identified as either therapeutic trials or preventive trials. Therapeutic trials are based on the principles of secondary prevention. They attempt to determine the ability of interventions to decrease or prevent recurrence of symptoms and to improve outcomes for individuals with specific states of health. Preventive trials are based on principles of primary prevention. They seek to reduce the risk of acquiring a specific health problem among a group of people who do not have that health problem at the onset of the study.

In designing intervention studies, consideration must be given to the selection of the sample. Random selection of the sample and random assignment of study subjects to the intervention and comparisons groups will produce a study sample that is representative of the experimental population the majority of the time. It is important that study participants comply as carefully as possible to study protocols. Baseline and outcome data are collected for all intervention and comparison groups with the primary objective to collect equivalent and uniform information for all groups. In the analysis, the rates of the outcome variables in the intervention group are compared with the corresponding rates in the comparison group. Potential biases from threats to both internal and external validity must be addressed at every stage of the research. All research studies should address the benefits and risks associated with the research, obtain informed consent if appropriate, and protect the human rights of participants.

CRITICAL THINKING QUESTIONS

1. From the literature, select an epidemiologic intervention study.
   a. Evaluate the results of the study by the cause-and-effect criteria outlined in this chapter.
   b. Identify the target population.
   c. Identify the experimental population.
   d. Were the study subjects selected randomly from the experimental population? If not how were they selected?
2. Explain how random selection and random assignment help to reduce threats to internal validity.
3. Explain how the size of the sample affects the study results.

REFERENCES

Burns N, Grove SK: *The practice of nursing research, conduct, critique and utilization,* ed 2, Philadelphia, 1993, WB Saunders.

DeMets DL and others: Statistical aspects of early termination in the beta-blocker heart attack trial, *Controlled Clin Trials,* 5:362, 1984.

Hennekens CH, Buring JE: *Epidemiology in medicine,* Boston, 1989, Little, Brown.

Hennekens CH, Buring JE, Mayrent SL: Smoking and aging in coronary heart disease. In Bosse R, Rose CL, editors: *Smoking and aging,* Lexington, MA, 1984, DC Health, pp 95-115.

Kleinbaum DG, Kupper LL, Morgenstern H: *Epidemiologic research,* Belmont, CA, 1982, Lifetime Learning Publications.

Lando H and others: Brief supportive telephone outreach as a recruitment and intervention strategy for smoking cessation, *Am J Public Health* 82(1):41-46, 1992.

Mausner JS, Kramer S: *Epidemiology—an introductory text,* ed 2, Philadelphia, 1985, WB Saunders.

Metzger BL, Therrien B: Effect of position on cardiovascular response during the Valsalva maneuver, *Nurs Res* 39(4):198-202, 1990.

Perry CL, and others: Communitywide smoking prevention: long-term outcomes of the Minnesota Heart Health Program and the class of 1989 study, *Am J Public Health* 82(9):1210-1216, 1992.

Urdang L, Swallow HH: *Mosby's medical and nursing dictionary,* St. Louis, 1983, Mosby.

7

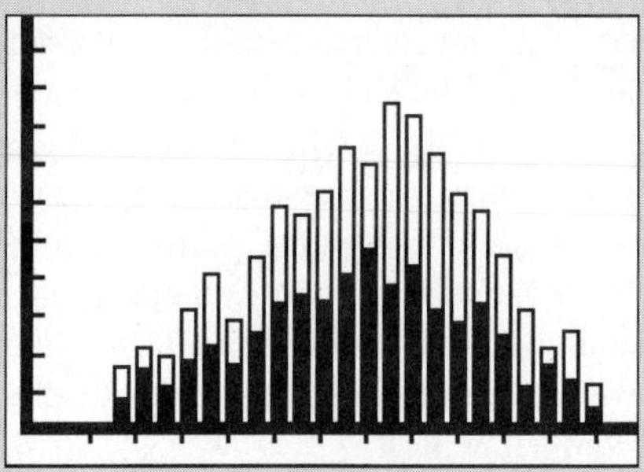

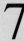

Epidemiology of Infectious Processes

Objectives

1. Comprehend the evolution of infectious disease epidemiology from the nineteenth century to the present time.
2. Conceptualize infectious diseases in terms of agent, host, and environment.
3. Discuss the effect of the host and the environment on the infectivity, pathogenicity, virulence, and immunogenicity characteristics of the agent.
4. Relate the pathogenesis of infection to the process of transmission of agent.
5. Differentiate between colonization, inapparent infection, and clinical illness.
6. Explain the relationship between reservoirs and the means of transmission of microorganisms.
7. Identify the nurse's use of principles of infectious disease epidemiology when initiating primary, secondary, and tertiary prevention strategies.
8. Define the principles of epidemiology used in investigation of an epidemic.

Key Terms

airborne transmission
biologic vector-borne
carrier
colonization
common-source epidemic
communicable disease
direct contact
droplet nuclei
epidemic
endemic
fomites
herd immunity
immunogenicity
inapparent infection
incubation period
index case
indirect contact
infectious agent
infectious disease
infectivity
infection
infestation
mechanical vector-borne
outbreak
pandemic
pathogen
pathogenicity
propagated epidemic
reservoir
source
vector
vehicle
virulence
zoonoses

Epidemiology originated in the latter part of the nineteenth century as a result of the need to prevent and control epidemics of infectious diseases, such as cholera and the black plague (Fig. 7-1). At that time, the leading causes of death were of infectious origin. During the twentieth century, great advances were made in the prevention and control of infectious diseases through the purification of drinking water, waste control, availability of a variety of foods, immunizations, and drug therapy. Today, the scope of epidemiology has broadened, reflecting the changes in health patterns throughout the world. Epidemiology now includes the study of all factors that affect the health of human beings.

Despite the remarkable success in reducing the impact of infectious diseases on the population, an ongoing program of infectious disease prevention and control must be maintained. There is increasing evidence that new and more resistant organisms are emerging. Lost workdays and school days per year due to infectious diseases pose a significant economic burden to society. Two infectious processes also pose significant morbidity and mortality threats to the health of people in the United States. These are respiratory infections, such as pneumonia and influenza, and the human immunodeficiency virus (HIV). Nurses are intricately involved in the identification, treatment, control, and prevention of infectious diseases in acute care, long-term care, and community settings.

THE INFECTIOUS PROCESS

The infectious process depends on the interaction between an infectious agent, a susceptible host, and the environment (see Fig. 2-4). *Infection* is defined as the presence and replication of an infectious agent in the tissues of a host, causing local cellular injury, secretion of one or more toxins, and/or an antigen-antibody reaction in the host. When the host is disrupted from an infection so that signs and symptoms of disease occur, an *infectious disease* is present (Benenson, 1990; Brachman, 1990). Microorganisms are transmitted from where they live and multiply to another person or place. The illness that is produced may range from mild to severe, and death may result. Although *communicable disease* is often used synonymously with infectious disease, communicable disease is transmitted from one person (or animal) to another. Not all infectious diseases are communicable.

There are essential links in the chain of events that produce an infection in a human being. These involve interaction between the agent, host, environment, and a means of transmission of the agent from an infected host to a susceptible host (Fig. 7-2).

Agent

The *infectious agent* is an organism that is capable of producing an infection or an infectious disease (Benenson, 1990). Usually the infectious agent is a microorganism, such as a bacteria or virus, and is often called a pathogen. Infectious agents are classified as bacteria, viruses, rickettsias, fungi, protozoa, and helminths. Arthropods, such as lice, on the surface of the body are often identified as communicable diseases, although they are considered *infestations* rather than infections.

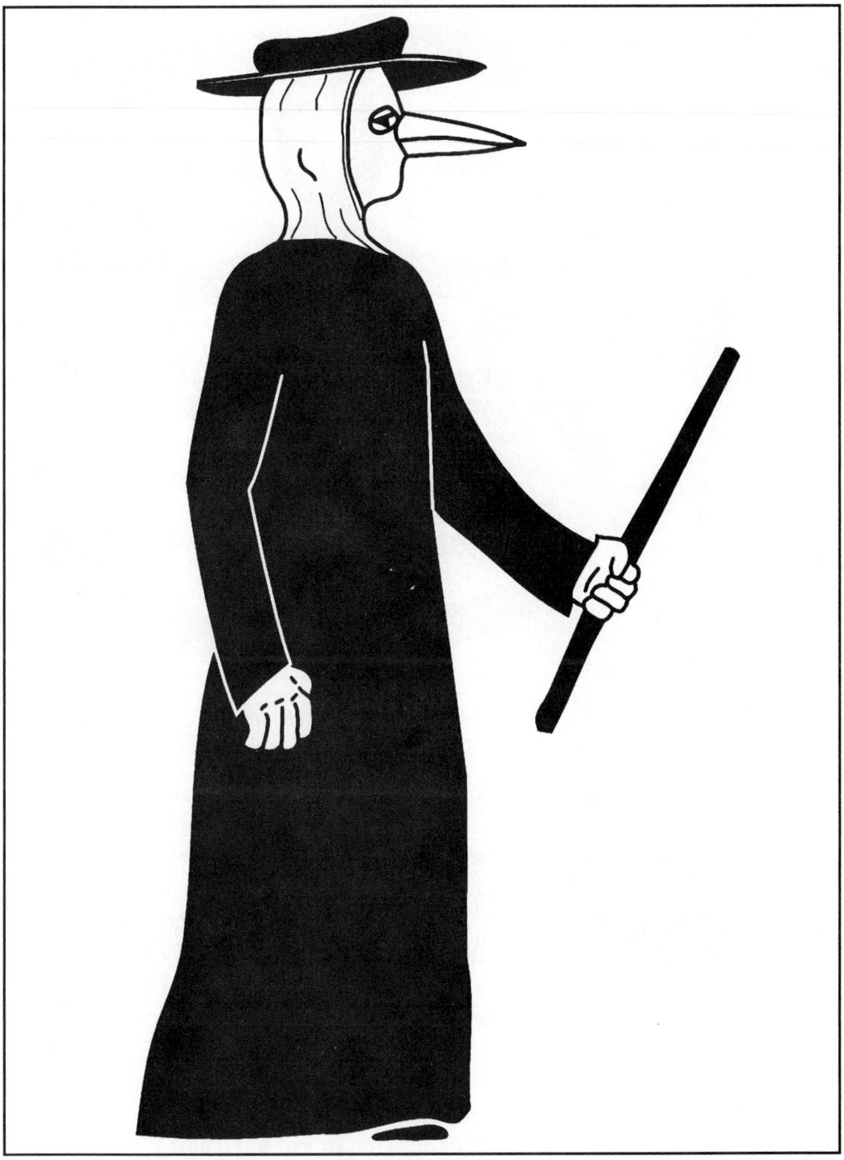

Fig. 7-1 Leather garb worn by care givers during the seventeenth century black plague epidemic. The eyepiece was made of glass and the beak-like nose was stuffed with perfumes.

All infectious agents have intrinsic properties that are unique but vary considerably between organisms. Examples of these characteristics include size, chemical composition and structure, requirements for growth, antigenic properties, and the abilities to produce toxin, develop resistance to environmental fac-

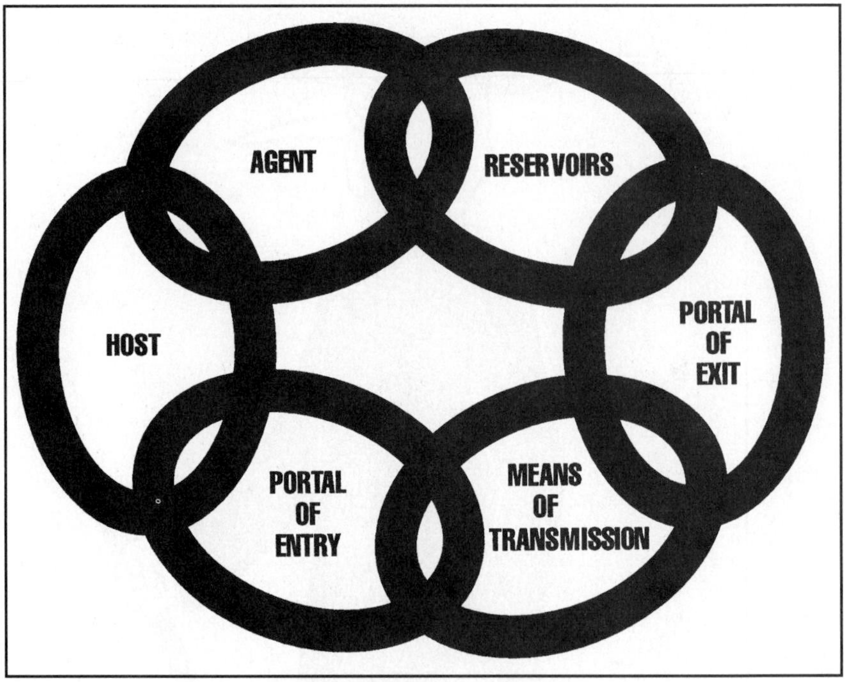

Fig. 7-2 Chain of infection.

tors, acquire new genetic information, and live for a period of time outside of the host. The reproductive cycle of the microorganism also influences the effect of the infectious agent on the host. The rate of reproduction of a microorganism is related to the body's ability to stimulate an inflammation and immune response that will counteract the effects of the agent. Knowledge of the reproductive cycles give clues to the prevention and control of the infectious disease. For example, some organisms require a warm, moist, dark environment for a breeding ground; others can survive in a variety of states until the proper conditions exist for them to grow and multiply. Interruption of these states at strategic times can decrease the possibility of transmission of the agent. Knowledge of these intrinsic properties is essential to public health officials, nurses, physicians, and other health care personnel in planning and implementing prevention and control measures for infectious diseases. Examples of agents of infectious disease are found in Table 7-1.

There are properties that have been described as characteristics of infectious agents that are not necessarily intrinsic to the agent itself but result instead from an interaction between the agent, host, and environment. These properties include the infectivity, pathogenicity, virulence, and immunogenicity associated with a particular infectious agent (Mausner and Kramer, 1985). Each agent has a normal range of these properties, however, host factors, such as age, nutritional status, and underlying illness, can result in an increased or decreased resistance to the agent. Also, environmental conditions surrounding exposure, such as the amount

Table 7-1 Selected agents of infectious disease

Type of agent	Specific agent	Disease
Bacteria	*Streptococci*	Streptococcal sore throat Scarlet fever Rheumatic fever
	Staphylococci	Impetigo Skin and wound lesions Toxic shock syndrome Staphylococcal food poisoning
	Mycobacterium tuberculosis	Tuberculosis
	Neisseria gonorrhoeae	Gonorrhea
	Treponema pallidum	Syphilis
	Borrelia burgdorferi	Lyme disease
Virus	Hepatitis A virus (HAV)	Viral hepatitis A
	Hepatitis B virus (HBV)	Viral Hepatitis B
	HIV	Acquired immunodeficiency syndrome (AIDS)
	Herpes simplex virus (HSV)	Herpes
	Varicella-zoster virus (V-Z virus)	Chickenpox
	A, B, and C Influenza virus	Influenza
	Measles virus	Rubeola, measles
	Rubella virus	Rubella, German measles
	Paramyxovirus	Mumps, infectious parotitis
	Rhinovirus, coronavirus	Acute upper respiratory infection
Rickettsia	*Rickettsia rickettsii*	Rocky Mountain spotted fever
	Typhus exanthematicus	Typhus fever
Fungi	*Trichophyton rubrum*	Athlete's foot
	Histoplasma capsulatum	Histoplasmosis
	Aspergillus fumigatus	Aspergillosis
Protozoa	*Entamoeba histolyticia*	Amebic dysentery
	Plasmodium falciparum	Malaria
Helminths	*Necator americanus*	Hookworm
	Ascaris lumbricoides	Ascariasis (roundworms)
	Enterobius vermicularis	Pinworms

of the dose or the means of entry into the host, can vary the ability of the agent to produce an infection.

Infectivity is the ability of the agent to invade the host and replicate. Infectivity can vary with the route of entry, source of the agent, and host susceptibility. For example, the gonococcus bacteria that causes gonorrhea, *Neisseria gonorrhoeae,* has a higher infectivity than the tetanus bacillus, *Clostridium tetani.* The gonococcus enters the host easily through sexual contact with infected persons, susceptibility is general, and reinfection can occur. However, the tetanus bacillus gains entry only through a contaminated puncture wound of the skin, and active immunity through immunization has decreased the availability of susceptible hosts.

Pathogenicity is the ability of the agent to produce an infectious disease in a susceptible host. A microorganism's potential to produce disease depends on its ability to invade and destroy body cells, produce toxins, and produce immune reactions. Not all pathogens have an equal probability of producing infectious disease (Relman and Falkow, 1990). Many host and environmental factors may alter the pathogenicity of a specific agent. For example, staphylococci often colonize the skin and also can be found in the gastrointestinal tract as normal body flora. However, staphylococci in the abdominal cavity can cause a severe illness. The staphylococci have a higher pathogenicity than the tubercule bacillus that causes infectious disease in only a small number of the susceptible, exposed individuals.

Virulence describes the severity of the infectious disease that results from exposure to the agent. It is a quantitative measure of pathogenicity or the likelihood of causing disease (Relman and Falkow, 1990). The case fatality rate is one measure of virulence. Virulence, such as infectivity and pathogenicity, depends on a combination of factors, such as dose, route of infection, and host factors. Fig. 7-3 illustrates the difference in virulence between the tubercule bacillus where inapparent infection is frequent, the measles virus where clinical disease is frequent

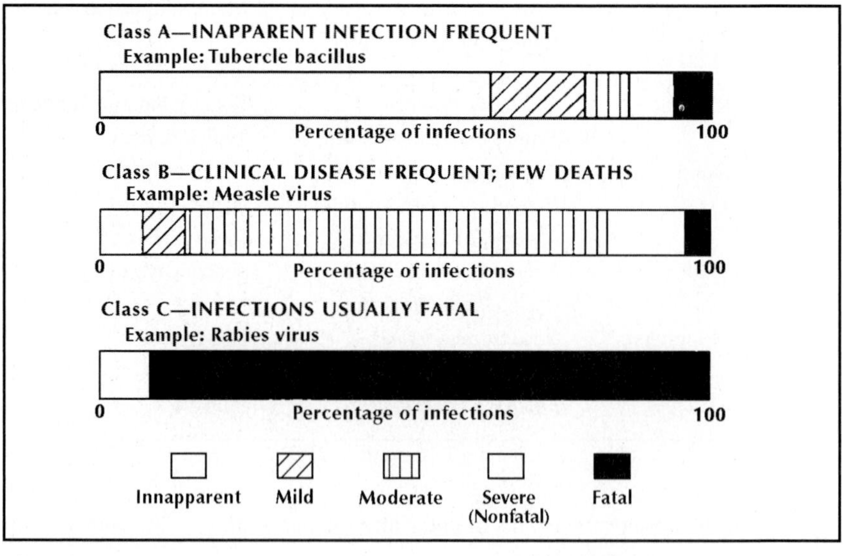

Fig. 7-3 Distribution of the clinical severity for three classes of infections (actual statistics not represented). (From: Mausner JA, Kramer S: *Epidemiology—an introductory text,* Philadelphia, 1985, WB Saunders, p 265.)

but few deaths occur, and the rabies virus where infections are usually fatal (Mausner and Kramer, 1985).

Immunogenicity is the ability of the agent to produce specific immunity within the host. Some infections, such as the measles virus, produce a life-long immunity within the host. Others, such as the gonococci, do not have strong antigenic properties, and reinfection can occur. Immunogenicity is affected by age, nutrition, other characteristics of the host, and factors, such as the virulence, dose, and route of infection.

Host

Presence of an infectious agent is not sufficient to produce an infectious disease. A susceptible host must be present. Many underlying host factors determine whether the individual will develop an infection or an infectious disease. Age, race, sex, physical and emotional health, and immune status are the most common host factors that determine susceptibility to infectious agents. Host susceptibility can be reduced through administration of vaccines and other immunizations that stimulate the immune system to counteract the infectious agent (primary prevention). As a result, there is less probability that the individual will acquire the disease. A summary of vaccines available in the United States is found in Table 7-2. Host susceptibility can also be reduced through early identification and reduction of risk factors for specific diseases (secondary prevention). Unfortunately, some diseases, such as cancer and HIV infection, can suppress the immune system causing the individual to become increasingly susceptible to infectious diseases.

There have been ongoing attempts in the United States to immunize the population against the common childhood infectious diseases. If enough of the population becomes immune to the diseases, the few susceptible people in the population are not likely to come in contact with the agent and, subsequently, develop the disease. The presence of a large proportion of immune individuals in a community decreases the chances of contact between any infected people and susceptible individuals. This phenomenon is called *herd immunity.* For example, epidemics of measles are likely to occur only when the number of susceptible people increase and herd immunity decreases. An entire population does not have to be immune to prevent an epidemic of a disease.

Once an infectious agent enters the host and begins to multiply, an infection has occurred. The time period between initial contact with the infectious agent and the appearance of the first signs or symptoms of the disease is called the *incubation period.* During this time, multiplication of the microorganism occurs within the host until the number of microorganisms are large enough to produce symptoms. Each infectious disease has a characteristic incubation period, however it will vary within individuals. A wide variety of clinical effects can be produced.

Colonization indicates the presence of an organism without a clinical or subclinical disease. An *inapparent* or *subclinical infection* indicates that the relationship between the agent and the host has been limited to an immune response that can only be detected by laboratory means or a positive reaction to a skin test. The

Table 7-2 Vaccines available in the United States, by type and recommended routes of administration

Vaccine	Type	Route
BCG (bacillus of calmette and guerin)	Live bacteria	Intradermal or subcutaneous
Cholera	Inactivated bacteria	Subcutaneous or intradermal*
DTP (D = diphtheria) (T = tetanus) (P = pertussis)	Toxoids and inactivated bacteria	Intramuscular
HB (Hepatitis B)	Inactive viral antigen	Intramuscular
Haemophilus influenzae b		
—polysaccharide (HbPV)	Bacterial polysaccharide	Subcutaneous or intramuscular†
—or conjugate (HbCV)	or polysaccharide conjugated to protein	Intramuscular
Influenza	Inactivated virus or viral components	Intramuscular
IPV (inactivated poliovirus vaccine)	Inactivated viruses of all three serotypes	Subcutaneous
Measles	Live virus	Subcutaneous
Meningococcal	Bacterial polysaccharides of serotypes A/C/Y/W-135	Subcutaneous
MMR (M = measles) (M = mumps) (R = rubella)	Live viruses	Subcutaneous
Mumps	Live virus	Subcutaneous
OPV (oral poliovirus vaccine)	Live viruses of all three serotypes	Oral
Plague	Inactivated bacteria	Intramuscular
Pneumococcal	Bacterial polysaccharides of 23 pneumococcal types	Intramuscular or subcutaneous
Rabies	Inactivated virus	Subcutaneous or intradermal‡
Rubella	Live virus	Subcutaneous
Tetanus	Inactive toxin (toxoid)	Intramuscular§
Td or DT‖ (T = Tetanus) (D or d = diphtheria)	Inactivated toxins (toxoids)	Intramuscular§
Typhoid	Inactivated bacteria	Subcutaneous¶
Yellow fever	Live virus	Subcutaneous

* The intradermal dose is lower.

† Route depends on the manufacturer; consult package insert for recommendation for specific product used.

‡ Intradermal dose is lower and used only for preexposure vaccination.

§ Preparations with adjuvants should be given intramuscularly.

‖ DT = tetanus and diphtheria toxoids for use in children age <7 years. Td = tetanus and diphtheria toxoids for use in persons age ≥ 7 years. Td contains the same amount of tetanus toxoid as DTP or DT but a reduced dose of diphtheria toxoid.

¶ Boosters may be given intradermally unless acetone-killed and dried vaccine is used.

(From Centers for Disease Control: ACIP: general recommendations, *MMWR* 38(13):207, 1989.)

host's immune system has been able to combat the infection without producing symptoms of the disease. People with inapparent infections may be capable of infecting others without having evidence of the disease themselves. They are potential sources of the disease and are called *carriers*. Carrier states may be of long or short duration. Early HIV infection often produces carriers with inapparent infection and has produced great problems for the prevention and control of its spread throughout the world. The communicability of infectious agents varies with agent characteristics, but an average length of time is from 3 to 7 days with the more common viral or bacterial infections. Infection with other agents like HIV can result in a carrier state that is undetermined in length.

Environment

The third element in the epidemiologic triad is the physical, biologic, and socioeconomic environment. The environment includes all external influences that affect living organisms. The physical environment includes the characteristics of the place, such as the geography of the region, the climate, and the seasons. The biologic environment includes the living plants and animals that surround us. The socioeconomic environment refers to the effects of social and economic conditions on the quality of our lives. Social and economic conditions determine the availability of uncontaminated drinking water, sanitary facilities, a variety of foodstuffs, and medical care. Public health measures like these have been responsible for the dramatic increase in the life expectancy during the twentieth century.

Transmission of infectious agents from a reservoir or a source to a susceptible person occurs within the environment. A *reservoir* is the location where an agent lives and reproduces under normal circumstances. A *source* of an infectious agent is the location from which the organism is immediately transmitted to the host (Brachman, 1990).

Reservoirs. The normal habitats of infectious organisms can be human beings, animals, insects, plants, or environmental inanimate matter, such as soil or water. The reservoir, a place to live and multiply, is an essential link in the transmission cycle of an infectious agent. Infected people are the reservoirs for most bacterial and viral infections that affect humans, such as staphylococcal and streptococcal infections and the common childhood diseases. Humans can be both hosts and reservoirs for many infectious agents.

Humans are also subject to infections acquired from infected animals that serve as reservoirs for human infection. These infections, transmitted from vertebrate animals to humans under normal conditions, are known as *zoonoses*. Humans are the susceptible hosts for these infections, but humans are not a part of the life cycle or a reservoir of the agent. Leptospirosis is an acute generalized infection, resembling meningitis or encephalitis, that results from infection with a bacterial spirochete normally found in domestic and wild mammals (reservoirs). It has a worldwide distribution, although it is rare in the United States. Humans are exposed through indirect or direct contact with the urine of an infected animal. It is an occupational hazard to workers in rice and sugarcane fields, farmers, veterinarians, dairymen, and military troops in countries where the disease is common. The infection can last from a few days to 3 weeks or longer and can be treated successfully with antibiotics. Humans are usually dead-end hosts, since further transmission to other people is rare. Other infectious diseases are characterized by complex life cycles that may include more than one reservoir and different developmental stages of the infectious agent in more than one host. Lyme disease, malaria, and tapeworm infestations are examples.

Mechanisms of transmission. There are three mechanisms through which transmission occurs: *direct contact, airborne transmission,* and *indirect contact.* Transmission by direct contact occurs when the infectious agent exits from the reservoir and is transferred to a portal of entry into a susceptible host through touching, biting, kissing, sexual intercourse, or droplet spray. For example, an outbreak of impetigo in a nursery school usually involves direct transmission of the staphylococcus organism from person to person through touch. Similarly, the HIV virus is transmitted through the exchange of body fluids that occurs during sexual intercourse.

Direct-contact transmission can occur through droplets that contaminate the conjunctiva or mucous membranes of the eye, nose, or mouth during sneezing, coughing, spitting, or talking. This usually occurs within a distance of approximately 1 meter. These droplets are large particles that do not enter the lungs unless they are reduced in size from evaporation. The mucociliary action of the respiratory passages inactivate and remove droplets from the respiratory tract.

Airborne transmission involves the dissemination of particles suspended in air that contain microorganisms. These are called *droplet nuclei.* Droplet nuclei are particle residues resulting from evaporation of fluid from droplets disseminated by an infected person. Coughing, or talking for approximately 5 minutes, can release more than 3000 droplet nuclei into the air (Des Prez and Heim, 1990). Sneezing will produce even more. Droplet nuclei can remain suspended in air in a dry state for long periods of time. The particles are quite small (1-5 μm) and can be easily breathed into the lungs where they are retained (Benenson, 1990). Once the terminal air passages are reached, multiplication occurs and infection begins. Pulmonary tuberculosis is the most common illness that is transmitted by droplet nuclei.

Other aerosols can be created commercially or accidently in laboratories. Dust particles containing microorganisms can also become airborne and, subsequently, breathed into the lungs. Contaminated clothes, bedding, and other objects in the environment can create dust that disseminates some microorganisms through airborne transmission.

Transmission by indirect contact occurs through either a *vehicle* or *vector.* Vehicles include substances or objects that have become contaminated with infectious organisms. *Fomites* are contaminated objects that include such things as toys, handkerchiefs, dishes, soiled clothing, bedding, and surgical instruments. Vehicles also include food, water, milk, and biologic secretions. The agent may or may not have multiplied on or within the vehicle before it is transmitted to another person (Benenson, 1990). Organisms on objects can be transferred through hand-to-mouth contact to the susceptible person.

Vectors are carriers of infectious agents, usually animals or arthropods, such as mosquitoes. Insects, such as flies, can transmit organisms that are picked up on its feet or proboscis to food or water. This is called *mechanical vector-borne* transmission. Multiplication or development of the infectious agent within the carrier is not required. Alternatively, a mosquito that is carrying an organism, such as the malaria parasite, in its body fluids can transmit microorganisms through its bite (inoculation). This is called *biologic vector-borne* transmission. Multiplication and development of the organisms occurs in the arthropod before it can transmit the infective form of the agent to humans (Benenson, 1990).

Lyme disease is an example of an epidemic illness in the United States that is transmitted by a small tick vector. The complex life-style of *Ixodes dammini*—the tick that acts as a reservoir for the agent of Lyme disease, *Borrelia burgdorferi*—is shown in Fig. 7-4. The larval or nymphal tick becomes infected with *B. burgdorferi* as it feeds on infected mice or deer. At this stage, ticks are most likely to bite humans. If the tick feeds for several hours on a human, transmission of the bacterial spirochete can occur (biologic vector-borne transmission).

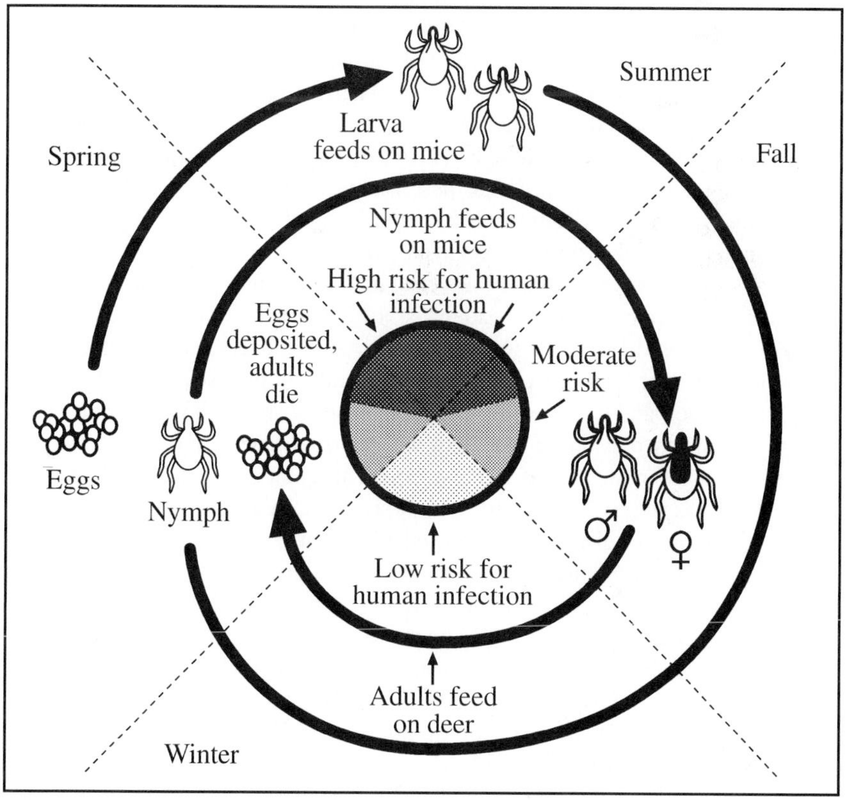

Fig. 7-4 Life cycle of the *Ixodes dammini* tick. The tick is a reservoir for *Borrelia burgdorferi,* the agent that produces Lyme disease in humans.

Knowledge of these intertwining life cycles provides clues as to the possible interruption of transmission as a measure to control the disease. For example, educating the public about means for personal protection (primary prevention) and symptoms that indicate early infection requiring treatment (secondary prevention) have been successful in decreasing the incidence of the disease in some communities.

PREVENTION AND CONTROL

The development of infection is multifactorial, resulting from interactions among many factors related to the agent, host, and environment. Since multiple factors must be assessed in the process of developing and implementing interventions, designing specific prevention and control measures is complex. The goal is to prevent the spread of the infectious agent from its reservoir or source to susceptible hosts, breaking the chain of infection (Fig. 7-2).

There are two basic principles for the prevention and control of communicable diseases. First, intervention strategies should be based on the epidemiologic characteristics of the disease. The factors involved in the development of the infection require modification for successful control and prevention. These factors will vary from one infectious disease to another. Second, intervention strategies should be directed toward the link in the chain of infection that is the most susceptible to interruption. However, cost effectiveness, time constraints, staffing requirements, and possible adverse effects of intervention measures must also be considered. Prevention and control activities are often compromises among many competing elements. All of these interrelated factors affecting the occurrence of the specific infectious disease should be identified and analyzed when prevention and control measures are planned (Brachman, 1990).

Nurses are constantly involved in assessment of patients or clients for factors that indicate whether a patient is at high risk for infection. Primary prevention strategies then can be initiated to prevent the occurrence of infections. Ongoing assessment for signs and symptoms of infectious disease results in prompt identification and treatment of infectious disease should it occur. These activities are secondary prevention strategies that interrupt the chain of infection at the link between infectious agent and reservoir. The agent is inactivated. Rapid and accurate identification of organisms and appropriate treatment can decrease or eliminate reservoirs in the environment, whether that environment is an acute care, long-term care, or home setting. Disinfection, sterilization, and environmental sanitation can also interrupt the normal habitat of infectious organisms.

When an infectious disease exists, proper precautions with excretions and secretions, handwashing, and trash and waste disposal will interfere with transmission from the portal of exit (Fig. 7-5). Each infectious agent has its own specific means of transmission. For example, staphylococci infections occur primarily through direct contact with purulent discharge. Hepatitis A virus is transmitted from person to person by the fecal-oral route often through contaminated food as a common vehicle. Tuberculosis occurs following exposure to inhalation of airborne droplet nuclei from the sputum of an infected person. Interruption of the

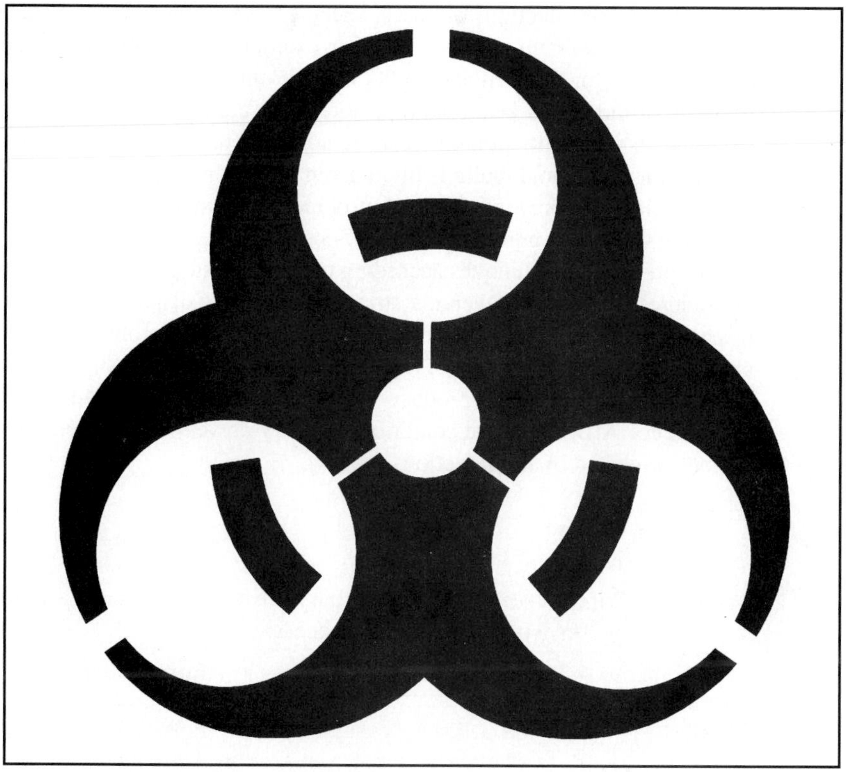

Fig. 7-5 Biohazard symbol.

chain of infection requires specific measures based on these epidemiologic characteristics.

The portals of entry for susceptible hosts are usually mucous membranes, the gastrointestinal or respiratory tracts, and broken skin. While normal defense mechanisms protect these areas, medical treatment can bypass these defenses. Intubation bypasses the respiratory mucous-membrane protective mechanisms. Catheters provide a direct pathway from the environment to internal structures as do drains placed in wounds. Unprotected portals of entry can easily be contaminated with pathogenic microorganisms. Aseptic technique and proper care when invasive devices are used will interfere with the transmission of infectious agents in these situations.

People with proper nutrition and who engage in exercise and other positive life-style behaviors are the least susceptible to infectious diseases. Conversely, those with immunosuppression from underlying conditions, such as diabetes, cardiopulmonary disease, cancer, burns, or exposure to surgery, are the most likely to develop infections. The treatment of underlying disease is paramount in interruption of the infectious process. Increasing the resistance of the host can be achieved through recognition of high-risk people and strengthening their defense mechanisms. For some infectious diseases, vaccines and toxoids produce active stimulation of the host's immune system. For example, influenza immunizations are recommended for children and adults with chronic disorders, healthy individuals 65 years of older, and health care personnel having extensive contact with high-risk patients. Immune globulins can be administered for temporary passive immunization. Immunoglobulin is often given to persons exposed to viral hepatitis.

It is clear that prevention and control measures involve principles of both primary and secondary prevention. Table 7-3 summarizes common primary and secondary prevention techniques according to the stage of the infectious process and also addresses tertiary prevention strategies. Residual disabilities from infectious diseases that require tertiary prevention strategies are not common, however disabilities do occur. For example, repeated ear infections can result in hearing loss, chronic Lyme disease can produce cardiovascular problems, and HIV infection can produce AIDS. In these conditions, tertiary prevention is specific to the limitations produced by the infectious process.

Table 7-3 Primary, secondary, and tertiary prevention measures according to the stage of the infectious process

Prevention level	Stage of infectious process	Interventions
Primary	Interaction between agent, host, and environment	Promotion of healthy life-styles Nutrition counseling Adequate housing and sanitation Immunizations Correcting environmental hazards Inactivation of known reservoirs of agents Employee health programs
Secondary	Infectious agent becomes established in host Multiplication of agent occurs Early physiologic changes occur	Screening Case-finding Early diagnosis and treatment
Tertiary	Clinical recognition of disease Signs and symptoms develop Disability and/or chronic state develops Death is possible	Treatment to arrest infectious process Minimize disability Promote adaptation to limitations

INVESTIGATION OF AN EPIDEMIC

The investigation of an epidemic is an example of the epidemiologic process in action. An *epidemic* occurs when there is a significant increase in the number of new cases of a disease or illness than past experience would have predicted for that place, at that time, among a specified population (Morton, Hebel, and McCarter, 1990). It is an increase in incidence beyond that which is expected. The term *outbreak* is synonymous with epidemic. *Endemic* refers to the constant or usual prevalence of a specific disease or infectious agent within a population or geographic area. A *pandemic* is an epidemic that occurs over a wide geographic area, often world-wide.

The epidemiologic process of investigating an epidemic includes (1) establishing the existence of the problem, (2) gathering data to describe the problem by person, place, and time, (3) formulating and testing hypotheses as to the most probable causative factors, (4) implementing a plan for control of the outbreak, including prevention of future outbreaks, and (5) evaluating results, preparing reports, and conducting further research as necessary. Although these activities are crucial to the proper investigation of outbreaks, it is not necessary that they be accomplished in order. The sequence may be altered based on the specific characteristics of the outbreak. For instance, it may be necessary to implement control measures to prevent further cases before all the data have been gathered. The ultimate purpose of the investigation is to identify the measures necessary to control the outbreak and prevent similar outbreaks from occurring.

Establishing the existence of an epidemic

To establish the existence of an epidemic it is necessary to have some estimates of past incidence rates. The background occurrence or endemic nature of the infectious disease must be known to judge whether this new information is a normal variation in rates or is the onset of an epidemic. The reported data should be a distinct departure from the normal incidence or prior occurrence of the infectious disease, and the observed rates should be greater than the expected rates. For example, an increase in *Salmonella* infections in the summer may be a normal increase for the season and therefore does not indicate the onset of an outbreak (Brachman, 1990). However, the emergence of one case of methicillin resistant *Staphylococcus aureus* (MRSA) in a hospital where none has previously existed signals the beginning of an epidemic. In making such judgments, the reliability of the reporting source is an important aspect to consider.

It is also essential to develop the criteria that will be used to define a case. The case definition should be broad enough to include all the cases that are relevant to the investigation. Some of these may be classified as noncases as the investigation proceeds. After more information is available, the case definition may need to be revised. The diagnosis should be verified. Sometimes this may require only a brief review of clinical findings, but more often laboratory tests will be necessary. There can be discrepancies between clinical observations and laboratory tests. Either one may be incorrect due to a multiplicity of factors. When complex, costly laboratory tests are required for diagnosis, the cost-effectiveness of the investigation becomes a factor in decision-making processes. Once the defining criteria have been developed, the suspected cases are often grouped into definite, probable, and suspected (possible) categories. Table 7-4 illustrates the criteria used to differentiate between definite, probable, and possible cases in a prospective epidemiologic investigation of a *Streptococcus pyogenes* outbreak in a hospital for the chronically ill (Harkness and others, 1992).

Describing the outbreak

Describing the outbreak by person, place, and time will provide valuable information about the magnitude and distinguishing features of the epidemic (see Chapter 4). Individual case data are gathered and then combined for the analysis. Specific attack rates in the population exposed to the infectious agent are calculated according to age, sex, occupation, exposures, and other relevant attributes. This information identifies what groups have acquired the infection. The population at risk often is identified by geographic location. However, the population at risk may be difficult to identify, particularly in community settings. For example, it may be difficult to identify the population at risk for a suspected epidemic linked to a specific restaurant. The people at a restaurant at a given time often do not know each other and may be from a wide geographic area. Even if a significant number later become ill, it may go undetected. In circumstances such as this, it may be necessary to conduct a survey to determine the population at risk.

More data may need to be gathered as the investigation proceeds. Surveys, laboratory analyses, environmental analyses, and epidemiologic studies may be required to understand the events that are occurring. People may need to be reexamined, and a search for missing cases may be required. The case definitions may need to be revised. Case-control studies are commonly used to compare the characteristics of those who have developed the illness with those who have not been affected (see Chapter 5). The results of these investigations should suggest, confirm, or challenge tentative hypotheses that attempt to explain the outbreak.

Table 7-4 Case definitions—*Streptococcus pyogenes* outbreak in a long-term care facility

Case type	Description
Definite	Positive culture for *S. pyogenes* Characteristic clinical manifestations present: cellulitis, pharyngitis, bronchitis, pneumonia, septicemia
Probable	Culture not obtained or negative for *S. pyogenes* Characteristic clinical manifestations present Antibody titer to Streptozyme was equal to or greater than 300 units/ml
Possible	No culture obtained before antibiotic therapy was initiated Characteristic clinical manifestations present Antibody titer to Streptozyme not done or not elevated

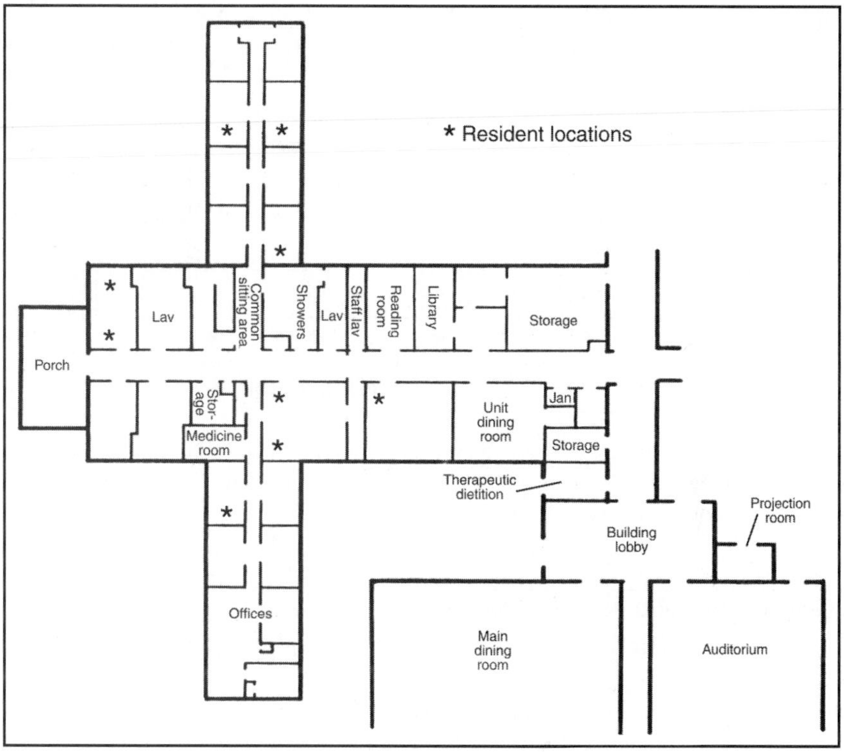

Fig. 7-6 Location of cases of *S. pyogenes,* Unit A, and vicinity.

Describing an epidemic by place involves plotting the cases by location on a spot map to determine concentrations within given areas. The characteristics of the place where the epidemic is occurring dictate the type of map to be used. For example, in the investigation mentioned above of the outbreak of *S. pyogenes* infection in a long-term care facility, Harkness (1992) diagrammed the location of nine of the total 14 cases. The proximity of these nine cases who were residing on Unit A where the outbreak began is demonstrated (Fig. 7-6). The outbreak began when two male residents of the same room developed cellulitis. Within 4 weeks the infection spread to three other residents of Unit A and, subsequently, to other units in the facility.

Describing an epidemic by time involves the creation of an epidemic curve. The number of cases of illness are plotted by the chronologic time of onset, usually expressed by hours, days, weeks, or months. Fig. 7-7 represents the epidemic curve generated from the *S. pyogenes* outbreak described by Harkness and others (1992). A total of eight definite cases, five probable cases, and one possible case occurred during the outbreak period. Both the median and mode of the outbreak occurred during Week 11. The relationship between time of onset, number of cases, and residence on Unit A is also shown.

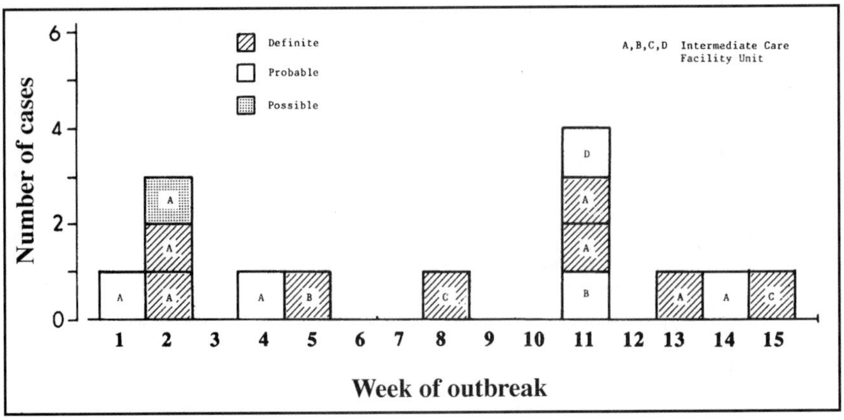

Fig. 7-7 Epidemic curve of the propagated *S. pyogenes* outbreak. (From Harkness GA, and others: *Streptoccus pyogenes* outbreak in a long-term care facility. *Am J Infect Control,* 20(3):142-148, 1992.)

Formulating and testing hypotheses

The examination of data regarding person, place, and time provides information about the agent, the source or reservoir, the means of transmission, and host factors. From this information tentative hypotheses or explanations that fit the data and identify the most probable source(s) of infection are developed. The type of epidemic should be identified. There are two primary types of epidemics, common source and propagated or progressive epidemics.

Common source epidemics. *Common source* epidemics are characterized by exposure to a common, harmful substance. Foodborne outbreaks such as the outbreak of *Escherichia coli* in January and February 1993 that involved 477 people in the state of Washington is an example. The *E. coli* strain identified in the outbreak was first determined to be a cause of illness in 1982 and was associated with the development of acute renal failure in children. The epidemic curve is presented in Fig. 7-8. On January 13, 1993, a physician reported a cluster of children with hemolytic uremic syndrome and bloody diarrhea to the Washington Department of Public Health. Preliminary investigations included a case-control study that compared 16 of the first cases with age-matched and neighborhood-matched controls. Cases were linked to the consumption of hamburgers from one fast-food restaurant chain during the week before onset of symptoms (Centers for Disease Control and Prevention [CDC], 1993). The hypotheses generated from the data indicated an *E. coli* contamination of hamburgers resulting in human infections. The hypotheses were tested and confirmed through laboratory tests. Although there was a multistate recall of unused hamburger patties from that restaurant chain, the outbreak continued through February 1993, and cases were reported from three other states. Although most common source outbreaks are infectious in nature, it is important to note that they also can result from noninfectious exposures, such as toxic spills or polluted air.

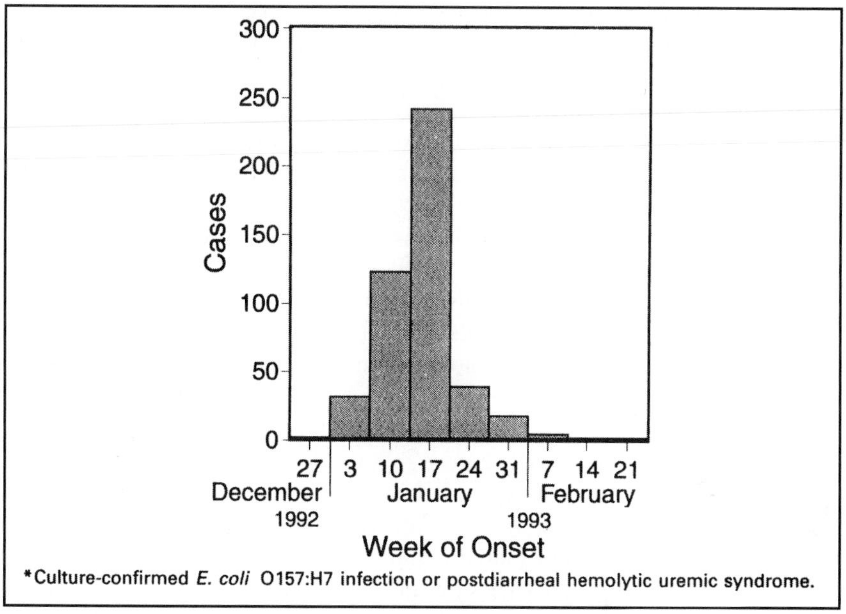

Fig. 7-8 Cases of *Escherichia coli* 0157:H7 meeting the case definition* by week of onset of illness–Washington, December 27, 1992 to February 21, 1993. (From Centers of Disease Control and Prevention: Update: multistate outbreak of *Escherichia coli,* 157:H7 infections from hamburgers–Western United States, 1992-1993, *MMWR* 42(14): 258-263, 1993.)

Propagated epidemics. *Propagated epidemics* result from direct or indirect transmission of an infectious agent from an infected person to a susceptible host. Simple person-to-person transmission can be involved, or more complex cycles involving vectors can occur. When the herd immunity is low enough, childhood infectious diseases can result in propagated epidemics.

The streptococcal outbreak in a long-term care facility described earlier is an example of a propagated outbreak (Harkness and others, 1992). Direct person-to-person transmission through contact with large droplets of saliva or nasal secretions is the primary means of transmission for this organism (Bisno, 1990). The two *index* (original) *cases* of the *S. pyogenes* infection in this outbreak were male roommates who previously had been cared for by a nursing assistant with an acute streptococcal pharyngitis. It was hypothesized that transmission of the organism occurred from the nursing assistant to the two men. However, by the time the events had been discovered, it was not possible to fully test this hypothesis through laboratory means.

After examination of the available data, it was further hypothesized that transmission could have occurred by direct contact between infected residents and uninfected residents. Most of the residents who became infected lived in proximity to one another and had frequent contact with other residents who became infected. A third hypothesis proposed that some residents experienced asymptomatic nasopharyngeal carriage and spread *S. pyogenes* to their associates. These hypotheses fit the data and were consistent with current knowledge about the organism. However, data to support these hypotheses were not gathered during the investigation. Documentation of the path of transmission is difficult to obtain during an outbreak. In discussing the conclusions from the investigation, the authors noted that the increased chances for direct contact between residents in long-term care facilities is a potential route for transmission of dangerous nosocomial pathogens. This rarely exists in the acute care setting.

Implementing control and prevention measures

Based on the hypotheses, plans should be developed for care of the sick, control of transmission, and prevention of the illness. These measures depend greatly on the facts found from describing the outbreak. Sometimes it is clear early in the investigation what control measures should be taken. Other times, it requires careful analysis of all facts before reasonable control measures can be identified. Ultimately, if the control measures that are introduced are successful in reducing the number of cases, there is evidence that the hypotheses are correct.

In the common-source outbreak involving contaminated hamburger meat (CDC, 1993), control measures involved a multistate recall of unused hamburger patties and a directive to cook meat at a higher temperature. Only 20% of these hamburger patties were recovered. A CDC epidemiologic investigation team traced the source of the contaminated meat. Five slaughter plants in the United States and one in Canada were identified as likely sources for the contaminated meat. Points were identified in the process where control measures could potentially reduce the likelihood of contamination. Surveillance is ongoing in an attempt to prevent further outbreaks.

In the propagated outbreak of *S. pyogenes* in a long-term care facility (Harkness and others, 1992), the infection control nurse initiated specific control measures as soon as the outbreak was observed. For all residents who experienced skin infections, drainage/secretion precautions were begun immediately and cultures were obtained. Appropriate antibiotic regimens were begun, and follow-up cultures were obtained 1 week after the end of the treatment. Residents with compromised immune systems, such as end-stage renal disease, were transferred off the unit where the outbreak began. The general hygiene of the unit was evaluated and improved, and shared fomites, such as bar soap and an electric razor, were removed.

Evaluating the results

An evaluation of the effect of the control measures and a report to the proper agency or officials are important final aspects of the investigation. Final reports usually include a summary of the factors leading to the epidemic, the effect of measures used to control the epidemic, and recommendations for prevention of similar episodes in the future.

In the *S. pyogenes* outbreak, the control measures were ultimately effective in limiting the transmission of the organism (Harkness and others, 1992). No further cases were identified after Week 15. None of the residents with compromised immune systems acquired the infection. Several recommendations for prevention of further outbreaks of *S. pyogenes* were made based on the results of the investigation. Ongoing surveillance for these infections among both residents and staff was recommended due to the severity of the illness that occurred. Suspected infections should be cultured, and all close associates of residents with suspected infections should be examined. Prompt specific treatment should be initiated and contact isolation should be considered if draining lesions are present. The importance of educating personnel about the disease and encouraging personnel to accept responsibility for decreasing transmission of infectious organisms was stressed.

SUMMARY

The science of epidemiology resulted from the need to control and prevent infectious diseases that were killing people throughout the world in the nineteenth century. Today most infectious diseases have been controlled, and the scope of epidemiology now includes the study of all factors that affect the health of human beings. However, infectious diseases still pose a significant economic burden to society in the form of lost workdays and school days. Respiratory infections and infection with HIV produce significant morbidity and mortality. Also, there is increasing evidence that new and more resistant infectious diseases are emerging.

Infection is the presence and replication of an infectious agent in the tissues of a host. Infectious disease is the illness that results. The infectious process involves interaction between the agent, a susceptible host, and the environment. Agents of infectious disease include bacteria, viruses, rickettsias, fungi, protozoa, and helminths. Infectivity, pathogenicity, virulence, and immunogenicity are characteristics of the agent that are influenced by the characteristics of the host and the environment.

A susceptible host must be present to produce an infectious disease. Many factors influence the susceptibility of the host. The most common factors include age, sex, race, physical and emotional health, and immune status. Once the agent enters a susceptible host there is an incubation period during which the microorganism begins to multiply. An inapparent or subclinical infection may occur that is limited to an immune response, or clinical illness may occur. People with inapparent infections often are carriers or potential sources of the disease.

The environment includes all external influences that affect living organisms: the physical, biologic, and socioeconomic environment. A reservoir is the location where an agent is usually found. Normal habitats of infectious organisms are human beings, animals, insects, plants, or inanimate matter, such as soil or water. The three mechanisms of transmission of infectious agents include direct contact, indirect contact, and airborne transmission. Airborne transmission involves dissemination of contaminated particles suspended in air.

Prevention and control measures should be based on the epidemiologic characteristics of the disease and directed toward the link in the chain of infection that is the most susceptible to interruption. Primary prevention interventions are helpful in disrupting the interaction between the agent, host, and environment. Secondary-prevention interventions are effective when the agent is becoming established in the host. Early diagnosis and treatment will prevent further complications. Tertiary prevention interventions promote adaptation when disability or chronic disease occurs. The epidemiologic process of investigating an outbreak includes several interrelated steps: (1) establishing the existence of the epidemic, (2) describing the outbreak, (3) formulating and testing hypotheses, (4) implementing control and prevention measures, and (5) evaluating the results.

Critical Thinking Questions

1. Explain how knowledge of microbiology assists in controlling pathogens that cause infectious illness.
2. Discuss the infectivity, pathogenicity, virulence, and immunogenicity of acute viral rhinitis.
3. Explain why a health care provider with a nasal culture positive for *Staphylococcus aureus* is potentially dangerous to the population of a newborn nursery.
4. Consider a typical acute care hospital; identify as many principles of infectious disease epidemiology as possible that are used to prevent or control infectious diseases.

REFERENCES

Benenson AS: *Control of communicable diseases in man,* Washington, DC, 1990, American Public Health Association.

Bisno AL: *Streptococcus pyogenes.* In Mandell GL, Douglas RG, Bennett JE, editors: *Principles and practice of infectious diseases,* ed 3, New York, 1990, Churchill Livingstone, pp 1519-1528.

Brachman PS: Epidemiology of infectious disease. In Mandell GL, Douglas RG, Bennett JE, editors: *Principles and practice of infectious diseases,* ed 3, New York, 1990, Churchill Livingstone, pp 147-155.

Centers for Disease Control and Prevention: ACIP: general recommendations, *MMWR* 38(13):207, 1989.

Centers for Disease Control and Prevention: Update: multistate outbreak of *Escherichia coli* 0157:H7 infections from hamburgers—Western United States, 1992-1993, *MMWR* 42(14):258-263, 1993.

Des Prez RM, Heim CR. In Mandell GL, Douglas RG, Bennett JE, editors: *Principles and practice of infectious diseases,* ed 3, New York, 1990, Churchill Livingstone, p 1880.

Friedman GD: *Primer of epidemiology,* ed 3, New York, 1987, McGraw-Hill.

Harkness GA: *Unit A and vicinity, Group A Streptococcus outbreak in a long-term care facility,* unpublished raw data, 1992.

Harkness GA and others: *Streptococcus pyogenes* outbreak in a long-term care facility, *Am J Infect Control* 20(3):142-148, 1992.

Last JM: *A dictionary of epidemiology,* New York, 1983, Oxford University Press.

Mausner JS, Kramer S: *Epidemiology—an introductory text,* ed 2, Philadelphia, 1985, WB Saunders.

Morton RF, Hebel JR, McCarter RJ: *A study guide to epidemiology and biostatistics,* Rockville, MD, 1990, Aspen.

Relman DA, Falkow S: A molecular perspective of microbial pathogenicity. In Mandell GL, Douglas RG, Bennett JE, editors: *Principles and practice of infectious diseases,* ed 3, New York, 1990, Churchill Livingstone, pp 25-32.

Turner JG, Chavigny KH: *Community health nursing—an epidemiologic perspective through the nursing process,* Philadelphia, 1988, JB Lippincott.

8

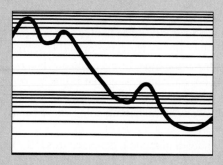

Epidemiology of Noninfectious Processes

MICHAEL D. MERRILL

Objectives

1. Examine leading threats to health from noninfectious processes according to epidemiologic data.
2. Contrast the characteristics of infectious and noninfectious diseases.
3. Define the prevalence of chronic diseases.
4. Identify methodologic problems in investigating the etiologic factors of chronic and psychosocial disorders.
5. Discuss the leading causes of death from noninfectious process.
6. Suggest prevention strategies for noninfectious conditions that involve health planning and health-policy changes.
7. Analyze the impact of world population trends on the health of individuals, health resources, and the health care delivery system.

Key Terms

- actual causes of death
- Behavioral Risk Factor Surveillance System (BRFSS)
- chemical agent
- chronic illness
  - clinical stage
  - disability stage
  - preclinical stage
  - susceptibility stage
- comorbidity
- demographic transition
- Healthy People 2000
- latency period
- lifetime prevalence
- physical agent

One of the most significant accomplishments of the twentieth century has been the control of communicable diseases. Those born in the United States at the beginning of the century had an average life expectancy of 47.4 years. Tuberculosis accounted for 25% of all deaths at the time. Life expectancy is now more than 75 years, and our population is not only increasing, but is also growing older. Public health measures, such as clean drinking water, control of waste, availability of a variety of foods, and medical advances in immunology have been largely responsible for this remarkable change.

With the exception of pneumonia and human immunodeficiency virus (HIV) infection, diseases of noninfectious origin have replaced infectious diseases as the leading causes of morbidity and mortality in the United States. Atherosclerosis, the process that underlies heart attacks and strokes, and conditions such as cancer, diabetes, emphysema, and arthritis now comprise the majority of the health burden in the United States. In 1990, 65.4% of all deaths were related to cancer, stroke and chronic diseases of the heart, and another 7% were related to accidents, suicide, and homicide (Centers for Disease Control, 1990). These illnesses are lengthy, require continuing monitoring and care, and therefore have contributed to the increase in health care costs that has occurred in the latter part of the century. These transitions represent challenges and opportunities for the profession of nursing as health care increasingly moves from acute care institutions into the community. Table 1-3 illustrates the changes in the leading causes of death between 1900 and 1990.

DIFFERENCES BETWEEN INFECTIOUS AND NONINFECTIOUS PROCESSES

As with infectious diseases, the prevention and control of noninfectious conditions involve understanding the interaction of the agent, host, and environment. Noninfectious diseases include both acute and chronic conditions resulting from pathophysiologic processes that are stimulated by a variety of agents. Chronic diseases are characterized by pathologic changes that are nonreversible, permanent, and result in disabilities. As a result they require rehabilitation of the patient and may require long periods of observation and care. Noninfectious diseases also include disorders of psychosocial and behavioral origin.

In contrast to infectious diseases, there is no single necessary agent to produce noninfectious illness. A wide variety of agents produce noninfectious diseases. Injurious *physical agents* include temperature extremes, changes in atmospheric pressure, radiation, trauma, noise, and prolonged vibration. *Chemical agents* can cause cellular injury, and highly toxic substances are known as poisons. Chronic exposure to air pollutants, insecticides, and herbicides and ingestion of lead from lead-based paint has caused significant morbidity in the United States. Gaseous substances like carbon monoxide can asphyxiate or irritate the respiratory system. Excesses or deficits of *nutrients* can also cause injury. *Genetic factors* can be etiologic agents for a variety of illnesses, as can exposure to psychologic *stress.* Even the physiologic processes of inflammation and the immune response can occasionally cause injury in the body (McCance and Huether, 1990).

Usually the etiology of noninfectious diseases is multifactorial. Several factors may react together additively, or they may react with each other synergistically to produce illness. For instance, smoking and occupational exposure to asbestos act synergistically to produce lung cancer in the host. This combination has been found to increase the risk of lung cancer 90 times that of nonsmoking, unexposed individuals (Selikoff, Hammond, and Chung, 1968). The life-style choices that we all make affect our exposure to noninfectious agents. These choices, such as smoking, lack of physical activity, or excessive alcohol intake, are risk factors that increase our probability for developing health problems of noninfectious origin.

The length of time between initial exposure to the agent(s) and development of illness is usually short for infectious diseases (incubation period) but long for noninfectious diseases (latency period). If a host is susceptible to an infectious disease, the infectious organism will begin to multiply until illness occurs. There is little time for a long-term adaptive response, other than stimulation of the acute inflammatory and immune processes, and recovery usually occurs. In contrast, agents of noninfectious diseases usually require multiple and often low doses of exposure to result in illness (Table 8-1). As this occurs over time, the body will often make adaptive changes. Although these changes may be beneficial at first, as the condition progresses the adaptive responses may be detrimental to the health of the individual. This can produce long-term disability that requires ongoing treatment and supervision.

For example, chronic exposure to low doses of a toxic substance like alcohol can stimulate a mild irritation or inflammation of the liver parenchyma. The extent of the inflammation is related to the amount (dose) of toxin present. The mild inflammation gradually produces fibrosis, and cirrhosis may develop slowly over a period of years. Ultimately, the fibrosis, degeneration, and necrosis result in derangement of the lobular architecture of the liver. It is important to note however, that acute stages of noninfectious disease can also occur. Damage to the body is more severe with increased exposure to the agent, resulting in the onset of acute signs and symptoms. An acute alcoholic hepatitis can result from excessive alcohol intake within a short period of time.

These differences create some methodologic problems in the study of illnesses of noninfectious etiology. The lack of a single agent, additive effects of multiple agents, and the synergism between some agents make the study of any

Table 8-1 Differences between noninfectious and infectious diseases

Noninfectious disease	Infectious disease
Usually multiple agents, nonliving	Single living agent
Multiple low-dose exposures to single or multiple agents often required	Single exposure may be sufficient
Latency period	Incubation period
Chronic illness often occurs	Acute illness often occurs
Immunity rare	Immunity can be acquired

single exposure factor difficult. These problems are compounded by a long latency period and an indefinite onset. As a result, measuring exposure accurately can be a challenge. There are many stages of illness in noninfectious diseases, and setting the criteria for identification of cases may be problematic. Criteria often involve a series of clinical symptoms, and laboratory data may not be helpful. This is particularly true when psychosocial disorders are investigated. Therefore the distinction between diseased and nondiseased people, or defining a precise outcome, may be difficult to establish. It is best to view noninfectious illness as a result of a breakdown of a multiplicity of factors. These factors can include biologic, cultural, economic, psychologic, and social factors. Identification of the multiple related factors that lead to a noninfectious disease are often illustrated in a web of causation (see Fig. 2-7).

CHRONIC ILLNESS

Characteristics

The phrase *chronic illness* encompasses diseases or conditions that produce signs and symptoms within variable periods of time, are long-lasting, and are often associated with some degree of disability. This contrasts with acute illnesses that result soon after exposure to the agent(s), often run a short course, and full recovery or death occurs. However, if acute illnesses do not completely resolve, they may become chronic. There are a large number of individual illnesses that potentially can be included under the category of chronic illness. It has been only in the last 30 years, that chronic illnesses have become a priority area in the health care system. Measuring the morbidity, mortality, and impact of these diseases has not been an area of concern in the past.

Chronic illnesses extend over a period of time and often are manifest in a sequence of stages. The natural history of chronic disease is a continuum that involves stages of susceptibility, presymptomatic disease, clinical disease, and disability. In the *susceptibility stage,* the disease has not developed, but risk factors are present. Primary prevention measures are focused on people with environmental or behavioral risk factors that are amenable to change. In the *preclinical stage,* no manifestation of the disease is present, but pathologic changes have begun. Secondary prevention like the initiation of screening procedures is particularly successful when directed toward people with presymptomatic disease. Early detection of the disease is followed by prompt treatment (see Chapter 9). When the *clinical stage* of disease is present, pathologic changes have occurred to the extent that signs and symptoms are present. Prompt treatment is essential to prevent disability. The *disability stage* has widespread implications for the individual, family members, and the community. Psychosocial roles change, income may be reduced, and community resources strained. Tertiary prevention measures are directed toward the restoration of optimal functioning and the prevention of further complications.

A major source of relevant data regarding chronic illness in the United States is the National Health Interview Survey. Fig. 8-1 shows 1989 figures of self-re-

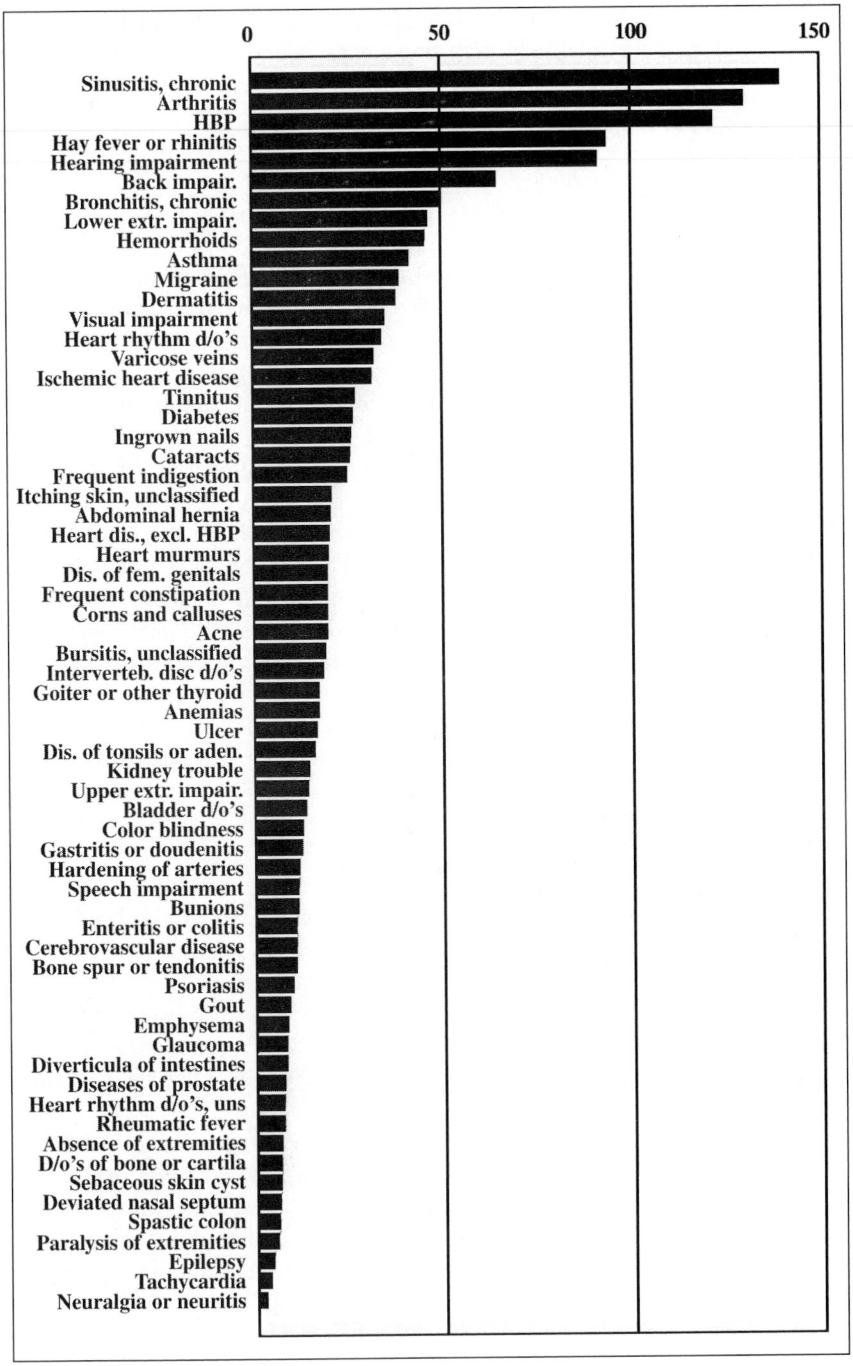

Fig. 8-1 Number of chronic conditions per 1000 persons—United States, 1988. (From US National Health Interview, Department HHS, 1989.)

ported chronic conditions in the U.S. population. A small number of chronic conditions have relatively high prevalence rates in the U.S. population, such as chronic sinusitis, arthritis, hypertension, hay fever, rhinitis, hearing and back impairment, and bronchitis. However, the majority of the conditions listed in the survey have lower rates, pointing to the complex nature of the chronic illness pattern in the population and the resultant difficulty in quantifying these problems.

Most chronic illnesses that affect American populations are nonfatal (Verbrugge, 1989). For example, arthritis is the leading chronic condition for women over age 45, with a rate of 339 per 1000 for women age 45 to 64, 528 per 1000 for women 65 to 74, and 566 per 1000 for women over 75. For men, arthritis is either the number one or number two chronic condition, with rates of 254, 371, and 405 per 1000 in the three respective age groups indicated above. The significance of non–life-threatening conditions should not be underestimated. These are problems that erode an individual's quality of life for a lifetime, and that take up a significant portion of both health care practitioners' time and the health care budget.

Another perspective of the extensive prevalence of chronic illness can be drawn from a report of age-specific percentages of the U.S. population who were limited in the performance of a major activity due to chronic illness in 1985 and in 1990 (Table 8-2). These data are based on household interviews of a sample of the civilian, noninstitutionalized population. In chronic illness the focus of care moves away from keeping the patient alive in an acute sense and toward establishing and maintaining a normal life-style despite adversity. Therefore activity limitation is a major concern. Although some progress has been made between 1985 and 1990, those persons age 45 years and older continue to have a substantial health burden that is manifested through limitations in daily living.

Comorbidity

Comorbidity is the presence of more than one illness or abnormal condition. The chronically ill patient frequently suffers from numerous diseases, each incrementally contributing to the individual's eventual death. As such it may be meaningless to ascribe such a patient's death to a single cause (Rothenberg and Koplan, 1990). This viewpoint suggests the necessity of revamping the concept of mortality rates as an epidemiologic measure when used in the study of chronically ill patients.

A Centers for Disease Control study (1989) based on the National Health Interview Survey looked at comorbidity of nine common chronic conditions: arthritis, hypertension, cataracts, heart disease, varicose veins, diabetes, cancer, osteoporosis/hip fracture, and stroke. The study found that the proportion of the population age 60 and older with two or more of the chronic conditions increased with age and was higher for women than men (Table 8-3). In people age 80 or over, 70% of women and 53% of the men had two or more of the conditions.

Theoretic framework for chronic illness

Strauss and Corbin (1988) constructed the following theoretic framework for examining the phenomenon of chronic illness that serves as an excellent overview

Table 8-2 Age-specific percentages of people limited in activity due to chronic illness—United States, 1985 and 1990

Age	1985	1990
All	13.4	12.9
< 14	4.8	4.7
15-44	8.3	8.5
45-64	23.4	21.8
65 and over	39.6	37.5
65-74	36.7	33.7
75 and over	44.3	43.3

Source: Abstracted from National Center for Health Statistics: *Health, United States, 1991,* DHHS Pub No (PHS) 92-1232; Hyattsville, MD, 1992, Public Health Service.

of the problem. Chronic illnesses are currently the prevalent form of illness in developed countries. They usually occur in later life but can occur at any time. Therefore the patient and provider must think in terms of managing the illness for a lifetime.

The acute phases of chronic illnesses are managed in a hospital or nursing home by health care professionals, but the majority of ongoing care takes place at home. Home health care is usually delivered and monitored by nurses. However, the ultimate responsibility falls on the patient and whoever else is available. The emphasis in chronic illness becomes maintaining a stable quality of life with a high level of functioning in living skills. The chronic illness affects all aspects of the patient's and family's life. Since the effects of chronic illness may be extensive, their needs often exceed the available resources. It was concluded that home care services are woefully inadequate to meet these needs and that it will be necessary to develop reimbursement mechanisms directed toward this central work of the patient and family in the home.

Table 8-3 Percentage of population age 60 or older reporting chronic conditions by sex and age—United States, 1988

	Number of chronic conditions		
Sex/age	0	1	2 or more
Men			
60-69	30%	35%	35%
70-79	22%	31%	47%
80+	19%	28%	53%
Women			
60-69	23%	32%	45%
70-79	14%	25%	61%
80+	10%	20%	70%

From Centers for Disease Control: Current estimates from the National Health Interview Survey, 1988, *Vital Health Stat* 10(173), 1989, p 106-107.

Five phases of chronic illness have been identified through a lengthy study of the topic through multiple patient and family interviews (Corbin and Strauss, 1988). Their methods were qualitative as they sought to understand trajectories and impacts of chronic illness on daily life. The phases they identified were: acute, comeback, stable, unstable, and downward. These phases, acting together or in various sequences, form the shape of the trajectory of an individual's chronic illness.

In an acute phase, the patient's life is interrupted by the disease process. Medical care is usually necessary and the patient will probably be either in a hospital or nursing home. The goal at this time is to get the patient back into his or her everyday world and functioning at least to a minimal level. An example would be hospitalizing a patient with myocardial infarction or stroke.

The comeback phase is the phase of rehabilitation. It is characterized by uphill progress toward but not necessarily fully reaching a normal life for the patient. This involves physical healing, stretching of physical limitations, and reforming the individual's self-perception and daily habits to fit within new physical or mental limitations.

In the stable phase, the patient settles into routines around a chronic illness whose character is not changing. These routines consist both of managing the illness and participating in activities of daily living.

Unstable phases are characterized by disequilibrium in the illness process that requires considerable work in order to maintain the patient's daily living routines. These phases are distinct from acute phases in that normal life goes on and the patient stays out of the hospital or nursing home, but daily life is highly chaotic.

The downward phase of chronic illness involves deterioration and eventual death. The patient cuts back on activities as the disease worsens and must increasingly use wit and willpower to perform even simple tasks. In this phase, it becomes apparent that the organization and habits that chronically ill patients impose on their lives can be only temporary resting places against the downward trend.

Changes in mortality—1900-1990

In examining the emergence of chronic illness as a major concern in health care, three qualitative changes in death have occurred between the beginning of the century and the 1990s (Rothenberg and Koplan, 1990). First, there have been increases in crude death rates from diseases classified as chronic. For example, the cancer mortality rate for the people age 55 to 64 in 1901 was 268.3 per 100,000 people, and by 1986 this rate had climbed to 477.8 per 100,00 people (Fig. 8-2).

A second difference is a decrease in the randomness of death. In the early 1900s, deaths from acute processes, such as septicemia, pneumonia, and tuberculosis, struck people at all age levels with an inevitable randomness that distributed mortality across the age range. With the exception of pneumonia, which remains as a top ten cause of death, public health measures, antibiotics, sterile technique, and other modern medical developments have reduced these factors to low levels in developed nations. As a result, chronic causes of illness and subsequent mortality have increased.

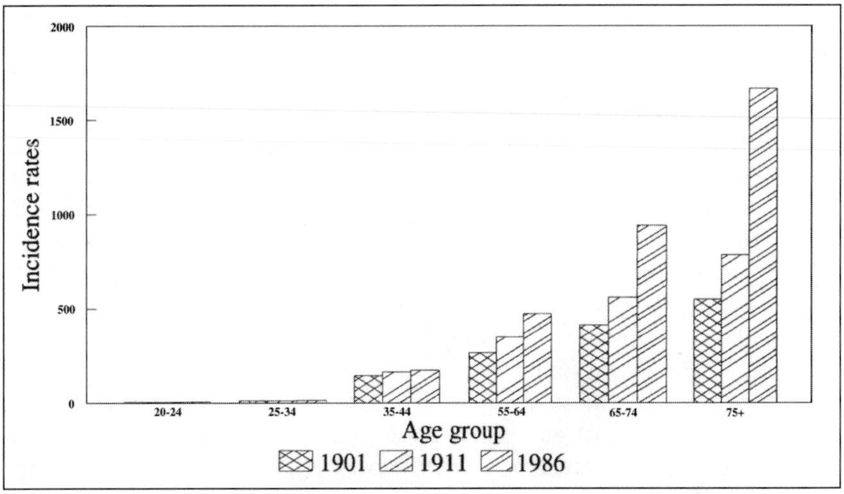

Fig. 8-2 Age-specific cancer rates, 1901, 1911, and 1986. (From Rothenberg RB, Koplan JP: Chronic disease in the 1990s, *Ann Rev Public Health* 11:267-296, 1990.)

A third difference in death rates from chronic illness between the early twentieth century and now is the significant relationship between certain risk factors and multiple diseases. For example, it is now clear that smoking tends to lead to heart disease, lung cancer, and chronic obstructive pulmonary disease. This link would not have been as clear to an epidemiologist studying populations in the early 1900s due to the clouding effects of the random deaths from the more immediate problem of acute disease.

Among life-threatening chronic conditions, a major public health trend in this century has been an epidemic of cardiovascular and cerebrovascular disease. Despite a decline in the mortality rates, these disease processes continue to be the leading causes of death in the United States. Two factors credited for the reduction in these diseases were a decrease in the prevalence of risk factors and improved medical techniques.

A number of the chronic illnesses that are endemic in the U.S. population, such as heart disease and cancer, are associated with the Western life-style (Hutt and Burkitt, 1986). This conclusion was based on the facts that prevalence rates of these illnesses are highest in industrialized countries and that prevalence is similar in black and white populations in the United States. Prevalence rates are lower in Japan, where there is still adherence to traditional, agrarian-style diets, and prevalence is lower among some groups in industrialized countries who are vegetarian and do not smoke. When people from developing countries migrate to the United States, the prevalence of these chronic diseases increases.

Particular risk factors for these diseases are the smoking and diet habits specific to developed and developing nations. Diet-related chronic conditions include Crohn's disease; carcinomas of the colon, rectum, breast, and prostate; chronic cholecystitis; and diabetes mellitus. Smoking-related chronic conditions include carcinomas of the lung and pancreas, chronic bronchitis, and emphysema.

In 1990, approximately 214,800 residents of the United States died due to heart disease, cancer, stroke, accidents, and other leading causes of death (see Table 1-3). Most diseases and many injuries are multifactorial in nature, resulting from a combination of intrinsic (genetic) and external factors. This is particularly true of noninfectious processes. Approximately 50% of the deaths in 1990 have been attributed to tobacco, diet and activity patterns, alcohol, microbial agents, toxic agents, firearms, sexual behavior, motor vehicles, and illicit use of drugs (McGinnis and Foege, 1993). Table 8-4 shows the estimated number of deaths attributed to these factors.

These statistics have significant implications for program priorities. Our ability to achieve the nation's health objectives for the year 2000 is dependent on our ability to identify and modify these contributors to mortality. Health care costs in 1993 are estimated to be $900 billion dollars, an average of $14,000 for each family of four (McGinnis and Foege, 1993). Most of these dollars have been targeted toward treatment of the leading causes of death after they have occurred. The national investment in preventive measures is estimate to be less that 5% of the national allocation to health care.

The top three contributing factors to death, tobacco, diet and activity patterns, and alcohol, are rooted in behavioral choices. Knowledge alone is not sufficient to change behaviors. Supportive social environments and availability of special services are also required. These services are clearly within the scope of nursing practice, particularly that of the primary health care nurse practitioner. Nurse practitioners provide primary health care to clients, emphasizing promotion of health and prevention of disease. Outcome criteria for nurse practitioner practice are that clients demonstrate knowledge of their state of health, including personal-health risk factors and develop skills to negotiate mutually acceptable goals and plans with health care providers (American Nurses Association, 1987).

Table 8-4 Estimates of *actual causes of death*—United States, 1990

Cause	Estimated no. of deaths	Percentage of total deaths
Tobacco	400,000	19
Diet/activity patterns	300,000	14
Alcohol	100,000	5
Microbial agents	90,000	4
Toxic agents	60,000	3
Firearms	35,000	2
Sexual behavior	30,000	1
Motor vehicles	25,000	1
Illicit use of drugs	20,000	<1
TOTAL	1,060,000	50

From McGinnis, JM, Foege WH: Actual causes of death in the United States, *JAMA* 270(18): 2207-2212, 1993.

Access to these services cannot be achieved without the nation changing its program emphases and appropriately allocating its social resources.

Behavioral risk factor surveillance

In the 1960s and 1970s the role of personal behaviors, such as cigarette smoking, excessive alcohol intake, and physical inactivity, became recognized as risk factors for the leading causes of morbidity and mortality in the United States. In addition, preventive practices, such as cholesterol screening and mammography, have been found to be effective in identifying preclinical abnormalities and instituting early treatment, thereby reducing the burden of disease.

In 1984, the *Behavioral Risk Factor Surveillance System* (BRFSS) was established to collect, analyze, and interpret state-specific behavioral risk factor data that could be used to plan, implement, and monitor health promotion and disease prevention programs (Siegel and others, 1991). The BRFSS program is a collaborative effort between the Centers for Disease Control and Prevention and state health departments. State-specific information is gathered about health behaviors, including obesity, lack of physical activity, smoking, and safety-belt use. Data about the use of preventive health services are also gathered. This includes screening for breast and cervical cancer and elevated blood cholesterol. These BRFSS data were used in the formulation of the national objectives for the year 2000 and are continuing to be used to measure the achievement of these objectives.

A summary of the *Healthy People 2000* objectives, the percent of increase or decrease that is targeted for the year 2000, and the median percent found in the BRFSS data in 1991 are summarized in Table 8-5. The data demonstrate that substantial state-to-state variations exist. Since the BRFSS data are presented as median percents, it appears that some states will be able to attain these objectives, while others may not. Clearly, a substantial effort should be made in the next few years to modify and decrease those behavioral risk factors that predispose people to noninfectious disease (CDC, 1991).

Control and prevention issues

In attempting to control the impact of chronic illness on the population, prevention is the strategy most likely to produce the greatest benefits. However, prevention largely means changing behavior on the personal level—quitting smoking, losing weight, and exercising regularly (Rothenberg and Koplan, 1990). It also means implementing primary prevention strategies and secondary prevention screening activities, and practicing clinical, preventive medicine.

A likely area of epidemiologic concern in the future will be patient willingness to accept the treatment and life-style regimens that are established to maximize an individual's state of health. A chronically ill person who does not take care of himself or herself will not reach the maximum level of health and personal function possible and will strain the health care system. Noncompliance is widespread. For example, noncompliance with dietary restrictions for diabetes ranged in various studies between 35% and 73%, and noncompliance rates for urine-testing ranged from 43% to 70% (Becker and Janz, 1985). The increasing body of

Table 8-5 Selected year 2000 health objectives for the nation and median Behavioral Risk Factor Surveillance System level of attainment—1991

Healthy People 2000 **objective**	**Year 2000 target percent**	**BRFSS, 199 median percent**
Obesity		
Ages ≥18	≤20%	23.4%
No leisure-time physical activity		
Ages ≥18	≤15%	28.0%
Ages ≥65	≤22%	42.3%
Cigarette smoking		
Ages ≥18	≤15%	23.0%
Reproductive-aged women (18-44)	≤12%	24.6%
Safety-belt use		
Ages ≥18	≥85%	58.2%
Cholesterol screening within preceding 5 years		
Ages ≥18	≥75%	63.7%
Clinical breast examination and mammogram within 2 years		
Women ages ≥50	≥60%	57.8%
Pap smear within 2 years (women with intact uterine cervix)		
Ages ≥18	≥85%	79.7%

From Centers for Disease Control and Prevention: *CDC Surveillance Summaries* 42*(SS-4)*:18-20, 1993.

knowledge regarding the relationships between personality factors, cultural influences, and health beliefs on health behaviors, like compliance with dietary limitations is essential in addressing these chronic disease issues.

As acute illness is increasingly conquered, chronic illness is likely to become the primary focus of health care in the twenty-first century. As the trend continues, it will be increasingly necessary to focus attention on people's functional status and daily lives to minimize the effect of chronic illnesses. This will have a significant effect on the practice of nursing. It is anticipated that nursing care in the future will focus on meeting the health care needs of the community-dwelling elderly. Understanding the epidemiology of common noninfectious chronic disorders is essential. This body of knowledge provides the basis for assessing individuals and populations at high risk, diagnosing actual or potential health problems, and formulating plans to meet individual and community needs.

PSYCHOSOCIAL FACTORS AND NONINFECTIOUS DISORDERS

Mental health

Those researchers attempting epidemiologic investigations of factors affecting mental health have always faced the problem of identifying disorders that the sufferers either do not know about or do not want to admit to. Prior to the 1950s, study of the distribution and determinants of psychiatric disorders was confined to research on patients who entered psychiatric hospitals. However, the validity of these studies began to be questioned when it was noted that people who lived closer to such hospitals were more likely to enter them. It became necessary to collect psychiatric data across larger geographic areas. Still, efforts to measure the correlates of psychiatric morbidity were hampered by the fact that those presenting for treatment were obviously a subset of the general affected population. The innovation of the diagnostic interview has allowed researchers to measure psychiatric morbidity in untreated populations. Such interviews, administered to a random population sample by "laymen," have been found to give fairly accurate and consistent results (Robins and others, 1984).

The *lifetime prevalence* of any psychiatric disorder, defined as the proportion of persons who have ever experienced such disorders up to the date of assessment, has been estimated to be between 28.8% and 38% (Compton and others, 1991; Robins and others, 1984). Robins and others (1984) examined data from the National Institute of Mental Health's Epidemiologic Catchment Area (ECA) program that was collected during the early 1980s in New Haven, Baltimore, and St. Louis. The ECA program used the Diagnostic Interview Schedule, a tool based on American Psychiatric Association's DSM-IIIR criteria for classification of psychiatric disorders. Respondents were asked if they had ever experienced symptoms corresponding to the 15 covered diagnoses at any time in their life. A positive answer to any of those questions triggered another set of probing questions designed to determine whether the complete criteria for a positive diagnosis were met at any point in the respondent's past. A summary of results from this study is found in Table 8-6. There is a remarkable similarity between the rates of psychosocial disorders among the population of these three cities. These statistics indicate that alcohol abuse and substance use are clearly major problems among our urban populations and substantiate the need for public health control and prevention measures.

Table 8-6 Lifetime prevalence rates of psychosocial disorders per 100 people, National Institutes of Mental Health, Epidemiologic Catchment Area

	New Haven	Baltimore	St. Louis
Any disorder	28.8	38.0	31.0
Affective disorders	9.5	6.1	8.0
Major depression	6.7	3.7	5.5
Manic episodes	1.1	0.6	1.1
Dysthymia (despondency)	3.2	2.1	3.8
Substance use	15.0	17.0	18.1
Alcohol abuse	11.5	13.7	15.7
Phobias	7.8	23.3	9.4
Antisocial personality disorder	2.1	2.6	3.3
Schizophrenia	1.9	1.6	1.0

Adapted from Robins, LN and others: Lifetime prevalence of specific psychiatric disorders in three sites. *Arch Gen Psychiatry* 41:949-58, 1984.

Table 8-7 Admissions to selected inpatient psychiatric facilities by selected primary diagnoses—United States, 1986

Primary diagnoses	State and county mental hospitals	Private psychiatric hospitals	Nonfederal general hospitals
Alcohol-related disorders	22.5	6.6	41.4
Drug-related disorders	8.7	6.1	20.2
Organic disorders	4.3	2.0	9.8
Affective disorders	22.8	41.9	121.9
Schizophrenia	49.7	9.9	63.3
All diagnoses	136.1	86.1	331.7

Adapted from National Center for Health Statistics: *Health, United States, 1991,* DHHS Pub. No. (PHS) 92-1232, Hyattsville, MD, 1992, Public Health Service.

However, another aspect of mental health can be determined by examination of rates of admission to inpatient psychiatric facilities by primary diagnosis (Table 8-7). The majority of patients with mental health problems are treated in general hospitals (331.7 admissions per 100,000 people). Further breakdown of these statistics showed that admissions were the highest in the 25 to 44 age group for all diagnoses and all facilities. The only exception was for organic disorders where admissions were more common in those 65 years and older (National Center for Health Statistics, 1992). Strategies for prevention are best directed toward this age group.

Suicide rates in the United States have been considerably higher for men than for women since 1900 with temporary increases occurring around the year 1910

HEALTHY PEOPLE 2000 OBJECTIVES FOR MENTAL HEALTH AND MENTAL DISORDERS

Reduce suicides to no more than 10.5 per 100,000 people

Reduce by 15% the incidence of injurious suicide attempts among adolescents age 14 to 17

Reduce to less than 10% the prevalence of mental disorders among children and adolescents

Reduce to less than 10.7% the prevalence of mental disorders among adults living in the community

Reduce to less than 35% the proportion of people age 18 and older who experienced adverse health effects from stress within the past year

Increase to at least 30% the proportion of people age 18 and older with severe, persistent mental disorders who use community support programs

Increase to at least 45% the proportion of people with major depressive disorders who obtain treatment

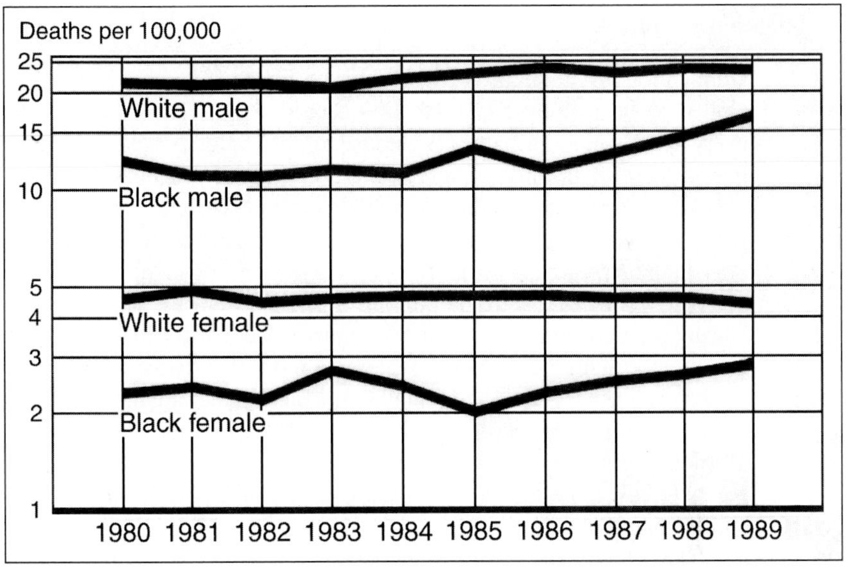

Fig. 8-3 Death rates for suicide among persons 15 to 24 years of age, according to race and sex—United States, 1980-1989. (From National Center for Health Statistics: *Health, United States,* 1991, DHHS Pub No [PHS] 92-1232, Hyattsville, MD, 1992, Public Health Service.)

and in the early 1930s. The latter was presumably due to the economy during the Great Depression (Monk, 1987). In 1990, the age-adjusted suicide rate for both sexes was 12.4 per 100,000 people. However, the rate for males was 19 per 100,000 people but only 4.5 per 100,000 for females (US Bureau of the Census, 1993). Suicide rates have been increasing in the 15 to 24 age group (Fig. 8-3). The rate in 1990 was 13.6 per 100,000 people, more than 8% higher than in 1980. This observation prompted creation of a national objective of 8.2 suicides per 100,000 youths for the year 2000. Higher suicide rates have been found for unmarried people and residents of western states, while lower rates were recorded for married people and residents of eastern states. A summary of the national mental health and mental disorders prevention objectives for the year 2000 are found in the box on p. 148.

All nurses are concerned with mental health promotion and maintenance. Patients with emotional problems are found in any health care setting. Psychiatric-mental health nurses work with individuals, families, groups, and communities to assess mental health needs and dysfunction, assist clients to regain or improve their coping abilities, and prevent further disability (American Nurses Association, 1994). Epidemiologic data regarding lifetime prevalence of psychosocial disorders, knowledge of trends in psychosocial problems, and an understanding of risk factors that predispose people to mental health problems assists nurses in their practices. These data enhance nurses abilities to assess and evaluate clients, target at-risk situations, initiate interventions, and prevent potential complications.

Unintentional injuries

Unintentional injuries or accidents are the fourth leading causes of death in the United States, killing about 100,000 people a year (NCHS, 1992). One out of every 10 hospital discharges is due to nonfatal injuries, and these injuries are a major cause of disability. Approximately one half of the deaths from unintentional injuries result from motor-vehicle crashes. Deaths from falls rank second, followed by deaths from poisoning, drowning, and residential fires (Committee on Trauma Research, 1988).

The young and older adults are at highest risk for unintentional injuries. During the first four decades of life, injuries account for more deaths than either infectious or chronic diseases. Males are more than twice as likely to die from motor-vehicle accidents than females, and black males are more likely to die from crashes than white males (Fig. 8-4). Alcohol use is a factor in about one half of all motor-vehicle fatalities and many drownings. These injuries have been estimated to cost more than $100 billion dollars annually (US Department of Health and Human Services [USDHHS], 1991).

The primary Healthy People 2000 objectives for unintentional injuries are to reduce these deaths to no more than 29.3 per 100,000 people, a 15% decrease, and increase automobile safety-restraint use to at least 85% of occupants, a 102% increase. Prevention of accidents will require changes in behavior, particularly on the part of parents and children. Nurses and other health providers need to identify behavioral and environmental risk factors and incorporate safety education and accident prevention into all health maintenance programs. Prevention will be

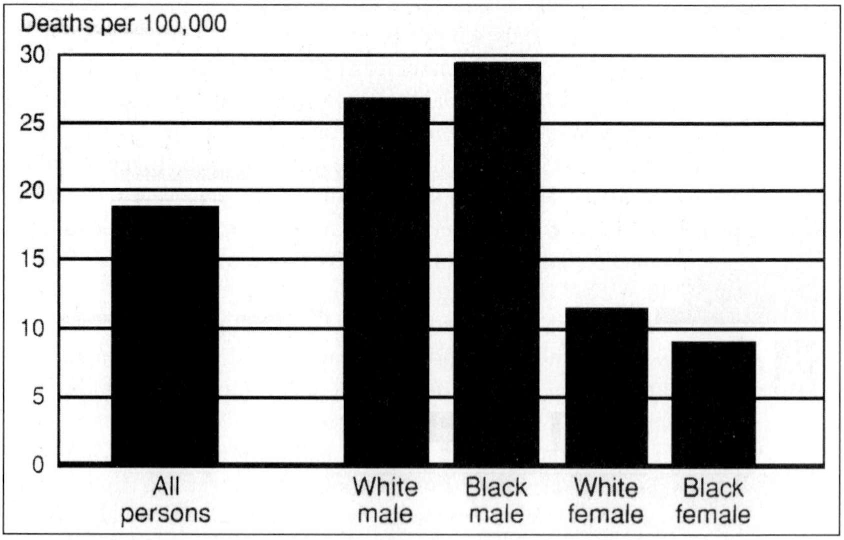

Fig. 8-4 Death rates for motor vehicle crashes, according to race and sex—United States, 1989. (From National Center for Health Statistics: *Health, United States, 1991,* DHHS Pub No [PHS] 92-1232, Hyattsville, MD, 1992, Public Health Service.)

achieved primarily through health education of the public.

Violence and abusive behavior

According to Freud, humans have an innate, independent, and instinctual tendency toward aggression. Although other scholars have challenged this belief, violence and abusive behavior (intentional injury) seem to be permanent parts of society. Child and spouse abuse and other types of family violence threaten the health of thousands of American families each year and have been increasingly recognized as an important public health problem (USDHHS, 1991).

Fig. 8-5 and 8-6 illustrate the extent of deaths from homicide and legal intervention. Males and blacks are at a higher risk than females and whites. As with motor-vehicle fatalities, about one half of all homicides are associated with alcohol use. More than half of all homicide victims are relatives or acquaintances of the perpetrators of the crimes (NCHS, 1992). Prevention objectives for violent and abusive behavior in the year 2000 are summarized in the box on p. 152.

An interesting contrast between intentional and unintentional injuries has been presented by the Centers for Disease Control in a study of deaths resulting from firearm and motor-vehicle–related injuries in the United States between 1968 and 1991. More than half (55%) of all injury-related deaths are caused by firearms and motor vehicles. The number of deaths from motor vehicles has consistently exceeded those from firearms. However, the deaths from motor vehicles have declined by 21%, while firearm-related deaths have increased by 60%. Based on these trends, by the year 2003 the number of firearm-related deaths will surpass the number of motor-vehicle deaths (CDC, 1994). Firearms will become

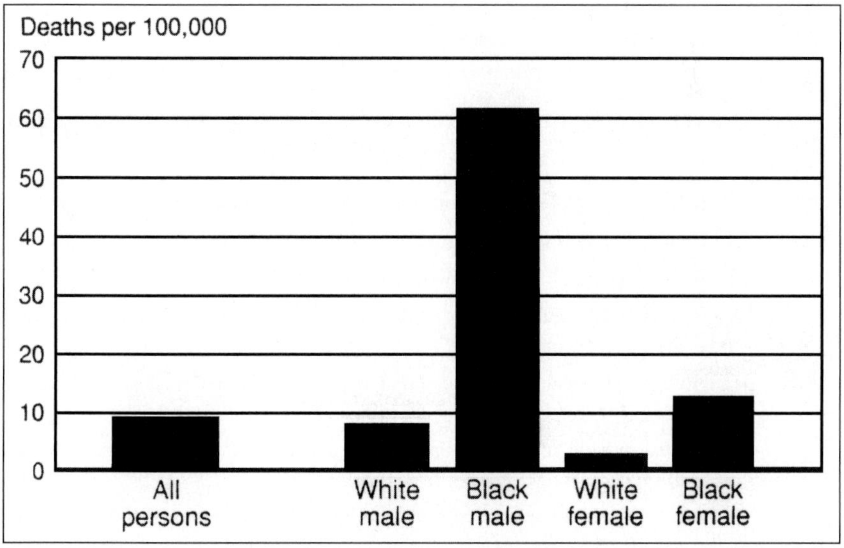

Fig. 8-5 Death rates for homicide and legal intervention, according to race and sex—United States, 1989. (From National Center for Health Statistics: *Health, United States, 1991,* DHHS Pub No [PHS] 92-1232, Hyattsville, MD, 1992, Public Health Service.)

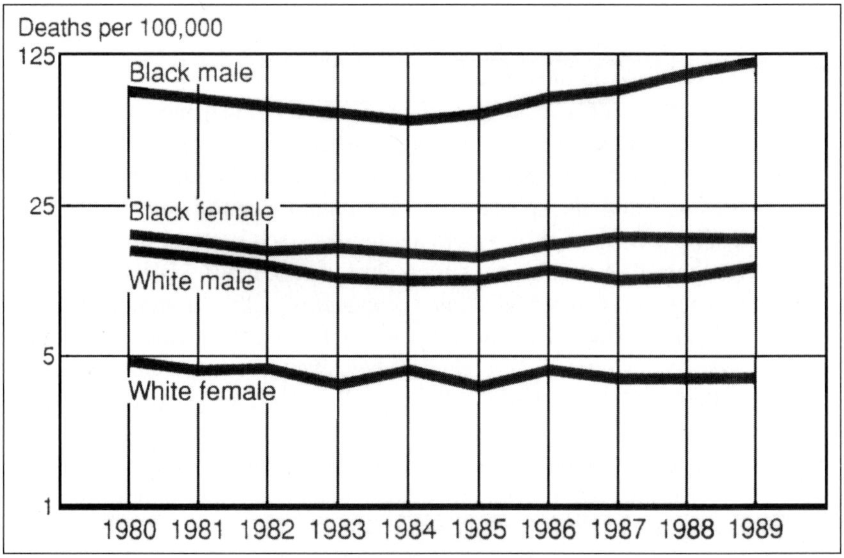

Fig. 8-6 Death rates for homicide and legal intervention among persons 15 to 24 years of age, according to race and sex—United States, 1980-1989. (From National Center for Health Statistics: *Health, United States, 1991,* DHHS Pub No [PHS] 92-1232, Hyattsville, MD, 1992, Public Health Service.)

HEALTHY PEOPLE 2000 VIOLENT AND ABUSIVE BEHAVIOR PREVENTION OBJECTIVES

Reduce homicides to no more than 7.2 per 100,000 people

Reduce suicides to no more than 10.5 per 100,000 people

Reduce weapon-related, violent deaths to no more than 12.6 per 100,000 people

Reduce to less than 25.2 per 1000 children the incidence of maltreatment of children age 18 and younger

Reduce physical abuse directed at women by male partners to no more than 27 per 1000 couples

Reduce assault injuries among people age 12 and older to no more than 10 per 1000 people

Reduce rape and attempted rape of women age 12 and older to no more than 108 per 100,000 women

Reduce by 15% the incidence of injurious suicide attempts among adolescents age 14 to 17

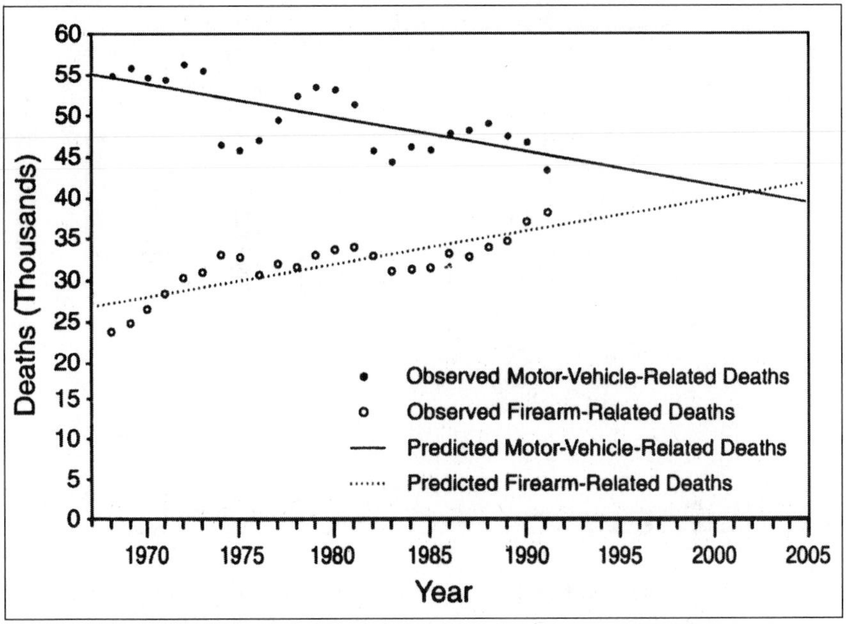

Fig. 8-7 Observed and predicted firearm- and motor-vehicle–related injury deaths, by year–United States, 1968-2005.

the leading cause of deaths from injuries (Fig. 8-7).

It is suggested that this trend may reflect differences in the approaches to preventing these injuries. Comprehensive and science-based interventions and policies have been developed for the prevention of motor-vehicle injuries. These have included public information programs, promotion of behavioral change, changes in legislation, rules, and regulations, and advances in engineering and technology. The combination of these approaches has resulted in safer vehicles and driving practices along with safer environments and improved medical services. In contrast, there have been limited efforts to develop a systematic framework for reducing the incidence and impact of firearm injuries. A multifaceted approach is proposed to reduce firearm injuries. This includes fostering changes in behavior by campaigns to educate and inform people about the risks and benefits of firearm possession and the safe use and storage of firearms. Legislative efforts can prevent access to or acquisition of firearms and regulate their storage, transport, and use. Engineering and technologic changes could modify firearms and ammunition to make them more safe to use. Because highway safety has been a national priority since 1966, it is estimated that 250,000 deaths have been prevented. A similar approach for firearms has the potential to reduce the public health impact and societal burden from the injuries they produce (CDC, 1994).

WORLD POPULATION TRENDS

Demographers expect world population to increase through most of the twenty-first century, making it increasingly difficult to maintain public health worldwide

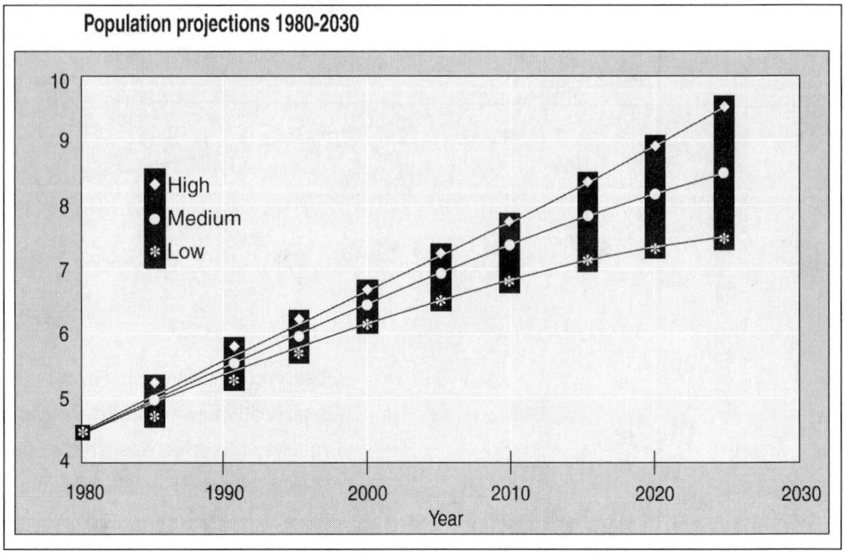

Fig. 8-8 Population projections 1980-2030. (From United Nations Population Fund: *The state of world population, 1991,* New York, 1991, United Nations.)

(Fig. 8-8) (Ehrlich and Ehrlich, 1990). In 1991 the United Nations Population Fund estimated that world population would increase through most of the twenty-first century, leveling off toward the year 2100 at about 11.6 billion, more than twice its current level. Of this growth, 95% will be in developing countries, especially Africa and southern Asia (United Nations Population Fund, 1991).

Industrial areas, such as North America, east Asia, and Europe, tend to have relatively low population-growth rates. For example, Japan and western Europe all have fertility rates of less than two births per woman. These countries' birth rates would maintain their populations at stable levels if there was no immigration. However, many industrial countries experiencing significant immigration rates have increasing populations, which give way to population-related health problems. According to the political organization Zero Population Growth, every year the United States population increases by 3 million people or half the population of the state of Massachusetts.

These industrial nations with low fertility rates have passed through what population biologists call the *demographic transition.* In the early stages of a nation's industrial development, both birth and death rates are high, and population is generally kept at a certain level by negative factors, such as disease, starvation, and war. As countries become exposed to modern medicine and food production techniques, death rates begin to fall and population increases. After a lag time, birth rates also begin to fall and population stabilizes.

In industrial countries like the United States, these demographic changes have led to an increasing proportion of populations consisting of the elderly (Fig. 8-9).

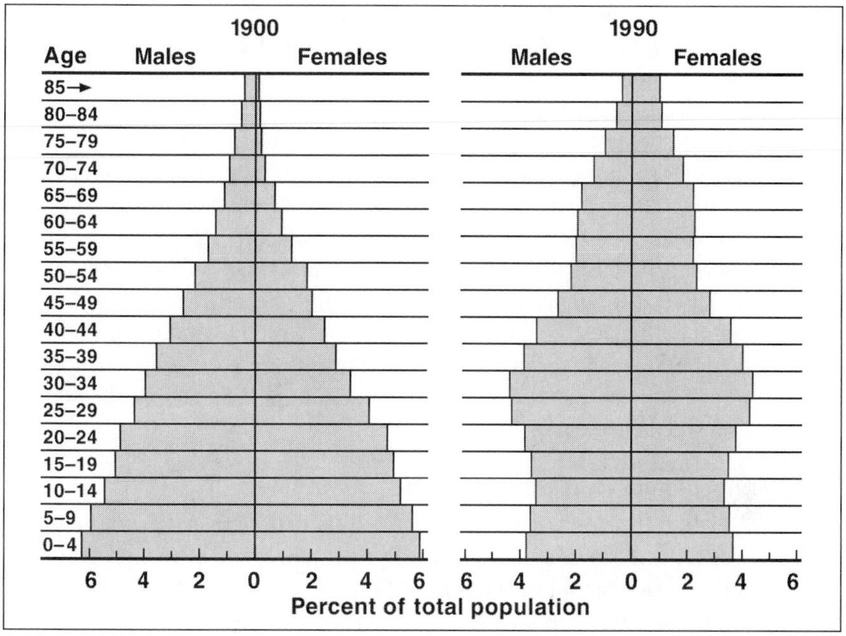

Fig. 8-9 U.S. population pyramids, 1900 and 1990. (Data adapted from US Bureau of the Census: *Historical statistics, colonial times to 1978,* series A 23-25, and current population reports, series P-25-1092.)

Demographers expect people age 65 and older to reach 16% of the population of these countries by the year 2000 (United Nations Population Fund, 1991).

The increasing number of elderly in the United States and the growing proportion of the US population they represent are due to an increase of 12 years in life expectancy since 1940. Lower overall birth rates in the past several decades and the fact that young adults are waiting longer before having children have also contributed to this change. (Califano, 1986). This trend will continue as the "Baby Boom" of the post-World War II years ages to create a "Senior Boom" in the early twenty-first century. In 1940, 7% of the population was 65 years old or more. By 2030, that figure is expected to reach more than 21%.

The increasing number of the elderly in the United States is expected to have a marked impact on the health care delivery system well into the twenty-first century. Specific areas of impact are expected to be an increased demand for nursing home beds and an increased need for community nursing services with an emphasis on maintaining self-sufficiency in chronically ill patients. Also, increased demand combined with a decreasing percentage of adult population producing income in the work force are expected to lead to more rationing of limited health care resources.

The decreased mortality from acute diseases has left most Americans spending their later years suffering from chronic illness. Nursing homes have been the fastest growing sector of the health care industry since 1965, yet nursing home beds have failed to keep up with demand. Between 1975 and 1984, the 85-and-older population grew at an average annual rate of 4%, while nursing home beds were increasing only at about 3% a year (Califano, 1986).

As the nation's health care system faces increasingly high numbers of chronically ill patients in coming years, it will be important for health care professionals to focus on keeping disability rates low (Manton, 1987). Traditionally, efforts have been focused on reducing mortality rates, but a focus on keeping patients active and functional would decrease health care use and spending and increase quality of life. Increased functioning of the chronically ill would also mean they could help care for each other in a future with a dwindling ratio of providers to demand. The health care delivery strategy of the health maintenance organization, in which incentives are built into the system to keep patients healthy, is expected to benefit the elderly.

Effect of population on malnutrition and starvation

As of 1992, there were at least one billion malnourished or starving people in the world or nearly one out of every five people. Some of that problem is caused by uneven distribution of food. Studies have shown that the world's croplands cannot produce enough food to feed everyone indefinitely. A Brown University study has shown that if everyone in the world ate a vegetarian diet, the world could feed six billion people, a level expected by the year 1998. If some agricultural products were fed to livestock (an indirect and inefficient way to feed humans) and everyone consumed 15% of their calories from animal products, there would be enough food for about four billion people. If everyone ate a typical American diet, consuming 35% of their calories as animal products, there would be enough food for about 2.5 billion people or one-half the 1990 population. Thus population levels affect world health by straining food resources and causing starvation, malnutrition, and related morbidity and mortality.

High birth rates and women's health

The World Health Organization estimates that 500,000 women die each year in connection with pregnancy and childbirth. Most of these deaths are in developing countries with high birth rates and where contraception is not readily available. The United Nations reports that if women in developing countries had contraception available to them when they wanted it, between 25% and 40% of these maternal deaths would be eliminated.

Stress-related morbidity associated with crowding

A number of empirical studies in the past few decades have supported the hypothesis that crowding and high population levels create stress and associated psychologic and social pathology. Overcrowding, as measured by high densities in living situations, high social demands, and a lack of privacy, has been associated with poor mental health, poor relationships within the home and poor child care.

A study conducted in the Netherlands in the early 1970s found that population density was positively correlated with overall mortality rates, medical and psychiatric hospital admissions, criminal behavior, and divorce (Levy and Herzog, 1974). A strong positive correlation was found between population density and heart disease deaths in males. However, a significant negative correlation was discovered between population density and female heart disease deaths. Criminal behaviors with the strongest correlations to population density were property and sexual crimes. Despite a seemingly obvious connection between crowding and violence, formal research on the topic has been inconclusive (Anderson, 1982).

Disease transmission effects associated with crowding

Numerous studies have documented a connection between crowded living conditions and increased morbidity and mortality in both developing and industrial nations. For example, Rahman and others (1985) showed that children born in two villages in Bangladesh during 1976 and 1977 were significantly more likely to die within 1 year if they lived in households with more than 10 residents. Crowded conditions have contributed to recent outbreaks of cholera and the plague in developing nations.

Environmental health problems exacerbated by population levels

A growing body of thought in the environmental movement has linked population levels with the world's increasing environmental problems. The argument is that every additional human in the world, especially one living in an industrial nation, increases the strain modern life-style puts on the environment. In these environmentalists' eyes, population is a major cause of such environment-linked illnesses as lung cancer and leukemia.

SUMMARY

The control of communicable diseases through public health measures and medical advances has increased life expectancy in the United States from 47.4 years in 1900 to more than 75 years today. As a result, chronic conditions of noninfectious origin have replaced infectious diseases as the leading causes of morbidity and mortality. Most chronic conditions are nonfatal, affect an individual's quality of life and ability to function independently, and require long-term care and monitoring. This is one reason why health care costs have risen in the latter part of the century. The care and monitoring of people with chronic conditions presents a challenge and an opportunity for the nursing profession.

Chronic conditions with the highest prevalence rates in the U.S. population include chronic sinusitis, arthritis, hypertension, hay fever and rhinitis, hearing impairment, back impairment, and bronchitis. Most chronically ill people are affected by more than one disorder, each incrementally contributing to an individual's eventual death. Injuries, violence, and mental health disorders also comprise a large share of the health care burden in the United States.

World population projections indicate an increase through most of the twenty-first century, leveling off toward the year 2100 at about 11.6 billion people or more than twice the current population of the world. Most of this growth will be in developing countries, especially Africa and southern Asia. Industrial nations have passed through a demographic transition, where death rates have fallen, birth rates have fallen after a lag period, and the population has grown older. Demographers expect that by the year 2000, 16% of the population of industrial nations will be age 65 and older.

These trends will impact the health of individuals, health care practitioners, and the health care delivery system. There is concern that the world's croplands cannot produce enough food to feed everyone indefinitely. Malnutrition and starvation will continue. Women are and will continue to die each year in connection with pregnancy and childbirth. Crowding contributes to stress-related, psychologic illnesses, social pathology, and transmission of disease.

Critical Thinking Questions

1. Identify at least five differences between infectious and noninfectious diseases.
2. Contrast the prevalence of chronic with infectious diseases in the United States.
3. Discuss the impact on nursing practice, given the difference in prevalence rates of chronic and infectious diseases.
4. Identify as least two methodologic problems investigating the incidence and prevalence of psychosocial disorders.

REFERENCES

American Nurses Association: *A statement of psychiatric-mental health clinical nursing practice and standards of psychiatric-mental health clinical nursing practice,* Washington, DC, 1994, The Association.

American Nurses Association: *Standards of practice for the primary health care nurse practitioner,* Kansas City, MO, 1987, The Association.

Anderson C: Environmental factors and aggressive behavior, *J Clin Psychiatry* 43:7, 1982.

Becker M, Janz NK: The health belief model applied to understanding diabetes regimen compliance, *Diabetes Educator* 11:41-47, 1985.

Califano JA, Jr: *America's health care revolution. Who lives? Who dies? Who pays?* New York, 1986, Random House.

Centers for Disease Control: Mortality patterns—United States, 1987, *MMWR* 39(12), 1990.

Centers for Disease Control and Prevention: *CDC surveillance summaries* 42(*SS-4*):18-20, 1993.

Centers for Disease Control: Comorbidity of chronic conditions and disability among older persons—United States, 1984, *MMWR* 38(46):788-791, 1989.

Centers for Disease Control: Current estimates from the National Health Interview Survey, 1988, *Vital Health Stat* 10(173), 1989.

Centers for Disease Control and Prevention: Deaths resulting from firearm- and motor-vehicle–related injuries, United States, 1968-1991, *MMWR* 43(3):37-42, 1994.

Committee on Trauma Research, Commission on Life Sciences, National Research Council and Institute of Medicine: *Injury in America: a continuing public health problem,* Washington, DC, 1988, National Academy Press.

Compton WM and others: New methods in cross-cultural psychiatry: psychiatric illness in Taiwan and the United States, *Am J Psych* 148:12:1697-1704, 1991.

Corbin JM, Strauss A: *Unending work and care; managing chronic illness at home,* San Francisco, 1988, Jossey-Bass.

Ehrlich P, Ehrlich A: *The population explosion,* New York, 1990, Simon & Schuster.
Hutt MSR, Burkitt DP: *The geography of non-infectious disease,* Oxford, 1986, Oxford University Press.
Levy L, Herzog AN: Effects of population density and crowding on health and social adaptation in the Netherlands, *J Health Soc Behav* 15(3):228-240, 1974.
Manton KG: The interaction of population aging and health transitions at later ages: new evidence and insights. In Schramm, CJ, editor: *Health care and its costs,* New York, 1987, WW Norton.
McCance KL, Huether SE: *Pathophysiology—the biologic basis for disease in adults and children,* St Louis, 1990, Mosby, pp 55-66.
McGinnis JM, Foege WH: Actual causes of death in the United States, *JAMA* 270(18):2207-2212, 1993.
Monk, M: Epidemiology of suicide, *Epidemiol Rev* 9:51-69.
National Center for Health Statistics: Health, United States, 1991, DHHS Pub No. (PHS) 92-1232, Hyattsville, MD, 1992, Public Health Service.
Rahman M and others: Impact of environmental sanitation and crowding on infant mortality in rural Bangladesh, *Lancet* 28-30 July 6, 1985.
Robins LN and others: Lifetime prevalence of specific psychiatric disorders in three sites, *Arch Gen Psych* 41:949-958, 1984.
Rothenberg RB, Koplan JP: Chronic disease in the 1990s, *Annu Rev Public Health* 11:267-296, 1990.
Ryan PM: Epidemiology, etiology, diagnosis and treatment of schizophrenia, *Am J Hosp Pharm* 48:1271-1280, 1991.
Selikoff, NJ, Hammond, EC and others: Asbestos exposure, smoking and neoplasia, *JAMA* 204:106, 1968.
Siegel, PZ and others: Behavioral Risk Factor Surveillance, 1986-1990, *MMWR* 40(SS-4):1-24, 1991.
Strauss A, Corbin JM: *Shaping a new health care system: the explosion of chronic illness as a catalyst for change,* San Francisco, 1988, Jossey-Bass.
United Nations Population Fund: *The state of world population, 1991,* New York, 1991, United Nations.
US Bureau of the Census: *Statistical abstract of the United States: 1993,* ed 113, Washington, DC, 1993, US Government Printing Office.
US Department of Health and Human Services, Public Health Service: *Healthy People 2000,* Washington, DC, 1991, US Government Printing Office.
Verbrugge LM: Recent, present and future health of American adults, *Annu Rev Pub Health* 10:333-361, 1989.

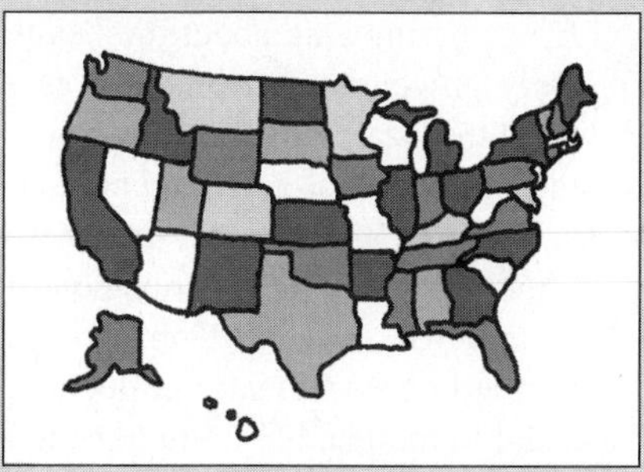

9

Surveillance and Screening

Objectives

1. Define surveillance.
2. Compare and contrast the four types of surveillance.
3. Diagram the surveillance process.
4. Define screening.
5. Describe how nurses use both surveillance and screening in their practice.
6. Compute the sensitivity, specificity, and predictive value of a screening test.
7. Discuss the effect of prevalence on the sensitivity, specificity, and predictive value of a screening test.
8. Discuss the criteria that should be used for evaluating a screening program.
9. Identify the types of epidemiologic studies that can be used to evaluate screening programs.

Key Terms

active surveillance
case-finding
mass screening
multiphasic screening
obligatory reportable epidemic
passive surveillance
predictive value
regularly reportable disease
reportable disease
screening
selective screening
selectively reportable disease
sensitivity
sentinel surveillance
special surveillance
specificity
surveillance
universally mandatory reportable disease

SURVEILLANCE

Surveillance is a continual, dynamic method for gathering data about the health of the general public for the purpose of primary prevention of illness. It is a process of monitoring emerging and endemic health hazards in the community setting. It entails (1) ongoing scrutiny of the states of health of a defined population through a recording and reporting process, (2) collating and analyzing these data, and (3) summarizing and publishing the findings, including a provision of feedback to the reporting sources. The Centers for Disease Control and Prevention (CDC) define surveillance as the "ongoing, systematic collection, analysis, and interpretation of health data essential to the planning, implementation, and evaluation of public health practice." (CDC, 1988).

Through the surveillance process, changes in the trend or distribution of various states of health in the population can be detected (Last, 1988; Thacker, 1983). Identifying these changes in trends provides increased awareness of health and disease patterns. Once unusual situations or problems are found, further investigation can be initiated. However, surveillance has little worth if action is not taken to control or prevent health problems. Timely feedback of these data to those persons who have need for information for planning control and prevention activities is essential. Surveillance data also can be used to evaluate previous actions that already have been taken to control or prevent health problems. Fig. 9-1 provides a model of an official surveillance system flow chart.

Nurses' roles in surveillance

Public health, community health, and primary care nurse practitioners use the process of surveillance in two ways. First, nurses *use* surveillance data in identifying the need for provider outreach services. Provider outreach services are primary prevention community interventions that are delivered in the client's environment, such as in the home, school, place of employment, or neighborhood center. Examples are well-baby, family-planning, and immunization clinics. Community-screening activities focused on identification of specific health problems are also considered provider outreach services. Screening activities are considered secondary prevention measures.

Second, nurses *engage* in surveillance activities as they monitor the health of individuals in their caseloads. Identifying individuals with health problems within families and community groups and planning early interventions to control or prevent illness, requires consistent monitoring. The burden of illness in the community can be reduced effectively and efficiently through these activities.

Characteristics of a successful surveillance system

There are several characteristics of successful surveillance systems. First, they involve health problems that are perceived to be important public health concerns. Second, some type of official reporting or unofficial recording of information is involved. However, reporting the existence of a disease or condition is only one step in the surveillance process. Third, successful surveillance requires frequent, sustained interaction with reporting sources, including feedback and follow-up of

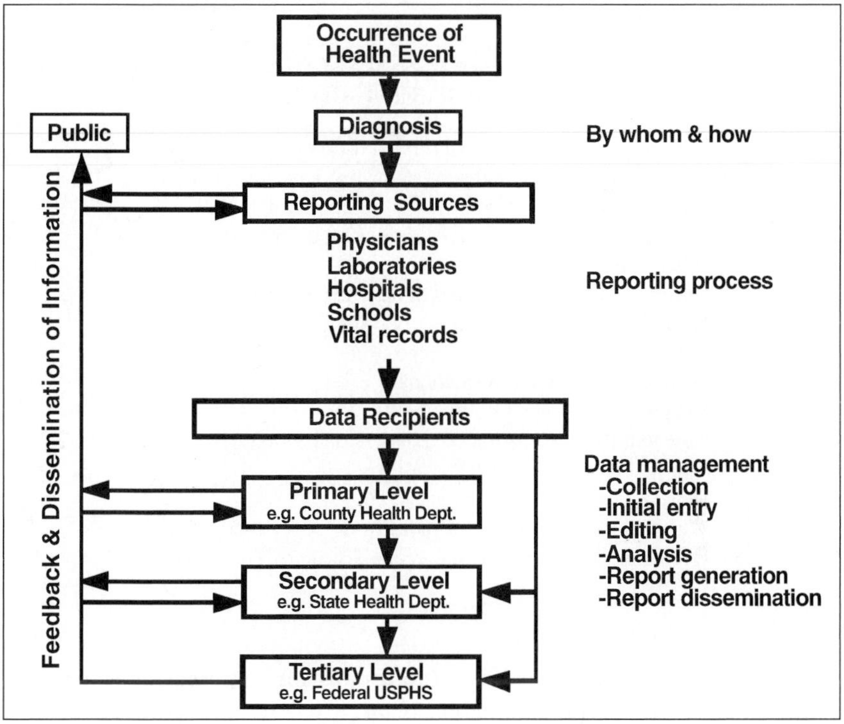

Fig. 9-1 Surveillance system flow chart. (From Centers for Disease Control: Guidelines for evaluating surveillance systems, *MMWR* 37:S-5, 1988.)

reported cases. This is referred to as the surveillance feedback loop. Fourth, the health care personnel who are involved in the process understand the importance of follow-up of cases (Istre, 1992).

When planning a surveillance system, there are several questions to be answered. Detailed, thoughtful answers to these questions will provide the components for a successful surveillance system (see the box on p. 164). It is helpful if a specific flow chart is designed that outlines the process of the surveillance system. Other factors that contribute to the success of a surveillance process include its simplicity, timeliness, flexibility, representativeness, ability to detect true cases, and acceptability to people outside of the sponsoring agency (Klaucke, 1992). These characteristics of successful surveillance systems form the basis for evaluation of surveillance programs. Public health resources are used efficiently when only important public health problems are under surveillance in a cost-effective process.

Types of surveillance

There are four general categories of surveillance programs: passive, active, sentinel, and special systems (Istre, 1992). Most local and state health departments use the most common form of surveillance, *passive surveillance.* Health care per-

QUESTIONS ADDRESSING THE COMPONENTS OF A SURVEILLANCE SYSTEM

Will the surveillance system serve a useful purpose?
Are there other surveillance systems that have a similar purpose?
What are the objectives of the surveillance system?
What are the characteristics of the health event?
What is the population to be surveyed?
During what period of time will data be collected?
What data will be collected?
Where will the information come from?
Who will report the information?
Who will collect the information?
How will the information be transferred and stored?
Who will analyze the data?
How and when are the data analyzed?
Who will receive reports of findings?
How and when will these reports be distributed?

sonnel use standardized report forms to submit information about cases of communicable disease. No action is taken unless the reports are received by the agency.

Active surveillance involves an ongoing search for new cases. This can be accomplished through such activities as telephone calls to health care personnel or laboratories or a review of hospital or clinic records. Active surveillance programs are more complete than passive surveillance programs but are more expensive to maintain (Istre, 1992).

Rather than conduct large-scale, active surveillance programs, *sentinel surveillance* systems are often used to identify trends in frequently occurring conditions. A random sample of physicians' offices or health care clinics are contacted and asked to report incidence of infectious diseases on a regular basis. For example, up-to-date information about the incidence of influenza and the specific strains of the organism that may be circulating in the community is gathered periodically by the CDC. Similarly, seroprevalence surveys, using data from clients attending sexually transmitted disease clinics, form the basis for the national sentinel surveillance system for human immunodeficiency virus (HIV)-1 infection in the United States. Recently, sentinel surveillance for HIV-2 infection in high-risk populations has been initiated (Onorato and others, 1993). Sentinel systems are not as useful for illnesses, such as meningococcal infections, that require specific follow-up measures for control purposes (Istre, 1992).

The Behavioral Risk Factor Surveillance System (BRFSS) program, a collaborative effort between the CDC and state health departments, is an example of a *special surveillance* system. A series of random telephone surveys are conducted periodically to track the progress of programs intended to affect health behavior. State-specific information is gathered about health behaviors, such as the prevalence of being overweight, cigarette and alcohol use, and seat belt nonuse, and the use of preventive health services, such as cholesterol screening and mammography. These data are being used to monitor progress toward achieving the nation's health objectives for the year 2000. Other types of special surveillance systems include microbiologic surveys and monitoring the emergence of antibiotic resistant organisms and presence of organisms, such as *Vibrio cholera* in sewage.

Sources of surveillance information

The World Health Organization (1968) has defined ten principal sources of surveillance information for general populations. All of these sources have a method of recording and reporting the data. The following box indicates sources of surveillance information from both general populations and specific populations. In the United States, surveillance of the health of the population is the primary responsibility of the CDC.

General populations

Reportable diseases. Morbidity data are usually gathered from case reports submitted to local or state health departments by health care personnel, although it can also be gathered from sentinel sites or sentinel health events. These data are dependent on the diagnosis that is made by the health care practitioner and are often supported by laboratory reports. Each state has a list of communicable diseases that must be officially reported to the state health department (see the box that follows). Most of these cases of communicable disease are then reported by state officials to the CDC. In addition, the American Public Health Association has established a classification system for reporting communicable diseases (see the box on p. 166). The major principles underlying this classification system are that official reporting is restricted to diseases that have procedures in place to control transmission of the illness or for which epidemiologic information is required for a definite purpose (Benenson, 1990).

SOURCES OF SURVEILLANCE INFORMATION

General populations	Specific populations
Morbidity data	Hospital or clinic records
Mortality data	Medical records
Case investigation	Insurance records
Epidemic reports	Patient or family interviews
Epidemic field investigation results	Provider office records
Laboratory reports	Worker's compensation records
Population surveys	Employee health records
Animal and vector population surveys	Personnel records
Biologic product use reports	Absentee reports
Demographic data	

AMERICAN PUBLIC HEALTH ASSOCIATION CLASSIFICATION SYSTEM FOR REPORTING COMMUNICABLE DISEASE

Class 1: Case report universally required

1 A. Diseases subject to international health regulations: plague, cholera, yellow fever, and smallpox

1 B. Diseases under surveillance by the World Health Organization: louse-borne typhus fever and relapsing fever, paralytic poliomyelitis, malaria and viral influenza

Class 2: Case report regularly required

2 A. Rapid reporting followed by weekly reports: examples are typhoid fever and diphtheria

2 B. Report by most practicable means: examples are brucellosis and leprosy

Class 3: Cases selectively reportable in endemic areas

3 A. Rapid reporting in specified areas: examples are scrub typhus Argentine and Bolivian hemorrhagic fever

3 B. Case report by most practicable means: examples are bartonellosis, coccidioidomycosis

3 C. Collective report weekly: examples are schistosomiasis, fasciolopsiasis

Class 4: Obligatory report of epidemics

Rapid report of pertinent data regarding outbreaks: staphylococcal food poisoning, adenoviral kerato-conjunctivitis, unidentified syndromes

Class 5: Official report not ordinarily justifiable

Includes diseases that are usually sporadic and uncommon or where the report would be of no practical value

From Benenson AS: *Control of communicable diseases in man,* ed 15, Washington DC, 1990, American Public Health Association.

The *universally mandatory reportable* diseases (plague, cholera, and yellow fever) require quarantine. Quarantine entails isolation of people with a communicable disease or those people who have been exposed to communicable disease during the contagious period. This is an attempt to prevent the spread of the illness. *Regularly reportable* diseases are differentiated according to their urgency for investigation of contacts, for identification of the source of infection or starting control measures. The *selectively reportable* diseases are those that are endemic only in certain areas of the world. Diseases included in this classification are often not reportable in many states and countries. *Obligatory report of an epidemic* normally requires rapid reporting of outbreaks but no case reporting. All other communicable diseases fall into the category of *official report not ordinarily justifiable.* Examples of diseases that fall under specific categories are found

COMMUNICABLE DISEASES REPORTABLE IN A MAJORITY OF STATES

AIDS	Malaria
Amebiasis	Measles
Anthrax	Meningitis, aseptic
Botulism	Meningitis, bacterial
Brucellosis	Meningococcal disease
Campylobacteriosis	Mumps
Chancroid	Outbreaks
Chickenpox-Zoster	Pertussis
Chlamydia	Plague
Cholera	Poliomyelitis
Diphtheria	Psittacosis
Encephalitis	Rabies
Food-associated illness	Reye syndrome
Giardiasis	Rocky Mt. spotted fever
Gonorrhea	Rubella
Granuloma inguinale	Rubella, congenital
Hemophilus influenzae; invasive	Salmonellosis
	Shigellosis
Hepatitis A	Syphilis
Hepatitis B	Tetanus
Hepatitis Non-A, Non-B	Toxic shock syndrome
Hepatitis unspecified	Trichinosis
Legionellosis	Tuberculosis
Leprosy	Tularemia
Leptospirosis	Typhoid fever
Lyme disease	Typhus
Lymphogranuloma venereum	Yellow fever

From Chorba and others: Mandatory reporting of infectious diseases by clinicians, *JAMA* 262:3081-3026, 1989.

in the box above. The reporting class for each communicable disease is found in the American Public Health Association publication *Control of Communicable Diseases in Man* (Benenson, 1990). Further information regarding morbidity and mortality statistics can be found in Chapters 1 and 3.

It is important to note that a number of states mandate laboratory reporting of some noninfectious conditions. For example, as of 1992, 18 states, representing approximately one half of the U.S. population, mandated reporting of elevated blood lead levels. Registries have been developed to investigate lead-poisoning cases, identify high-risk groups, examine trends, and target interventions at specific work sites (Maizlish and Rudolph, 1993).

National surveillance. The CDC conducts epidemiologic surveillance of all health events considered to be of high priority. These health events include both

ESTABLISHED SURVEILLANCE SYSTEMS

World Health Organization
U.S. Centers for Disease Control and Prevention
State Public Health Departments
American Hospital Association
Voluntary nonprofit organizations
(Examples: American Cancer Society
American Heart Association)

reportable diseases and other nonreportable conditions that contribute to the health burden of the United States. Data regarding reportable diseases are published weekly in the *Morbidity and Mortality Weekly Report (MMWR).* Surveillance summaries, recommendations, and reports on other nonreportable diseases and conditions are published either in the regular issues or in supplemental reports of the *MMWR.* Examples of these publications include infectious diseases, chronic conditions, infant mortality, injuries, occupational diseases, behavioral risk factors, suicides, and years of potential life lost. State-specific rates that are gathered as a part of the CDC's diverse surveillance systems are available to individual states. This information is then used for implementing control measures and planning preventive activities. Health care providers can access this information by contacting their state health department. Examples of established general population surveillance systems are shown in the box above.

Cases of certain diseases, such as those that produce a new or severe illness, will always be investigated by local or state health departments or the CDC. For example, cases of poliomyelitis and botulism will be carefully reviewed and analyzed. The onset of an illness in a group of people that indicates that the expected rate in the community has been exceeded may also be investigated. An outbreak or epidemic may have occurred. Although most epidemics are reported, not all epidemics are investigated. For example, once the influenza season is under way, epidemics will not be investigated unless unusual events occur. When information about the determinants or cause of an illness needs to be identified, field investigations that include population (community) surveys may be performed. The 1993 outbreak of *Escherichia coli* that caused episodes of acute renal failure in children in the state of Washington was linked to a fast-food restaurant chain through this type of investigative process.

Surveillance of animal and vector disease occurrence is an important means of gathering information about illnesses that can be communicated to humans. The CDC publishes the number of cumulative cases of animal rabies for the year in the *MMWR.* There has been a resurgence of rabies in animals, particularly on the east coast of the United States in recent years. Fig. 9-2 illustrates the secular incidence of rabies in wild and domestic animals in the United States and Puerto Rico that has been monitored by a mandatory reporting system. Other, more specific types

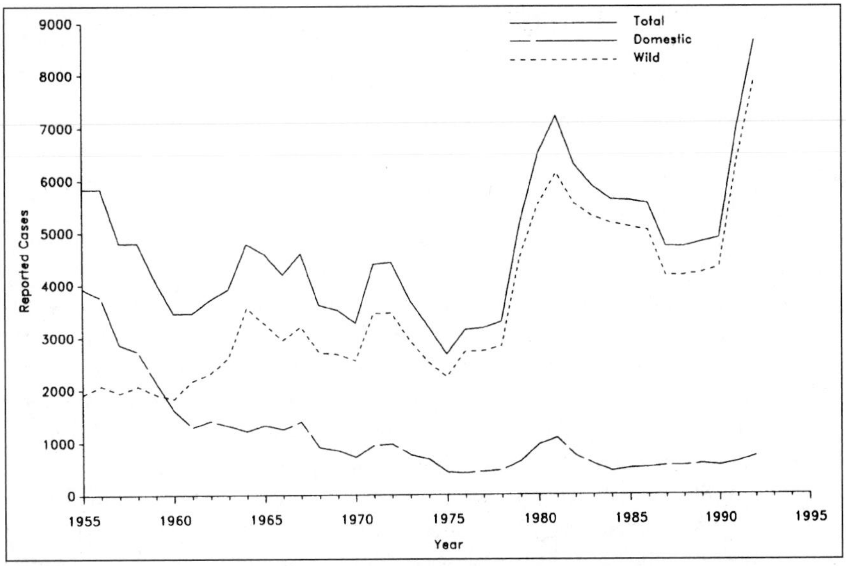

Fig. 9-2 Secular trends for rabies in wild and domestic animals—United States and Puerto Rico, 1955-1991. (From Centers for Disease Control: Summary of notifiable diseases, United States, 1991, *MMWR* 40(53), 1991.)

of general population surveillance can include the monitoring of requests for biologic products, such as human rabies immune globulin or botulism antitoxin.

Special populations. Nurses use the data from surveillance of general populations in providing outreach services. Nurses engage in surveillance activities when monitoring the state of health of special populations. Records that have been kept in hospitals, clinics, offices, or workplaces provide the source of surveillance data for special populations.

Good examples of epidemiologic surveillance are infection control programs in hospitals, long-term care, and other health care facilities. Infection control programs are coordinated by infection control practitioners, the majority of whom are nurses. The purpose of infection control surveillance is to establish and maintain a data base that describes the occurrence and distribution of infections acquired in institutions. The purpose of infection control surveillance is to (1) define the endemic or background rates of nosocomial infections, (2) identify increases in infection rates above this endemic level, (3) determine the risks associated with hospital care and specific procedures, and (4) to inform personnel of these risks so that control and prevention measures can be taken (Peri, 1993). Active, institution-wide or targeted surveillance is implemented through clinical rounds, monitoring laboratory data, and reviewing medical records. A more detailed description of the role and responsibilities of the infection-control practitioner is described in Chapter 12.

Nurses in specialty practice use surveillance data and engage in surveillance activities in their workplaces. For example, school health nurses perform physical, cognitive, and psychosocial evaluations for the children in their district and keep ongoing records of these activities. Primary prevention activities include emphasis on teaching students to be responsible for their own health. One of the fundamental objectives of programs established by occupational health nurses is to monitor health hazards in the environment and protect employees. Also, a major focus on primary prevention encourages personal health maintenance among all employees.

SCREENING

Screening is a process of active, presumptive detection of unrecognized disease, illness, or deficit in asymptomatic, apparently healthy individuals. It is a strategy for secondary prevention of disease in populations. Tests, examinations, or other procedures are applied to a large group of apparently well people. The intent is to identify those people in the group who have a high probability of having the health problem under study and to separate those who probably have the disease from those who probably do not. Those people who have a high probability of having the disease are then referred for a diagnostic workup and treatment, if warranted. The screening procedure alone does not diagnose the illness. Positive screening test results are always an indication for further diagnostics procedures (Thorner and Remein, 1961; Mausner and Kramer, 1985).

Illness is often diagnosed after people seek health care for an investigation of specific symptoms. Therefore many people are in a relatively late stage of an illness when diagnosis occurs and treatment is started. Often, the results of treatment are more effective in preventing death and disability if illness is detected prior to the development of serious symptoms—in the preclinical stage. This entails participation in ongoing surveillance programs that screen for specific health problems. In some circumstances, searching for early asymptomatic illness now is considered a routine and important aspect of good health care.

Types of screening

Screening procedures are available and are recommended for breast, cervical, testicular, colon, rectal, and skin cancers, diabetes, hypertension, tuberculosis, sexually transmitted diseases, and several other conditions. There are four types of screening procedures: mass, selective, multiphasic, and case-finding (Valanis, 1992). Nurses use screening procedures for clinical decision-making and the identification of people and populations at risk (see Chapter 1). These data are essential for planning and implementing health care for individuals and in meeting the needs of the community.

Mass screening is applied to entire populations. For example, since 1981, 15 states have established registries for surveillance of adult lead absorption, primarily based on reports of elevated blood lead levels from clinical laboratories (Baser, 1992). The CDC now recommends universal blood lead screening for all American children under age 6 except for children in communities that can demonstrate that they do not have a childhood lead-poisoning problem. Many mass screening programs have been incorporated into the health care system.

During the 1970s several states enacted legislation requiring that women admitted to hospitals be offered a Papanicolaou's (Pap) test to improve hospital screening for cervical cancer. Unfortunately, elderly and low-income women still remain underscreened (Klassen, Celentano, and Weisman, 1993). Phenylketonuria (PKU) testing of newborns is mandated in many states. This is a rare, congenital defect that affects metabolism of protein and can be effectively treated through diet therapy to prevent severe mental retardation.

Selective screening is applied to specific high-risk populations. For example, mammograms may be recommended more frequently for women with a strong family history of breast cancer, or tuberculin tests (PPD) may be done on hospital employees. Occupational health nurses often plan periodic selective screening activities to monitor employees' exposure to hazardous working conditions. Exposure devices are used to monitor personnel working with radiation, and pulmonary function tests, blood chemistries, and cytologic analysis of urine may be performed periodically for those exposed to toxic substances.

Multiphasic screening applies a variety of screening tests to the same population on the same occasion. For example, a series of tests are commonly performed on a single blood sample. These data are gathered as results of preoperative examinations, preadmission procedures, periodic health assessments, periodic surveillance of drug therapy, or for monitoring the stage of an illness. Collectively, the data can be used for the establishment of baseline data at a health care facility and risk factor appraisal (Valanis, 1992).

Case-finding involves a clinician's search for illness as a part of a client's periodic health examination. It is an established practice of advanced nurse practitioners as they monitor the health of individuals in their caseload. There are many screening tests available for health assessments. Pap smears, and breast examinations are part of routine examinations for women, and testicular examinations are routine for men. The United States Preventive Services Task Force has identified indications for the routine use of screening tests; these are summarized in Table 9-1 (US Preventive Services Task Force, 1989). Nurses frequently use the Denver Developmental Screening Test that provides a measure of the motor, personal-social, and language development of children. Further examples of routine screening of children are found in Table 9-2.

Characteristics of screening programs

Screening programs are not feasible for all health problems. Since a large number of apparently healthy people are evaluated, there are many factors that must be considered before establishing a screening program. To be appropriate for screening, a health problem should have serious consequences. The expenditure of resources for screening should result in positive outcomes or be cost-effective. For example, routine Pap smears for cervical cancer can ultimately result in a possible cure for a life-threatening disease. Screening for PKU and lead poisoning can prevent mental retardation. Health problems that are more compatible with life or are often asymptomatic in the general population, such as osteoarthritis, may not be suitable for screening programs (Hennekens and Buring, 1987).

Table 9-1 Indications for the routine use of selected screening tests*

Screening test	Indications for use
Blood typing	Pregnant women (first prenatal visit)
Blood lead level	Every few months in children at risk through age 6; adults at occupational risk
Blood pressure	Yearly beginning at age 3; each prenatal visit
Breast examination	Every 1 to 3 years for women in high-risk groups age 19 to 39; annually for all women over age 40
Chlamydial testing	Periodically for all sexually active persons with multiple sexual partners
Dipstick urinalysis	Yearly for persons over age 65
Electrocardiogram	Every 1 to 3 years for those at risk; every year for those over age 65
Fasting plasma glucose	Periodically for those at risk; every year for those over age 65
Fecal occult blood/colonoscopy or sigmoidoscopy	Every 1 to 3 years for those at risk from age 19 to 64; yearly for those over age 65
Gonorrhea culture	Periodically for all sexually active persons with multiple sexual partners; pregnant women
Hearing	Initially at 18 months for high-risk infants, age 3; all persons exposed to high noise levels; those 65 and older
Height and weight	At birth, 2, 4, 6, 15, and 18 months, and when seen for immunizations to age 6; during periodic exams to age 18; every 1 to 3 years to age 65, then yearly; each visit for pregnant women
Hemoglobin and hematocrit	Once during infancy; pregnant women
HIV testing and counseling	Every 1 to 3 years for those at risk from age 19 to 64; pregnant women in high-risk groups (initial visit and 28 weeks)
Mammogram	Every 1 to 2 years for women over age 35 with a family history of premenopausal breast cancer and all women aged 50 to 75
Oral cavity examination	Every 1 to 3 years for those at risk from age 19 to 64; every year for those over age 65
Palpation for thyroid nodules	Every 1 to 3 years for persons at risk from age 19 to 64; every year for those over age 65
Pap smear	Every 1 to 3 years for sexually active females age 18 or older
Rubella titre	Females of childbearing age lacking evidence of immunity; pregnant women (first prenatal visit)
Skin examination	Every 1 to 3 years beginning at age 13 for persons at risk; every year for those over age 65
Testicular examination	Every 1 to 3 years for males age 13 to 39 in high-risk groups
Total serum cholesterol	Every 5 years; more frequently for those at high risk

Table 9-1 Indications for the routine use of selected screening tests *(cont.)*

Tuberculin skin test	Children between ages 2 and 12; yearly for household contacts who remain tuberculin negative or members of groups at high risk
Ultrasound examination	Pregnant women (36 weeks)
Urinalysis for bacteriuria	Periodically for preschool children and for persons with diabetes; pregnant women
VDRL/RPR	Periodically for all sexually active persons with multiple sexual partners; pregnant women

*Indications for routine screening only.

For screening to be beneficial, the treatment given during the preclinical phase should result in a better prognosis for the individual than the treatment given after the symptoms have developed. The screening process should be effective in reducing both morbidity and mortality. If early diagnosis and treatment has no better prognosis than treatment after the disease is established, then screening is not feasible. At present, lung cancer has a very poor prognosis whenever it is diagnosed and treated. Therefore screening programs for lung cancer are not considered cost-effective at this time. Also, screening is of no benefit if there is no treatment that can alter the course of the illness (Hennekens and Buring, 1987).

Screening is more cost-effective if the prevalence of the health problem is high in the population and if the screening tests are available at low cost. Screening tests also should be acceptable to the people being screened. They should be administered quickly, easily, without discomfort, and of a noninvasive nature, if possible. Provision for follow up of people with positive results is es-

Table 9-2 Routine screening tests for children

Age	Test
Birth	PKU
	T4/TSH
6 months	Lead
	Hematocrit and hemoglobin
9 Months	PPD
2 Years	Hematocrit and hemoglobin
3-12 Years	Hematocrit and hemoglobin
	Lead
	Blood pressure
	Vision
	Hearing
	Dental
	Tuberculin test
	Urinalysis
9-12 Years	Scoliosis

sential. Failure to provide for follow up for positive screening tests can constitute malpractice. A summary of the criteria for establishing screening programs is found in the box below.

The results of screening tests should be valid. Validity indicates how well a test represents reality or the truth. Those people with a preclinical condition should be identified as test-positive, and those without the preclinical condition should be identified as test-negative. In other words, the test should be accurate. If a screening test is valid, it is also reliable. Reliability means that the test has consistent results and that findings can be repeated or replicated. Validity is measured by the sensitivity, specificity, and predictive value of the test.

Sensitivity and specificity

Sensitivity is the ability of the test to correctly identify people who have the health problem. It is the probability of testing positive if the health problem is truly present. *Specificity* is the ability of the test to correctly identify people who do not have the health problem. It is the probability of testing negative if the health problem is truly absent. The relationship between screening test results and a true diagnosis is found in Table 9-3, and the calculations of sensitivity and specificity values are found in Table 9-4.

Increasing the sensitivity of a test will cause a decrease in specificity. Conversely, increasing the specificity of a test decreases sensitivity. A classical example is a hypothetical distribution of intraocular pressures in glaucomatous

CRITERIA FOR ESTABLISHING AND EVALUATING SCREENING PROGRAMS

The health problem should:
- Have a high prevalence in the population
- Be relatively serious
- Be able to be detected in early stages
- Have an effective treatment that improves outcomes

The screening test should be:
- Cost-effective
- Simple, safe, and easy to administer
- Of minimal discomfort
- Sensitive enough to detect most cases
- Specific to the health problem
- Valid and reliable

The group to be screened should:
- Be identifiable
- Be assessable
- Accept the screening procedures
- Be willing to seek treatment
- Accept follow-up procedures

Table 9-3 Relationship between screening tests and a true diagnosis

Screening test results	Health problem present	Health problem absent	Total
Positive	True-positives (TP)	False-positives (FP)	TP + FP
Negative	False-negatives (FN)	True-negatives (TN)	FN + TN
Total	TP + FN	FP + TN	TP + FP + TN + FN

and nonglaucomatous eyes as measured by tonometer (Thorner and Remein, 1961). Intraocular pressure normally varies during a 24-hour cycle, and variability is greater in those persons with glaucoma. In any given population, it can be expected that there will be more people with nonglaucomatous eyes than glaucomatous eyes (Fig. 9-3). These people, illustrated as group A, have an intraocular pressure ranging from 14 to 26 mm Hg. Group B people with glaucomatous eyes have intraocular pressures ranging from 22 to 42 mm Hg. The intraocular pressure distributions in the two groups overlap. Therefore anyone whose test results are between 22 and 26 mm Hg could either have or not have glaucoma. False positives and false negatives occur in the overlap. Therefore screening alone cannot determine whether such an individual is normal or has glaucoma. The degree of sensitivity and specificity may be changed by selecting a screening level at any point in the overlap area of 22 to 26 mm Hg.

In an ideal situation, a screening test would be able to identify the presence or absence of a health problem in every person screened. In this case, both sensitivity and specificity would be 100%. However, this is almost impossible to achieve in actual practice. Establishing various screening levels should be carefully analyzed by health care planners before screening projects are undertaken. Much depends on the consequences of leaving some cases undetected (false negatives) or classifying healthy people as having a health problem (false positives).

Table 9-4 Calculation of sensitivity, specificity, and predictive value

Sensitivity	$\dfrac{\text{True-positives}}{\text{True-positives + False-negatives}}$ (All with the health problem)	× 100
Specificity	$\dfrac{\text{True-negatives}}{\text{True- negatives + False-positives}}$ (All without the health problem)	× 100
Predictive value Positive test (PV+)	$\dfrac{\text{True-positives}}{\text{True-positives + False-positives}}$ (All positives)	× 100
Negative test (PV−)	$\dfrac{\text{True-negatives}}{\text{True-negatives + False-negatives}}$ (All negatives)	× 100

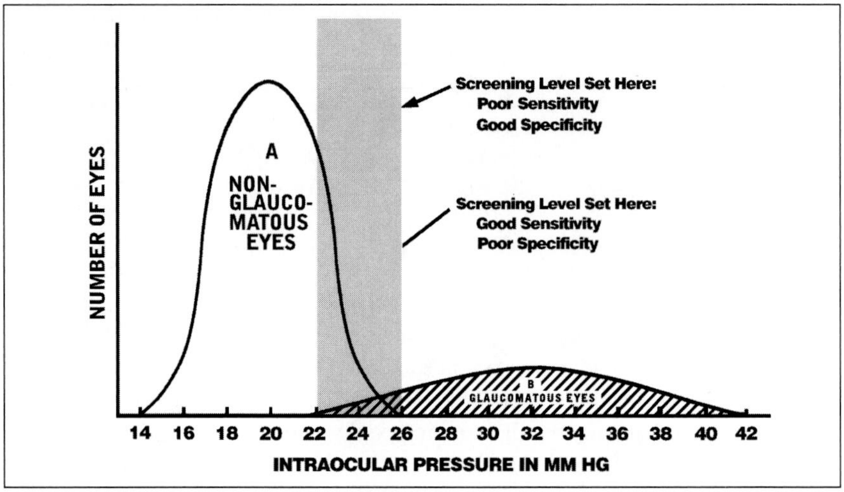

Fig. 9-3 Hypothetical distribution of intraocular pressures in glaucomatous and nonglaucomatous eyes as measured by tonometer. (Adapted from Thorner RM, Remein QR: Principles and procedures in the evaluation of screening for disease, US Department of Health, Education, and Welfare, *Public Health Monograph 67,* 1961.)

The choice of screening levels is subjective, based on the severity of the disease, cost, time factors, advantages of early treatment, and other screening criteria (see box, p. 174). One of the ways of addressing this problem is to use several screening tests to make decisions.

Predictive value

Predictive value measures the frequency with which the test results correctly identify the health problem among those who are screened. Predictive value positive (PV+) is the proportion of those testing positive who actually have the health problem. Predictive value negative (PV−) is the proportion of those testing negative who do not have the health problem. There is a relationship between sensitivity, specificity, and predictive value. As sensitivity increases, it is less likely that an individual with a negative test will have the health problem. Therefore the predictive value negative increases. Conversely, as the specificity increases, it is less likely that an individual with a positive test will be free from the health problem. Therefore the predictive value positive increases. The predictive value of a test is an indication of yield. Yield is defined as the number of previously unrecognized cases that are diagnosed and brought to treatment as a result of the screening process (Hennekens and Buring, 1987). The calculation of predictive values is found in Table 9-4.

Effect of prevalence on screening levels

Sensitivity, specificity, and predictive values vary according to the prevalence of the health problem in the population that is screened. When the prevalence of a health problem is low (1% of the population), as it often is for chronic diseases, most of the population will be free of the illness. Therefore positive screening test results from general population groups are likely to include a large proportion of false positives. Also, a small decrease in specificity of a test will greatly increase the number of false positives (Fig. 9-3). Alternatively, an increase in prevalence usually results in a small reduction in the number of false positives. The yield of new cases will increase however, in proportion to the increase in prevalence. When prevalence reaches 15% to 20%, an adequate predictive value is achieved (Mausner and Kramer, 1985). This is a principle underlying screening of high-risk groups. They are likely to have a higher prevalence of disease than the general population. This increases the predictive value of a positive test and increases the yield of new cases.

Evaluation of screening programs

Screening programs should be evaluated based on their feasibility and cost-effectiveness, as addressed in the box on p. 174. Effectiveness is also measured by determining whether the screening process reduces morbidity and mortality. Epidemiologic studies are often used to evaluate screening programs. For example, cross-sectional, correlational studies examine the relationship between morbidity and mortality rates and the frequency of screening. In case-control studies, the effect of past exposure to screening programs in compared for those with and without the health problem of concern. Cohorts can be followed forward in time to determine morbidity and mortality outcomes between those screened and those who were diagnosed after symptoms developed (see Chapter 5). Case-fatality rates are often compared. Randomized, controlled clinical trials usually provide the best method for evaluation (see Chapter 6). These studies compare the morbidity and mortality outcomes of a group of people who are screened for the health problem with a group of people who do not receive screening tests. Screening is the intervention in a clinical trial.

SUMMARY

Surveillance is a method of monitoring emerging and endemic health problems in the community for the purpose of establishing primary prevention programs. Nurses use surveillance data in establishing and implementing provider outreach services. They engage in surveillance activities as they monitor the health of clients in their caseloads.

Successful surveillance systems involve (1) health problems that are perceived to be important public health concerns; (2) a system of reporting and recording information; (3) frequent, sustained interaction with the reporting sources; and (4) health care personnel who are committed to the follow up of cases. There are four types of surveillance systems: passive, active, sentinel, and special systems surveillance. These categories are differentiated by the level of action taken and characteristics of the populations under surveillance. Sources of surveillance data can come from either general populations or specific population groups. The American Public Health Association has a classification system that is widely used for reporting communicable diseases. However, many other surveillance systems involve health problems that are noninfectious in nature.

Screening involves the presumptive detection of unrecognized health problems in asymptomatic, apparently healthy individuals. It is a strategy for secondary prevention of health problems in the community. The intent is to separate those who probably have the health problem from those who probably do not and refer them for diagnostic workup and treatment. Mass screening, selective screening, multiphasic screening, and case-finding are the four types that have been identified. Nurses in advanced practice use screening procedures as they monitor the health of the individuals in their caseload.

There are several criteria for establishing and evaluating screening programs that involve the nature of the health problem, the characteristics of the screening test, and the group to be screened. Basically, the screening program should be feasible, cost-effective, and result in a better prognosis for the individual than the treatment given to the individual after symptoms develop.

There are three measures of the validity of screening tests: sensitivity, specificity, and predictive value of the test. Sensitivity is the ability of the test to correctly identify people who have the health problem. Specificity is the ability of the test to correctly identify people who do not have the health problem. Predictive value measures the frequency with which the test results correctly identify the health problem among those who are screened. These values are related to the prevalence of the health problem in the population that is screened. Epidemiologic studies are frequently used to further evaluate the effectiveness of screening programs by comparing the outcomes of those screened with those who are not screened.

CRTIICAL THINKING QUESTIONS

1. Identify and describe a surveillance system for nosocomial wound infections that would be appropriate for a 200-bed community hospital.
2. Identify occupational health surveillance and screening programs that should be established in a hospital setting.
3. Discuss the role of surveillance and screening programs in quality control initiatives in health care facilities.

Results of a screening test

	True Diagnosis		
Test result	**Health problem present**	**Health problem absent**	**Total**
Positive	178	34	212
Negative	27	9761	9788
Total	205	9795	10,000

4. Based on the results of a screening program shown above, calculate the sensitivity, specificity, and predictive value of a positive test.
5. How would you evaluate the results of this screening program? Was it effective?
6. Suggest a health problem where screening that leads to early diagnosis has been shown to improve outcomes for the individual and general community.

REFERENCES

Baser ME: The development of registries for surveillance of adult lead exposure, 1981-1992, *AJPH* 82(8):1113-1118, 1992.

Benenson AS: *Control of communicable diseases in man,* ed 15, Washington, DC, 1990, American Public Health Association.

Centers for Disease Control: *CDC surveillance update,* Atlanta, 1988, The Centers.

Centers for Disease Control: Guidelines for evaluating surveillance systems, *MMWR* 37:S-5, 1988.

Centers for Disease Control: Summary of notifiable diseases, United States, 1991, *MMWR* 40(53):38, 1991.

Chorba TL and others: Mandatory reporting of infectious diseases by clinicians, *JAMA* 262:3018-3026, 1989.

Hennekens CH, Buring JE: *Epidemiology in medicine,* Boston, 1987, Little, Brown.

Istre GR: Disease surveillance at the state and local levels. In Halperin W, Baker EL, editors: *Public health surveillance,* New York, 1992, Van Nostrand Reinhold.

Klassen AC, Celentano DD, Weisman CS: Cervical cancer screening in hospitals: The efficacy of legislation in Maryland, *AJPH* 83(9):1316-1320, 1993.

Klaucke DN: Evaluating public health surveillance systems. In Halperin W, Baker EL, editors: *Public health surveillance,* New York, 1992, Van Nostrand Reinhold.

Last JM: *A dictionary of epidemiology,* New York, 1988, Oxford University Press.

Maizlish N, Rudolph L: California adults with elevated blood levels, 1987 through 1990, *AJPH* 83(3):402-405, 1993.

Mausner JS, Kramer S: *Epidemiology—an introductory text,* Philadelphia, 1985, WB Saunders.

Onorato IM and others: Sentinel surveillance for HIV-2 infection in high-risk US populations, *AJPH* 83(4):515-519, 1993.

Peri TM: Surveillance, reporting and the use of computers. In Wenzel RP, editor: *Prevention and control of nosocomial infections,* ed 2, Baltimore, 1993, Williams & Wilkins.

Thacker SB, Choi K, Brachman PS: The surveillance of infectious diseases, *JAMA* 249:1181, 1983.

Thorner RM, Remein QR: *Principles and procedures in the evaluation of screening for disease,* US Department of Health, Education, and Welfare, Public Health Monograph 67, 1961.

US Preventive Services Task Force: *Guide to clinical preventive services,* Baltimore, 1989, Williams & Wilkins.

Valanis B: *Epidemiology in nursing and health care,* ed 2, Norwalk CT, 1992, Appleton & Lange.

World Health Organization: The surveillance of communicable diseases, *WHO Chron* 22:439.20, 1968.

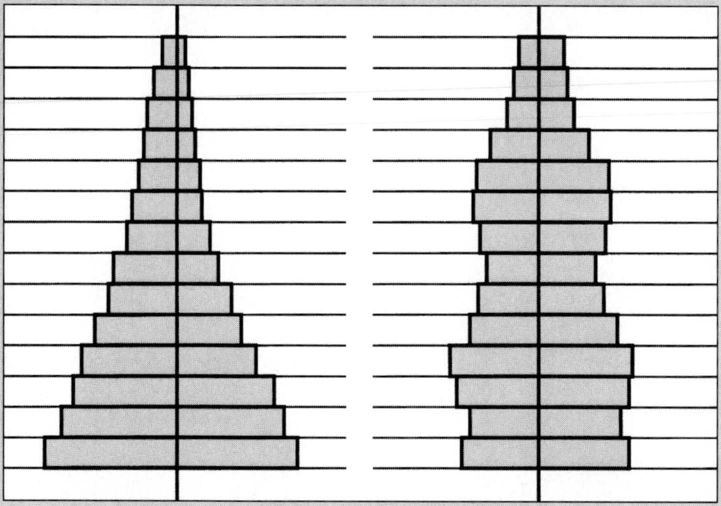

Part II

Epidemiology Applied to Nursing Practice

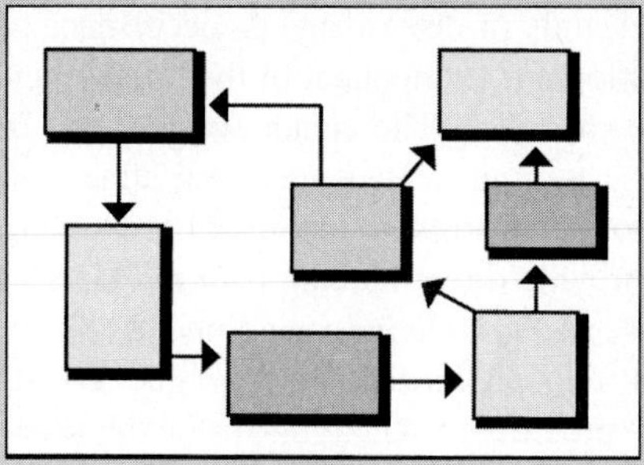

10

Epidemiology in a Nurse-Managed Center

ELIZABETH O. DIETZ

Objectives

1. Describe the application of epidemiologic principles in a nurse-managed center.
2. Differentiate types of nursing care in a nurse-managed center according to primary, secondary, and tertiary levels of prevention.
3. Determine the epidemiologic methods used within the nurse-managed center.
4. Specify the models of causation used in the nurse-managed center, giving examples of each.

Key Terms

community health assessment
levels of prevention
- primary
- secondary
- tertiary

nurse-managed center
risk assessment
screening
web of causation

Epidemiology, the art and science of the study of disease and its occurrence in human populations, is a major foundation and component of the nurse-managed and nurse-run health center, the Health Place. The center was created in 1983 for the express purpose of providing a clinical placement and education training site for gerontology nurse practitioner students in the School of Nursing at San Jose State University, and was to provide direct nursing care to elders in the community. It was created by the faculty as a vehicle for providing health care using nursing models, rather than medical models, in direct and indirect client-centered care. Principles of epidemiology provide a foundation for health planning that guides the interaction between nursing faculty, nurse-managed–center staff, students, and clients. The characteristics of the clients and the many different types of health problems seen at the center are continually assessed and measured as a part of nursing care. Since its inception, the Health Place has experienced many philosophic and organizational changes. It continues, however, to function as a nurse-managed clinic.

The Health Place functions as a home health service and a walk-in clinic that provides social and health care services to people age 55 and older. Clients eligible for services through the clinic are not presently eligible for insurance-reimbursed services because their needs are for nonacute, episodic care. Church groups and similar organizations are the only other organizations that provide free services in the home. The Health Place specializes in support for the activities of daily living, such as bathing, hygiene, diet and nutrition counseling, health care assessments, and medication monitoring. Assistance is also provided to relatives and friends who provide support and/or care to clients.

Presently, organizational goals include provisions of clinical placement and training sites for undergraduate and graduate nursing students. Graduate students focus on (1) integrating community health and gerontology nursing; (2) functioning as role models to the undergraduate nursing students; and (3) providing direct and indirect client care for clients over the age of 55 who are not eligible for reimbursable care. The catchement or service-provider area, called the West Valley area, includes the towns of Los Gatos, Monte Sereno, Saratoga, and parts of the bordering cities of San Jose and Campbell, California. No elderly client living within the catchement area of the clinic is rejected for service, all are treated.

Los Gatos, CA, is a small, independent town of affluent Silicon Valley residents located 60 miles south of San Francisco and 60 miles north of Monterey. The ethnic and racial profile does not match the neighboring large, multicultural city of San Jose. Most of the original settlers were transplanted San Franciscans who spent summers in Los Gatos. The housing was mostly nonpermanent, non-winterized homes. Social welfare and public safety services were not provided in the early history of the town. Most of the services were obtained from the neighboring city of San Jose. Gradually, a permanent structure was created in Los Gatos with its own government, police and fire departments, and public schools. The original cost of housing was approximately $4000 to $5000 per home. Today, these same homes and land average around $700,000.

The Health Place is located in the Los Gatos Neighborhood Center. This center was built to house multiple services for the elderly. Due to changes in the philosophy of the town and the need for space, other groups and services are also housed in the building. Other social services available in the center include Transit Assist, an independent transportation service; the Los Gatos Senior Coordinating Council, an independent agency that provides social and social welfare services; and the Teen Counseling Place, an independent emotional counseling for teens in need.

The clients of the Health Place could not afford to buy their homes today. Most would not be able to afford the costs of a mortgage, city taxes, and home owners insurance. Currently, the senior clients using the center have difficulty with the high cost of property and city taxes.

Most individuals of Los Gatos obtain their social welfare and health services from neighboring cities of San Jose, Campbell, and Santa Clara. County public health clinics are located at the Santa Clara Valley Medical Center in San Jose. The Community Hospital and Rehabilitation Center of Los Gatos maintained a gerontology center for 2 years but suspended the services, since most of the clients receive health care and hospitalization outside of the community. The facility failed to obtain physician support, and the hospital was unable to be reimbursed by California Medicaid. The physicians at the hospital were not accepting of the advanced practice roles of the gerontologic nurse practitioner.

Physical space at the Health Place presents certain challenges to delivering health care. The office is a single room with a sink, examining table, secretary's desk, and filing cabinets. Active client charts are stored in this office, while inactive and deceased client charts are located in a filing cabinet in an adjacent office. The office often reminds clients of a one-room school house. Medical and office supplies are located in or on top of cabinets and under and around the examining table and desk. Every inch of space is used in the center. People passing by an open door are surprised at the number of items crowded into the office. Former Naval personnel say the clinic reminds them of a submarine health center.

The health center computer and its database are located in the Senior Coordinating Council's staff office next door. The Health Place has arranged to perform home health visits for the Los Gatos Senior Coordinating Council, and they, in turn, allow their case-management employees and social workers to provide social services to clients. Collaborative relationships with other agencies help stretch our budget dollars and extend the work area. The Senior Coordinating Center boasts a long and excellent history of proper use of resources and services for seniors in the area. Students do not have that resource knowledge base. The case-management staff has also been in position for many years, while our students change each semester. Continuity helps bring students' knowledge base quickly into place so as to provide necessary home health services.

During the clinical days when the students are present in the Health Place, the neighborhood center's lounge is used to conduct clinical conferences, update charts, and provide other clinical activities and clinics.

A client is never discharged from the center service. Often, they temporarily may not need service but are likely to need active services in the future. Three client lists are maintained at the clinic. These lists are labeled as: active, inactive, and deceased. Active client rosters include all admitted clients who are visited once a week to once a month. Clients who do not need care are placed on the inactive status list. As new health problems arise these inactive clients are reactivated. Finally, the deceased roster provides a listing of clients who have died.

Since home health care services are free, funding must be secured and administered. However, foot care, regular injections like vitamin B_{12}, and blood pressure monitoring require a small fee. Over the years, the Health Place has survived by obtaining small grants, donations, and through the personal fortitude of the students and faculty. Presently, services are provided throughout the year, even during student vacation periods. Registered nurse graduate students and other nursing students are hired to provide the high priority care outside the normal academic year. Their services are paid for by a variety of the funding sources.

The undergraduate nursing students at the Health Place are in their community health—public health senior semester. Classes include a didactic theory lecture class for 4 hours per week, a clinical seminar for 2 hours per week, and a clinical practicum experience in the center for 12 hours per week. Each group of students will attend these classes for the entire 15-week semester.

Two nursing department faculty members are assigned to the Health Place clinical rotation. Two groups of students are assigned to the Health Place clinical rotation. Each student actually spends 6 hours per week in the Health Place, and 6 hours per week delivering nursing care in a traditional public health nursing department located a few miles away from the Health Place. During this experience, the students are responsible for completing nursing department-created learning packages to validate their clinical experiences. The content of the learning packages includes exercises in epidemiology, nutritional assessment for families, community assessment through epidemiology, identification of populations at risk, family assessment (epidemiology of the family and their strengths and weaknesses), newborn assessment, Denver Developmental Screening Tests (DDST) exercises, specialized elderly assessments, home assessments for seniors and children, and record-keeping using the Problem-Oriented Record (SOAP) format.

Students assigned to this clinical placement are responsible for matching resources and helping their clients use the appropriate community resources. Students are also responsible for examining their clients through the life cycle or developmental conceptual framework and from the individuals at risk framework. During this clinical experience, students should be able to function independently and make independent clinical family decisions.

The theory component of the course includes content on the legislative and/or political process. The link between health policy and clinical practice is emphasized. Students are encouraged to become politically active through participation in professional nursing associations, with the understanding that the regulatory processes allow students to use the epidemiologic process to its ultimate goal. That goal is to help the agency plan for the future and see the results of this process as it relates to client care.

LEVELS OF PREVENTION

The overall goal of the nursing care at the Health Place is to provide indirect and direct nursing services to allow the seniors and elderly clients to remain in their own living arrangements as long and as independently as possible. Prevention is a key concept used in all aspects of delivery of nursing care with our clients.

Primary prevention

Primary prevention is used to prevent health care problems. The main service of the Health Place is the provision of direct and indirect general health promotion for all homebound clients and those clients who seek services in the office as well. The Health Place uses specific primary prevention measures, such as provision of influenza immunization clinics for the center's clients and other senior citizens in the Los Gatos Neighborhood Center. The students visit five other senior nutrition centers and/or housing complexes to provide health-promotion nursing services to the participants at these community senior sites.

Secondary prevention

Secondary prevention focuses on early identification, treatment, and monitoring of exisitng health problems. Active disease cases are referred to local physicians for diagnosis and treatment. Since relationships with local physicians and hospitals are generally excellent, reports and assessments are quickly and efficiently dealt with by the physicians and family members. Students making home visits are charged to employ the nursing process and perform the nursing assessments to identify health care issues and problems.

Throughout the year, the clinic provides a regular schedule of clinics for hypertension monitoring, medication monitoring, and blood-glucose monitoring for clients who have had normal readings and for those diagnosed with diabetes. Foot care clinics are also held on a regular schedule. Clients are welcome to the center for periodic visits for medication monitoring, questions and answers on health care problems, and resources counseling.

Clients are turned over to licensed agencies that can make visits on a more regular basis when new health problems are discovered or chronic conditions worsen. Students can only visit one time per week rather than on a daily basis as might be needed. MediCal (Medicaid for California) and Medicare allow for reimbursable care to the licensed agencies who are certified to receive reimbursement. The Health Place temporarily steps aside and does not provide direct service, while the clients are able to obtain the licensed home health benefits. These benefits from the licensed home health agencies provide care as many times per week as medically ordered for the clients. The Health Place supplements the licensed home health nurse and therapist visits to the clients. Because good communication with the licensed home care agencies has been established, clients are referred back to the Health Place on discharge from the licensed care agencies. In a number of instances, the Health Place will begin service to a new client who has been referred by another licensed health care agency in cases where the agency believes that on-going care is necessary but not reimbursable.

Tertiary prevention

Tertiary prevention is a primary focus of the Health Place. These are the services that allow clients to be assisted with activities of daily living care and rehabilitation principles for as long as the clients can stay at home. It is believed that clients increase their independence through the facility's focus on activities of daily living. The potential result is decreased health care costs. The cooperation of family members and agencies working together is the key to the managed care principles that guide services. The facilitation of the clients' abilities to remain in their own homes, thereby avoiding placement in nursing homes or skilled nursing facilities, depends on the cooperation of other agencies and family members. Although no formal evaluation research has been conducted on the Health Place, many clients, in fact, remain in their own homes until death.

EPIDEMIOLOGIC METHODS

Since the Health Place was created for the purpose of educating nursing students, the epidemiologic model is formally applied to the practice of nursing care given through the center. All agency care involves the theoretic foundations of epidemiology. Student assignments include individual client assessments of lifestyle factors and health system factors. As the students care for the individual clients, they must continue to focus not only on the client, but also on the local, regional, and state environments as they relate to the entire community. The student groups are expected to use the teaching and assignment package of materials and report on the overall community surrounding the Health Place from the perspective of the epidemiologic model. These learning packages are created by the nursing department. Many different sources of data are used to provide a wider and varied knowledge base for the students. Selected indices of health care and descriptive epidemiology are used.

The Health Place uses the *web of causation* epidemiologic model (Friedman, 1987). The web of causation speaks to predisposing factors and the complex relationships with one another resulting in the final outcome of a disease or health problem. This web is a complex concept but allows for both noninfectious (noncommunicable disease) and infectious disease processes. The students conduct a community health assessment using the web of causation model or the conceptual framework for the assessment.

The students begin their community assessment with a windshield survey of the community. The students take still photographs of key geography and specific locations within the community. They also videotape clients in their homes (with permission) and points located in Los Gatos and Santa Clara County. One part of the students' responsibilities is to obtain actual statistics from the disease registers and other morbidity/mortality surveys in the area. Students analyze statistics from the local Los Gatos area, the neighboring city of San Jose, Santa Clara

County, and state statistics for California. Charts and graphs are prepared using all of the usual indices: birth and death/mortality rates, illness/morbidity rates, location type and varieties of health and nonhealth-related services, along with other cause-specific disease and death/mortality rates. When graduate students use the Health Place for a clinical placement, they continue the study of demographic and health statistics, including a state, national, and international perspectives. These assignments allow the students to practice an application of epidemiology to health and health care.

During the early part of the fall semester, the Health Place uses the traditional causation pattern of agent-host-environment as the guiding conceptual framework to participate in a city-wide program for influenza prevention. This program highlights and identifies clients at risk for the disease. It is believed that these programs decrease disease in clients, and it has been possible to increase the numbers of persons participating in the program.

An example of how this conceptual framework is used was the increase in adult abuse and neglect directly after the October 1989 Northern California earthquake. The academic semester had begun in August/September 1989, and the students had settled into providing care to their clients and completing written and oral assignments. The earthquake struck on Tuesday, October 19, 1989. A university decision closed the campus and classes were canceled for the remainder of the week. At the same time, the public safety officials of Los Gatos decided to close the town to nonresidents until Saturday, October 23, 1989. The Health Place students have clinicals on Wednesday and Thursday. Therefore no one was supposed to visit clients. However, every student called or visited their clients during the week. It is a credit to the devotion of the students who personally could not wait until the next week to check on their clients.

Not one client lost their home or sustained major physical harm. Many clients had structural or cosmetic damage to homes along with damage to wall hangings and collectables. However, that could not be said of the clients' family members. During the next few weeks, the students were amazed to find that tensions within the families had increased. Many of the clients were having more difficulty obtaining services. Additional communication was maintained through the adult protection and case-management services through the Los Gatos Senior Coordinating Council. During the end of November 1989, the entire crisis situation of the earthquake and its effects were examined through the eyes and analysis of epidemiology and causation.

Primary causes of the increased incidents of elder abuse and neglect were discussed as well as the secondary causes, such as the earthquake, fear of dying, and inability to care for themselves. Through these clinical discussions the students were able to provide counseling and support to the clients and family members. Not one client had to leave home as a direct or indirect result of the earthquake.

The Health Place continues to focus on its dual role as practice arena for nursing students and service arena for elderly clients in their own homes. The future is ensured for at least 3 more years, since a new federal nursing grant has been obtained to examine the outcomes of nursing care in this center as well as two other nurse-managed centers at San Jose State University. The clients and students may change, but the basic philosophy to implement the epidemiologic model in providing care to elders in the community continues as the overall arching goal of the center.

SUMMARY

Principles of epidemiology underlie the interaction between clients, students, and staff in nurse-managed centers. The assessment, measurement, and subsequent analysis of actual or potential health problems is a continual process, forming the basis for nursing care. The Health Place, located in Los Gatos, CA, and managed by the faculty of San Jose State University, models a nurse-managed center with two purposes:(1) to provide educational experiences for gerontology nurse practitioner students; and (2) to provide direct nursing care to elders in the community. The Health Place was created by the faculty as a vehicle for the provision of health care, using nursing models rather than medical models in the direct and indirect client-centered care.

The overall goal of the Health Place is to provide indirect and direct nursing services that allow the elderly clients to remain independently in their own living arrangements as long as possible. Prevention is a key concept used in all aspects of delivery of nursing care. Primary prevention is practiced through health-promotion activities, such as influenza immunization clinics. Secondary prevention is practiced through health screening. When new problems are discovered, the Health Place refers the client to local physicians and licensed agencies if home health care is needed. Tertiary prevention services allow clients to be assisted with activities of daily living and rehabilitation for as long as the clients can stay at home. This entails cooperation between the staff of the Health Place, other health care agencies, and family members.

There are two epidemiologic models that are used at the Health Place. The traditional epidemiologic interactive model of agent, host, and environment is the guiding conceptual framework for programs, such as the city-wide program for prevention of influenza. The web of causation model forms the conceptual framework for community health assessments, where morbidity and mortality data are analyzed according to indices of community health.

Critical Thinking Questions

1. In the past 10 years, the nursing literature has provided descriptions of nurse-managed centers. Select one of the descriptions and apply the principles of epidemiology outlined in this chapter to the description.
2. Give three examples of health-promotion topics that might be presented in an educational session to the older adults who are clients of a nurse-managed center.
3. Identify three screening programs that might be offered to older adults who are clients of a nurse-managed center.

4. Give four examples of indirect or direct nursing services offered by a nurse-managed center that would allow older adults to remain living in the community as long and as independently as possible.
5. Choose a community in your county, and plan a nurse-managed center to help meet the health care needs of the population.
6. Outline the steps in the process that you would use to identify the health needs of the residents in an independent-living housing project for elderly people.
7. Use the components of an epidemiologic model to plan a program to reduce exposure and transmission of the tuberculosis organism in a group of elderly living in a community.

REFERENCES

Clark M: *Nursing in the community,* Norwalk, CT, 1992, Appleton & Lange.

Friedman G: *Primer of epidemiology,* ed 3, New York, 1987, McGraw-Hill.

Mausner J, Kramer S: *Epidemiology—an introductory text,* ed 2, Philadelphia, 1985, WB Saunders.

Stanhope M, Lancaster J: *Community health nursing: process and practice for promoting health,* ed 3, St Louis, 1992, Mosby.

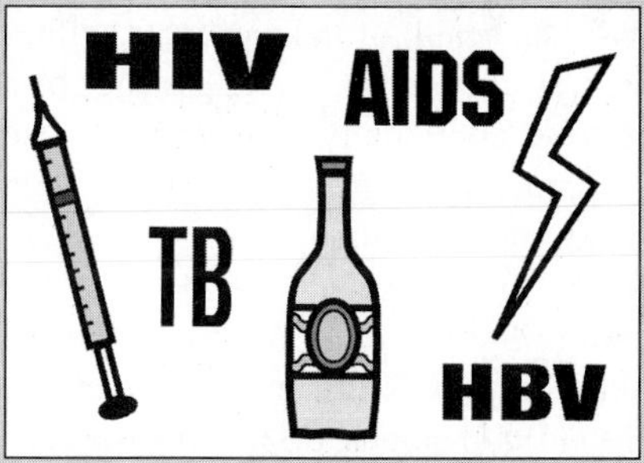

11

Epidemiology in Community Health Nursing Practice

HENRIETTA BERNAL

Objectives

1. Explain the difference between community health nursing practice and practicing in a community-based agency.
2. Give two examples of the historic traditions of community health nursing.
3. Apply the principles of epidemiology in the delivery of community health nursing care in the school, home, workplace, and with special populations.
4. Use epidemiologic principles as a basis for assessment, planning, intervention, and evaluation.

Key Terms

aggregate
community assessment
community health nursing
levels of prevention
  primary
  secondary
  tertiary
occupational health nursing
school nursing

THE CONTEXT OF COMMUNITY HEALTH NURSING PRACTICE

Community health nursing is concerned with the health of individuals, families, and population aggregates. While the specialty focuses on the aggregate, or a population group with common characteristics, community health nurses also provide care to individuals and families in community settings. Involvement with both the individual and family levels provides the opportunity for a clearer understanding of the aggregate (Zerwekh, 1992).

Definitions of community health nursing offered by the American Nurses Association (ANA) (1980) and the Public Health Nursing Section of the American Public Health Association (APHA) (1981) emphasize the link between the two disciplines of nursing and public health. The ANA definition highlights the general nature and comprehensiveness of community health nursing practice (ANA, 1980, p. 2):

> Community health nursing is a synthesis of nursing and public health practice applied to promoting and preserving the health of populations. The practice is general and comprehensive. It is not limited to a particular age group or diagnosis, and is continuing, not episodic. The dominant responsibility is to the population as a whole; nursing directed to individuals, families or groups contributes to the health of the total population. Health promotion, health maintenance, health education, and management, coordination, and continuity of care are utilized in a holistic approach to the management of the health care of individuals, families, and groups in the community.

The APHA definition was presented in a position paper in 1981 with the purpose of presenting a clear statement of public health nursing with an emphasis on public health nursing rather than community health nursing. However, similarities with the ANA definition are evident, since they both emphasize a wide scope of practice and prevention and a view of the *aggregate* as the unit practice. The APHA definition is given below (APHA, 1981, p. 4):

> Public health nursing synthesizes the body of knowledge from the public health sciences and professional nursing theories for the purpose of improving the health of the entire community. This goal lies at the heart of primary prevention and health promotion and is the foundation for public health nursing practice. To accomplish this goal, public health nurses work with groups, families, and individuals as well as in multidisciplinary teams and groups. Identifying the sub groups (aggregates) within the population which are at high risk of illness, disability, or premature death and directing resources toward these groups is the most effective approach for accomplishing the goal of public health nursing. Success in reducing the risk and improving the health of the community depends on involvement of consumers, especially groups experiencing health risks and others in the community in help planning and self help activities.

The central theme in community health nursing is a problem-solving approach that links the nursing process and the epidemiologic process. One of the factors that distinguishes a community health nurse (CHN) is the ability to use these two processes. Community health nursing practice includes a view of the community and the population at risk that goes beyond the skilled care provided by a home care nurse to a hospice client. A CHN, whose population focus is hospice patients, would use the knowledge gained from the individual observations made in the care of specific clients to understand the needs of the group. Intervention would be aggregate-based and include services, such as support groups for clients and families. The CHN would also advocate for additional services, such as volunteer services in the home. It is true that CHNs face many challenges that prevent them from a purely population-based practice (Anderson, 1991; Zerwekh, 1992). Nevertheless, knowledge of the basic epidemiologic process, supported by a systematic approach to assessment, planning, intervention, and evaluation, can help to make the connection between the individual, family, and population group. As pointed out by Zerwekh (1992, p. 1), these associations should proceed in both directions:

> . . . those of us who spend our careers rescuing individuals as clients, who are continually found downstream and drowning, should be encouraged to look upstream to stop aggregate level forces from hurling people into raging stream. Likewise, those of us seeking to stop the collective forces that drown vulnerable populations will grow in wisdom through discovering the extraordinary clinical wisdom developed by going to the people.

The key point in this statement is that CHNs, regardless of setting, will benefit from understanding both the population factors that contribute to health and illness of individuals and families and the data obtained by providing individual and family care. Aggregates may be better understood through the insight that is gained from individual experiences and life patterns that CHNs, such as home care nurses, obtain on their daily visits. However, these insights must be organized and channeled effectively. One way to accomplish this task is to provide models of practice that incorporate epidemiologic principles.

EPIDEMIOLOGIC TRADITIONS OF COMMUNITY HEALTH NURSING

From a historic point of view, there are many examples of the use of epidemiologic principles by nurses. Florence Nightingale's work in Scutari is an excellent example of the use of epidemiology in the assessment and intervention at the aggregate level. Her observations of the total environment of the hospital in which the soldiers in the Crimean War were being treated, and her use of statistics to document observations was essentially a descriptive epidemiology study. Her findings (see Chapter 1) led to major reforms in the sanitary conditions of the military hospital resulting in a lower mortality rate of the soldiers under her care (Kopf, 1991). Nightingale was also instrumental in the development of district nursing in England. She saw the need and the value of nurses going into the home and caring for the sick as well as being concerned for their health. This concern for the effect of the social and physical environment on health status and the role of the nurse in bringing about changes both at the aggregate and individual level places Nightingale at the forefront of community health nursing. Her own words are a testament to this:

> "The work that we are doing has nothing to do with nursing disease, but with maintaining health by removing the things which disturb it . . . . dirk, drink, diet, damp, draughts, and drains" (Monteiro, 1985, p. 182).

In the United States, the work of Lillian Wald in the Henry Street Settlement House stands as the shining example for all CHNs. Her work is as relevant today as it was in the late nineteenth century and early twentieth century. Urban communities today would be well-served by the programs and initiatives that Wald developed in the Henry Street community. Wald was an astute observer of the environment around her. These observations led to a number of interventions. Playgrounds were established to keep children off the street and prevent childhood injuries; *school nursing* was established to keep children in school, while being treated for health problems; and home care nursing was developed to ensure healthy maternal deliveries and help families survive illness. Her concern for disease prevention, health promotion, and care of mothers and children extended far beyond the individual and family level. Wald was a political and community activist who saw the need to intervene at the social system level and change the environmental and socioeconomic factors that contributed to the health status of her community (Wald, 1938).

Both of these examples show the use of epidemiologic principles through the assessment of host, environment, and agent factors that contribute to health and illness. They also demonstrate problem-solving strategies in primary, secondary, and tertiary prevention within the context of a caring paradigm (see Chapter 2). In other words, Florence Nightingale and Lillian Wald demonstrated community health nursing at its very best.

EPIDEMIOLOGIC APPLICATIONS IN COMMUNITY HEALTH NURSING

In the school

Never in the history of community health nursing have so many challenges been present in the schools. Although the environmental conditions of crowded classrooms and lack of adequate facilities that characterized schools in the early part of the twentieth century have improved, the problems that children bring with them have become more challenging and complex.

Drugs and alcohol, acquired immunodeficiency syndrome (AIDS), teen pregnancy, and the threat of crime and violence in schools and neighborhoods make attending school a high-risk activity for many children. In addition, the movement toward integrating the disabled child into the mainstream educational process poses new responsibilities on the school health services (Zanga and Oda, 1987).

In one inner-city school in a northeastern region of the United States, the principal of an elementary school reported that 25% to 30% of the children entering that school came from substance-abusing homes. Many of these children displayed behavioral problems that could be attributed to fetal alcohol syndrome and/or that reflected the family problems associated with drug abuse. How does a nurse working in this environment practice community health nursing, using principles of epidemiology to improve the health conditions of the school community and beyond?

First and foremost, a school nurse must be able to assess the problems that are presented on a daily basis by the children. The nurse must also conduct a *community assessment* for factors that contribute to the health and illness conditions that children present in the school setting. Using assessment skills, the school nurse, can observe and document the physical, developmental, and behavioral problems of children with fetal alcohol syndrome. These cumulative observations can lead to a view of the aggregate that may provide the data needed to develop a community outreach program in the school. Using the descriptive data derived from individual assessments, the school nurse can gain the cooperation of the school principal in developing a task force that could include parents, teachers, and community leaders. The nurse's knowledge of epidemiology could direct the task force to develop strategies in *primary, secondary,* and *tertiary prevention.*

The school nurse practices as a CHN by incorporating the larger community or population group in the plan of care. Puerto Rican children living in inner-city communities have been found to have a higher-than-expected prevalence of asthmatic conditions (Guarnaccia, 1985). Understanding the risk factors that contribute to this high prevalence is of paramount importance in helping children and families prevent and ameliorate the condition. The health teaching that the school nurse can do at the individual, family, and community levels can be instrumental in raising awareness and influencing change. Furthermore, the school nurse involvement with other interested individuals can bring pressure to those people in political office resulting in policy change in the community. Conditions, such as poor housing and air pollution, that contribute to increased episodes of asthma can be addressed. These are *primary prevention* activities.

At the level of *secondary prevention,* the nurse can ensure that prompt treatment is initiated when a child experiences an acute attack of asthma. The nurse can advocate for clinic services in the school so that children are not kept waiting for appointments. Working with other members of the school team, the nurse can facilitate development of a school environment that increases the potential for achieving maximum success for the asthmatic child *(tertiary prevention)* by instructing teachers of the need to reduce risk factors in the classroom.

The school nurse uses principles of epidemiology in all aspects of nursing practice. These principles include disease surveillance, provision of routine immunizations, reporting safety hazards in the environment, and providing health education to children, parents, and teachers. The role of school nursing is central to the prevention of disease and disability and the promotion of health for a most important aggregate—school children.

CASE EXAMPLE

Lisa is a school nurse who works in a bilingual elementary school in a large, metropolitan area. The children that attend this school come from homes that have many social and economic problems. Her observations of the school's neighborhood and her many contacts with the parents and community agencies have made her aware of the increasing problem of substance abuse in the community served by the school. Lisa makes many referrals to the visiting nurse serving the same area and obtains feedback from her about the poor parenting skills and home life of the school children she has referred. Lisa has gained a reputation as a caring and knowledgeable individual and is asked to join a consortium of community agencies who want to bring changes in the neighborhood. Funds are obtained from a local foundation to conduct a community-based study that will identify the patterns of drug and alcohol use in the community. As a result of this study, collaboration of these groups, and her strong advocacy, major initiatives took place. A new residential program for drug addicts was instituted based on a well-known, long-term treatment program. A school-based preventive program for drug and alcohol abuse was initiated by a community-based agency. In-service programs for the teachers were organized to prepare them to cope with the behavioral problems presented by the children who came from these at-risk homes.

In this case example, the school nurse intervened at the aggregate level by collaborating with community groups and initiating a school-based drug and alcohol prevention program (primary prevention). She was instrumental in developing a treatment program for drug-abusing parents and other members of the target population (secondary prevention). Lisa showed additional concern by initiating an educational program with the local university to prepare teachers to deal with the children who had been affected by alcohol and drugs, thus improving the children's performance. This strategy had the potential for improving the children's functions in class and the home and preventing further cognitive disability (tertiary prevention).

In the workplace

The work environment presents an excellent opportunity for CHNs to apply principles of epidemiology. Working Americans spend at least one-third of their day in the workplace and workers represent about 80% of the population. Providing community health nursing services can have a positive influence on worker's health outcomes (Clark, 1992). It is in the self-interest of employers to have healthy employees who can work to their greatest potential, and who do not lose days of work because of illness or disability. The workplace provides an opportunity to prevent disease and disability and promotes healthy life-styles and a safe work environment. While other health care workers have the problem of motivating people to follow healthy-living recommendations, community health nurses working in industry have a captive audience who is motivated by the need to work. This presents a unique opportunity for applying the key principles of epidemiology.

Moreland (1989) has identified an epidemiology-based model of practice for occupational health professionals that involves four steps. These steps include (1) recognition of early warning factors for injury or disease; (2) evaluation of high-risk groups with health surveillance data; (3) provision of environmental controls to prevent disease and injury; and (4) coordination, implementation and re-evaluation of programs. The scope of practice of the *occupational health nursing* as presented by Rogers (1991) incorporates these concepts within the nursing process (see the box that follows).

RESPONSIBILITIES OF THE OCCUPATIONAL HEALTH NURSE

Assessing worker health and work environments, including identification of hazardous exposures at the work site and appropriate use of protective equipment
Providing direct care specifically related to occupational illness and injuries
Identifying potential and actual occupational health threats from biologic, physical, biochemical, chemical, and psychosocial agents
Planning, implementing, and evaluating worker health programs
Designing appropriate intervention strategies for health promotion and protection of the work force
Conducting research and improving the health of workers

From Rogers B: Occupational health nursing education, *AACHN,* 39(3):101-108, 1991.

Specific tasks that the occupational health nurse performs may include preemployment assessment including life-style risk assessments. These assessments provide counseling opportunities to help workers reduce high-risk behaviors both at home and in the workplace. The occupational health nurse may promote early detection of disease through screening tests, such as the monitoring of blood lead levels. A nurse may monitor hazards at work, such as exposure to radiation, noise, or heat; conduct health-promotion campaigns, such as stress reduction or self-breast examinations; and/or implement systems of injury and disease surveillance, such as monitoring blood levels of lead, the incidence of contact dermitis, and eye injuries.

The first step in the development of a primary accident prevention program includes assessment of the work environment in conjunction with other members of the occupational health team, and the development of a data base that can identify patterns of injury. For example, back injuries represent a major problem in such workplaces as hospitals, home care agencies, and heavy industry. The heavy lifting required in these settings places certain individuals at high risk for back injury. The occupational health nurse should collect data describing where, when and to whom the injuries are occurring. This assessment of the host and environment can lead to effective identification of the high-risk individuals and work areas. This epidemiologic investigation is the first step in effective program planning. Programs might include classes on proper body mechanics, changes in the environment contributing to injury, and the development of light work programs to return the injured worker back to work as soon as possible (Owen, 1991).

CASE EXAMPLE

Joe is a community health nurse working in an employee health clinic in a midsize urban hospital. He has been keeping records of the back injuries that have been reported during the past 6 months. It is time to analyze the data that he has been collecting for the purpose of identifying the individuals getting injured, and the patient units in which they work. Joe finds that the two areas with the highest reported rate of injuries is the neurointensive and general intensive care units; these are closely followed by the geriatric unit. Applying a patient classification system, he finds that patients in these units have the highest level of dependency and require assistance for most of their activities including turning in bed and transfers. His analysis of the characteristics of the personnel being injured reveal a high percent of nonprofessional personnel, such as nursing assistants and primary care nurses. This analysis prompted him to conduct some direct observations of the personnel in these high-risk units to observe their transfer techniques and the environmental factors contributing to the injuries. He noted that poor body mechanics were used, side rails were left up when trying to move patients, and the turning or transferring of heavy patients was done without help. Crowded areas around the patient's bed meant that nursing care personnel often used twisting and reaching body mechanics to take blood pressures on bed-bound patients. These observations, together with the other data he had collected, made a strong case to present to his employer. He was able to advocate for an injury prevention program that would include health education, environmental adjustments, and a light work program for injured employees.

In the above example, the nurse has used major principles of epidemiology. First, the nurse used a technique of data collection that focused on identifying high-risk individuals and environments. Secondly, the nurse identified specific factors that contributed to the injuries. The nurse then applied the levels of prevention framework with a plan of action that included primary prevention strategies, such as body mechanics classes for employees working in high-risk areas, and tertiary prevention through a light work program.

With special populations

The human immunodeficiency (HIV)/AIDS epidemic has demonstrated, in ways that never could have been imagined in modern times, how vulnerable human beings are to the effects of microorganisms and how important human behavior is in the prevention of disease. The complexities of AIDS has challenged the creative capacity of all health professionals to develop effective health education strategies to lower the incidence of the disease. Community health nurses working in the community have the opportunity to interact with special population groups that could benefit from their skill and knowledge in preventing the spread of HIV. Many population groups today present difficult challenges for applying basic epidemiologic principles and traditional community health strategies that could stem the tide of the AIDS epidemic. For example, certain behaviors, such as intravenous drug use and the practice of unsafe sex, place hard-to-reach individuals at higher risk for acquiring the infection. Lacking both an effective vaccine and a treatment for the cure of AIDS, the most effective method of controlling the epidemic has been health education preventive strategies. However, reaching some groups, such as intravenous drug users, and getting them to change some of their behaviors has been difficult to achieve.

HIV infection is increasing among female populations around the world. One high-risk group of women are prostitutes who do not practice safe sex. In some parts of the world women may augment their income to send their children to school by selling sex (Schoepf and Schoepf, 1988). Others may be forced by a drug habit to walk the streets in search of income to support their habit. Some become infected through their partners who are having sex with other women. In Haiti, for example, one study found that one in 10 pregnant women (not prostitutes) were infected by HIV (Palca, 1991). Even when women are aware of the dangers of practicing unsafe sex, lack of knowledge and control over their lives may place them at high risk. In a study conducted in Santo Domingo, women in the sex industry were found to lack knowledge on the appropriate way to apply condoms (Pareja and others, 1989). For the most part, these women were not making decisions about the use of condoms. Men were the final decision-makers. Therefore while the rate of AIDS is increasing among women, they are not in control of decisions that affect their health.

Whatever the reasons, women who sell sex, abuse drugs, and live with substance-abusing partners or partners who are not monogamous represent a special population in need of community health nursing intervention. Identifying and working with these women needs to be a high priority, since much more is at stake than their own health. In many cases, the health of their unborn or living children and the men with whom they come in contact are also at risk.

CASE EXAMPLE

Sue works in the city health department of a large, metropolitan area. Her district is known for the high levels of prostitution. Sue has seen many of these women at the sexually transmitted disease (STD) clinic and has decided to collect some data about their use of condoms. During the examination of these women she asks about their use of condoms. Slowly a picture begins to emerge that concerns her. Although all the women have heard of condoms, she discovers that a significant percent do not use them on a consistent basis, because either they do not carry them or their partners do not want them to use them. In fact, they may get paid a higher fee if they do not use them. In addition, when she asked them to explain how they apply the condoms she discovers that the majority were not using them properly. With this information, she alerted the health director who formed a committee to look further into this issue. The result of this investigation led to a policy, whereby every woman seen at the STD clinic was given an information session about condoms, including how to apply them correctly. The client was also given a supply of condoms. A community education campaign was implemented using outreach workers from the community. The emphasis was on not only giving out the condoms but also educating the women and men on the correct use of condoms.

In this case study, Sue has demonstrated that importance of using epidemiology as a framework for practice and assessing the high-risk behavior of a special population by implementing programs that could decrease their exposure to HIV.

USING KEY EPIDEMIOLOGIC CONCEPTS IN THE CLINICAL PRACTICE OF COMMUNITY HEALTH NURSING

Individual, family and community assessment

The assessment of individuals, families, and communities is the most important step in the nursing process for CHNs. The gathering of accurate data about the biologic, environmental, and sociocultural factors that may contribute to health and illness is essential to develop an appropriate plan of care from which primary, secondary, and tertiary prevention interventions will be derived. As shown in other examples, epidemiology principles can be used as an overall framework to direct the types of data to be collected. For example, at the individual level, the gathering of a family health history that reveals a genetic predisposition to hypertension can trigger screening of the rest of the family for evidence of hypertension. This, in turn, can direct health teaching to reduce the risks of hypertension through proper nutrition, exercise, and stress-reduction techniques.

There are a variety of ways that CHNs can gather data. As illustrated by the above example, data from health histories can provide clues for more data gathering through screening. Intake interview data that CHNs collect in a variety of settings can yield valuable data for understanding patterns of disease and disability. For example, having noticed that expectant mothers are entering prenatal care late in the pregnancy, a CHN can keep track of the number of women that respond in this way. With sufficient documentation of the number of cases within a certain time frame and the demographics of the cases, the nurse will be able to develop a more appropriate intervention and may advocate for greater support for the aggregate (Hood, 1985). The intervention may help individual women seek early prenatal care and prevent some of the complications that occur as a result of late entry into the health care system. It is this individual-aggregate-individual approach, which is most desirable in the practice of community health nursing. The community health nurse can also provide rich, contextual case data that help nurses and other health professionals to better understand the barriers that prevent these women from early prenatal care.

In addition to the collection of data through intake interviews, CHNs can gather observational data as they interact in the homes, neighborhoods, community centers, and other community environments. Most CHNs have stories to tell about the observations that they have made as they walk or drive through the community. The Windshield Assessment (Anderson and McFarlane, 1988) is a good observational approach that uses all of the senses to gather environmental data about the neighborhood and community where clients live. CHNs through their acute, observational skills, may notice the absence of screens in windows, broken banisters, unlit hallways, peeling paint, uncollected garbage, housing violations, rodent and pest infestation, and other environmental hazards. These hazards, if left unattended, can lead to accidents, disability, or illness.

CHNs can also participate in other forms of data gathering, such as the investigation of food-poisoning outbreaks. The CHN, as part of the public health department team, may be called on to conduct structured interviews to identify the common denominator present in all of the individuals who were sick in an outbreak of staphylococcal food poisoning. The nurse would look at such factors as the characteristics of the persons who were infected, environment or place where the outbreak occurred, characteristics of the agent, and time of day or season of the year when the outbreak occurred. For example, a series of interviews may reveal that all individuals who become ill had eaten chicken with white sauce from a particular fast-food place on a particular day in a given location. Investigating the food handlers may lead to an individual who prepared the meat and had an open, draining wound on the hand. In a large health department, other nonnurse professionals may be primarily involved in food-borne disease investigations. However, in small public health departments the community health nurse will do much of the interviewing and data gathering (Higgs and Gustefson, 1985).

CHN can also be involved in more formal community assessments in which data are gathered to better identify the problems, needs, and resources present in the community. The need may be triggered by a crisis event, such as an earthquake (Higgs and Gustefson, 1985), lack of data about the community, or changes occurring in the demographic profile that merit analysis. Identification of high-risk groups would be an important outcome of this assessment. Through this process more appropriate interventions are indentified as well as a plan for the use of existing resources.

CASE EXAMPLE

Changing demographics reveal a large increase of Hispanic people in an urban community. The local visiting nurse association has begun to notice an increase in the referrals for the care of newly diagnosed diabetic clients. A search of the literature revealed recent data from the Hispanic Health and Nutrition Examination Survey (HHANES) which indicates that Puerto Ricans and Mexican Americans have an 11.3% and 13.4% rate of diabetes as compared with 5% for the rest of the population (Perez-Stable and others, 1989). Further analysis of records revealed that most of the clients who have been referred were middle-age women who were first diagnosed due to an acute crisis, such as surgery, vaginal infection, or symptomatic hyperglycemia. Further investigation showed that most of this group of clients are being seen by hospital-based clinics due to poor health insurance coverage and reluctance on the part of private providers to see Medicaid clients. The nurses analyze these data and decide on a course of action to improve the early detection of diabetes in the Hispanic population. Interventions included a media campaign conducted in collaboration with an Hispanic advocacy group and highlighted the importance of early detection, weight control, and increased physical exercise. Other interventions included increased screening of family members of diagnosed diabetic clients and improved communication with the hospital-based clinics through the diabetic education nurse specialist.

In the above example, the nurses first observed a problem, but needed further data to validate their observation. The literature provided the support they needed to show that as an aggregate, the Hispanic community was indeed at higher risk for developing diabetes. In addition, the case data provided a key to the health care access issues for this population. These data highlighted the need for early detection, and so a media campaign was designed in conjunction with the Latino agencies to educate the public and promote early detection.

All nurses must guard against premature closure of problems due to lack of data. The assessment process that begins with the gathering of data and concludes with a nursing diagnosis or problem identification is time-consuming and complex. However, the alternative is not acceptable. Early closure of cases, unresolved problems, missed opportunities for prevention and health promotion, and

KEY ASPECTS OF THE PLANNING PROCESS

Categorizing
Prioritizing
Developing program objectives
Consumer involvement

failure to understand the risk profile of individuals, families, and communities is unacceptable.

Planning

Planning activities are key to the efficient and accurate delivery of care to clients. Many aspects of planning are presented in Chapter 14. However, it is important to point out the key steps and their relationship to the epidemiologic process (see the box above).

Categorizing. Both the nursing process and the epidemiologic process require that data be categorized to facilitate analysis and priority setting. Lacking a coherent format to look at the data, the nurse could easily miss the important information. Either through existing or new formats, data can be categorized in ways that can give clear direction for effective planning. Data on individuals and families could be organized into such categories as: life-style risk behaviors, environmental hazards, stressful life events, exposure to heavy metals, or immunization history. Having categorized data in this manner, the nurse discovers that 25% of the clients under his or her care have incomplete immunizations, 50% smoke cigarettes, and 10% have high blood pressure. These statistics provide valuable information for the next steps in the planning process.

Prioritizing. Determining priorities may initially seem simple, but it can be very complex when the cost/benefit ratio is considered. Whose priorities are considered—those of the group or health care system? What program will give the greatest benefit for the money spent? Should long-term or short-term results be of concern?

Developing program objectives. Setting priorities and objectives requires an overall framework that will direct the decision-making process. A levels of prevention model can give direction to the planning effort. Some would say that all of the risks that have been identified are equally important, but the community representatives may decide that primary prevention is more essential. Immunizations are available to protect the young who are the future of the community. Whatever the final decision, it is important to have a framework to help in the decision-making process. The levels of prevention model is one approach that can be effectively used.

Developing program objectives follows the establishment of priorities. Objectives need to be written that pertain to each priority and reflect measurable outcomes. Both long-term and short-term objectives may be necessary to guide the plan. Having decided that levels of prevention will guide the decision-making

PROGRAM OBJECTIVES FOR AN UNDER-IMMUNIZED COHORT OF CHILDREN

Primary prevention

All children entering school will have completed the required immunizations.

Of the parents of children attending primary grades, 50% will be contacted by the end of the first marking period and given information about immunizations schedules and resources.

Secondary prevention

School-based clinical services will be developed in this fiscal year to treat common health problems, such as otitis media.

Tertiary prevention

All hearing-impaired children through the first six grades will be provided with hearing evaluations and referrals on a yearly basis.

process, the objectives would also be influenced by this model. Objectives could be written that would reflect primary, secondary, and tertiary prevention for each priority. The box above reflects levels of prevention for an under-immunized cohort of children.

Consumer involvement. Consumer involvement, has proved to be difficult to achieve, although it is often recommended. However, to gain cooperation and collaboration from the target community or population group, grass roots participation by those who will be affected needs to occur at all levels of the planning process. This requires building coalitions with community groups that can help identify the reasons for poor immunization coverage in the community. Consumers can also be involved in establishing priorities and developing realistic, achievable objectives. The health professional team can educate the community regarding the benefits of prevention, screening, and prompt treatment to reduce disability and death. An involved consumer group can bring about change in the way services are delivered that will benefit the community as a whole. For example, having failed to gain the interest and concern over their plight, a group of Latino HIV-positive clients formed their own advocacy group. Aided by health professionals in a northeastern city, they formed a coalition with Latino health providers, health educators, and advocates and were incorporated. After obtaining funding, they conducted a variety of programs across all levels of prevention, including community health education and the provision of home-based treatment for Latino AIDS clients and support groups for partners and significant others.

Intervention

CHNs are engaged in significant interventions that can have a major impact on all levels of health for individuals, families, and aggregates. Community health nurs-

Table 11-1 Community health nursing interventions

Primary	Secondary	Tertiary
Teaching	Teaching	Teaching
Anticipatory guidance	Anticipatory guidance	Anticipatory guidance
Referral	Referral	Referral
Political action	Political action	Political action
Advocacy	Advocacy	Advocacy
Counseling	Counseling	Counseling
Examinations	Treatments	Rehabilitation
	Case finding	Case finding
	Assist families to provide care	Assist families to provide care
	Conduct support groups	Conduct support groups
	Provide respite care	Provide respite care
	Screening	Hospice

ing interventions can be categorized along the levels of the prevention continuum as shown in Table 11-1.

These interventions do not represent an exhaustive list. Some of the interventions could appear in more than one column, for example, examinations and treatments. This categorization is meant to illustrate that CHNs intervene at key points in the continuum of the disease process (prepathogenesis/pathogenesis/postpathogenesis) using primary, secondary, and tertiary interventions (see Chapter 2). In addition community health nurses intervene to reduce the agent, host, and environmental factors that interact to produce illness and disability.

CASE EXAMPLE

The local health department has contracted with a homeless center to provide community health nursing service to a homeless population consisting mostly of women and children. The CHN health nurse who has been assigned to serve the needs of this population realizes that he must assess the needs and develop programs that will address a variety of primary, secondary, and tertiary interventions. One of the needs that he sees quite readily is the need for better nutrition. Having observed the diet given to the women and children he concludes that the diet served at the shelter lacks certain essential nutrients, especially iron. He also observes that mothers are giving nonnutritious snacks to the children. A variety of interventions are carried out that can be categorized across the three levels of prevention. First, an education-information program is initiated for residents and staff, placing posters and other materials in strategic areas at the shelter. A nutritionist is consulted from the state health department, and menu review and consultation is provided. Hemoglobin/hematocrit screening is conducted on the children and women to screen for iron-deficiency anemia. Iron supplements are provided by a local pharmaceutical company.

In this example the nurse has used a variety of the interventions: education, referral, advocacy, screening, and treatment which promote prevention at all levels.

Evaluation

The final step in the nursing process is the evaluation of the outcomes of care using the planned objectives or criteria. Evaluation is a much easier process when clear outcome criteria have been established. In the example of the homeless center, the community health nurse could have established an outcome measure like: 100% of the children will be tested for iron-deficiency anemia within the first month of the program. This type of criteria provides a useful evaluation benchmark. Measuring program effectiveness can provide a stimulus for changing or revising the original program objectives. It could be that given the transient nature of the population, achieving the level of testing desired is not possible. Changes might need to be made regarding the timing of the testing. Keeping records that give data about the process would help to identify the location in the sequence of events, which one would need to make changes to test a majority of the children and mothers.

SUMMARY

Community health nurses, have had a long tradition of delivering care to individuals, families, and aggregates using principles of epidemiology. As community health nurses deliver care in schools, the home, the workplace, and homeless centers, they can be aided in their work by the use of models like the epidemiologic model. Understanding the natural history of disease, using biostatistics to analyze data, and using the levels of prevention as a framework for assessment, planning, intervention, and evaluation are tangible ways in which the work of CHNs are helped by a good understanding of key principles of epidemiology.

Critical Thinking Questions

1. Identify the major difference between community health nursing and working in the community.
2. Discuss the strategies Florence Nightingale and Lillian Wald used to assess and intervene at the aggregate level.
3. Give examples of two special populations—other than the ones cited in this chapter—to which community health nurses might deliver care.
4. Explain the techniques a community health nurse might use to assess, plan, intervene, and evaluate care for the identified, special population.

REFERENCES

American Nurses Association: *A conceptual model of community health nursing practice,* Kansas City, MO, 1980, The Association.

American Public Health Association: The definition and role of public health nursing in the delivery of health care, Washington, DC, 1981, The Association.

Anderson ET: A call for transformation (editorial), *Public Health Nurs* 8:1, 1991.

Anderson ET, McFarlane JM: *Community as a client: an application of the nursing process,* Philadelphia, 1988, JB Lippincott.

Clark JC: *Nursing in the community,* Norwalk, CT, 1992, Appleton & Lange.

Guarnaccia PJ, Pelto PJ, Schensul SL: Family health culture, ethnicity and asthma: coping with illness, *Med Anthropol* 9:203-223, 1985.

Higgs ET, Gufstafson DD: *Community diagnosis, community as a client: assessment and diagnosis,* Philadelphia, 1985, FA Davis.

Hood GH: Epidemiology. In Garvis LJ, editor: *Community health nursing: keeping the public healthy,* Philadelphia, 1985, FA Davis.

Kopf EW: Florence Nightingale as a statistician. In Spradley BW, editor: *Readings in community health nursing,* Boston, 1991, Little, Brown, pp 93-98.

Monteiro LA: Florence Nightingale on public health nursing, *Am J Public Health* 75:181-182, 1985.

Moreland RF: Epidemiologic considerations for the occupational health professional, *AAOHN J* 37(6): 215-220, 1989.

Owen BD: Reducing risk for back pain in nursing personnel. *AAOHN J* 39(1): 24-33, 1991.

Palca J: The sobering geography of AIDS, *Science* 252:372-373, 1991.

Pareja R and others: Santo Domingo female sex workers' use and handling of condoms: knowledge and skills, *Exchange* World Health Organization, 2:6-9, 1989.

Perez-Stable and others: Self-reported diabetes in Mexican Americans: HHANES 1982-1984, *Am J Public Health* 79: 770-772, 1989.

Schoepf BG and others: A view from Zaire. In *Aids in Africa,* Lewiston, New York, 1988, Edwin Mellen, pp 211-235.

Stanhope M, Lancaster J: *Community health nursing,* ed 3, St Louis, 1984, Mosby, pp 127-128.

Wald LD: *The house on Henry street,* New York, 1938, Henry Holt.

Zanga JR, Oda DS: School health services, *J School Health* 57:413-416, 1987.

Zerwekh J: Community health nurses—a population at risk (editorial), *Public Health Nurs* 9:1, 1992.

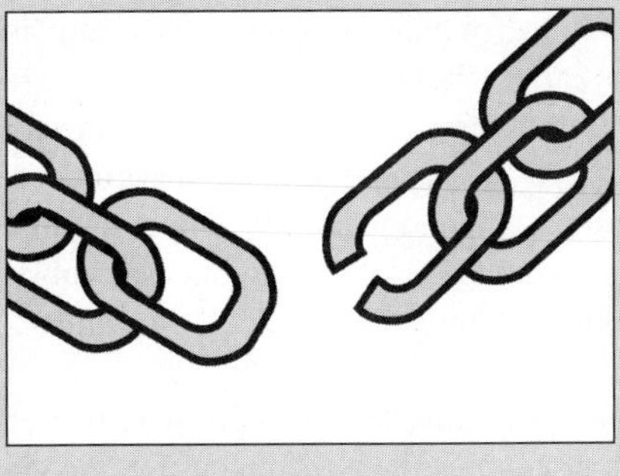

12

Epidemiology in Infection Control Practice

SANDRA BLAKE

Objectives

1. Define nosocomial infection.
2. Trace the evolution of hospital infection control programs.
3. List the functions of advisory and regulatory agencies.
4. Outline the structure and organization of infection control programs.
5. Explain the role of the infection control practitioner.
6. Describe the process of surveillance and reporting of nosocomial infections.
7. Differentiate between total house surveillance, priority-directed surveillance, and problem-oriented surveillance.
8. Diagram the process of analysis and reporting of nosocomial infection data.
9. Summarize the outbreak investigation process.
10. Discuss the expanded role of hospital epidemiology.

Key Terms

Centers for Disease Control and Prevention (CDC)
device-associated infection
hospital epidemiology
infection control committee
infection control practitioner
infection control program
Joint Commission on Accreditation of Healthcare Organizations (JCAHO)
National Nosocomial Infections Surveillance (NNIS)
nosocomial infection
Occupational Safety and Health Administration (OSHA)
priority-directed surveillance
problem-oriented surveillance
Study on the Efficacy of Nosocomial Infection Control (SENIC)
total house surveillance

EVOLUTION OF HOSPITAL INFECTION CONTROL PROGRAMS

Infection control practice as a specialty area for nurses began emerging in American hospitals in the late 1960s. By early 1980, most hospitals had employed an *infection control practitioner* (ICP) to coordinate a hospital-wide infection control program. Components of these programs included surveillance and analysis of nosocomial (hospital-acquired) infections and development and implementation of prevention and control measures. These programs probably represent the first application of epidemiologic methods by hospitals to evaluate adverse patient outcomes.

Although formal *hospital epidemiology* programs did not appear until the middle of the twentieth century, the need for such programs was identified much earlier by pioneers in health care. Ignaz Semmelweis is recognized as the father of hospital infection control because of his early use of epidemiologic techniques in documenting a hospital outbreak. Semmelweis was an obstetrician at the Lying-in Hospital in Vienna in 1847. The hospital was divided into two divisions. Division I was a teaching service staffed by medical students, and Division II was staffed by midwives. Semmelweis collected data regarding maternal deaths and noted that 10% of the women delivered by Division I died, while only 3% of the women in Division II died. Semmelweis noted that medical students of Division I generally entered the delivery room directly from the autopsy suite. He also noted that midwife trainees did not do autopsies. Semmelweis reasoned that the hands of medical students were contaminated by cadaveric materials and required that all students scrub their hands in chlorinated lime until the smell of cadavers was gone from their hands. Subsequently, he documented a dramatic decline in mortality from puerperal sepsis so that the mortality rate in the first division was similar to that in the second division staffed by midwives (LaForce, 1987).

Florence Nightingale is one of the first nurses to participate in hospital infection control. Teamed with William Farr, a British health statistician, Nightingale began to analyze mortality data from British hospitals. In her *Notes on Hospitals,* Nightingale suggested that a direct relationship existed between the sanitary conditions of a hospital and postoperative complications. She proposed a comprehensive reporting system for deaths in hospitals and suggested that ward sisters could maintain these statistical records. Her book also contains Farr's analysis of mortality among hospital employees, which suggests that mortality from contagious diseases was more common among hospital personnel than non-health care workers (LaForce, 1987).

Despite the work of these early pioneers, infection control in hospitals did not receive much attention until the 1950s when hospitals experienced epidemics of penicillin-resistant *Staphylococcus aureus.* Epidemics of staphylococcal infections in surgical and pediatric patients were the main impetus for the development of hospital epidemiology as a recognized discipline (LaForce, 1987). During the 1960s, infection control committees were formed in many hospitals, and various approaches to infection surveillance were initiated. However, early efforts tended to emphasize extensive environmental culturing, even though such microbiologic surveillance had not been shown to be effective in preventing hospital-acquired infections (Thompson, 1987).

In 1970, the First International Conference on Nosocomial Infections was sponsored by the *Centers for Disease Control (CDC),* the American Hospital Association (AHA), and the American Public Health Association. Out of this conference, two needs were identified: the need for surveillance and the need to document the efficacy of nosocomial infection control measures (Eickhoff, 1991). At this time, the hospital infection control movement was in its early development and professional organizations, such as the Association for Practitioners in Infection Control (APIC) and the Society for Hospital Epidemiologists of America (SHEA), were nonexistent. The only agencies calling attention to the problem of nosocomial infections were the Hospital Infections Branch of the CDC and the AHA's Advisory Committee on Infections within Hospitals (Eickhoff, 1991). One U.S. book on the subject of infection control had been published by the AHA in 1968. The Joint Commission for Accreditation of Hospitals (JCAH) had not yet developed standards specifically for infection control practice. In 1970, less than 10% of American hospitals had an ICP, less than 10% had policies requiring IV line changes, less than 10% had adopted closed urinary drainage systems, and slightly more than 10% had policies related to ventilator circuit changes (Haley and others, 1980). During this era, only 40% of U.S. hospitals had a surveillance program. By 1976, this percentage increased to 83%.

The Second International Conference on Nosocomial Infections sponsored by the CDC was held in August, 1980. By this time, the average U.S. hospital had an infection control program that was 5 years old (Dixon, 1991). Concerns identified at this meeting were the expanding use of invasive devices, patterns of antimicrobial use, sicker, hospitalized patients being discharged earlier, and personnel and resources being diverted from infection control (Dixon, 1991). The Third International Conference on Nosocomial Infections (1990) reemphasized these concerns and the emergence of resistant organisms. The 1990s present new areas of concern in terms of hospital infection control. Goals of current hospital infection control programs are focused in two areas: the safety of health care workers and the protection of patients from acquisition of nosocomial infections.

ADVISORY AND REGULATORY AGENCIES

The CDC has long been involved in the development of guidelines for infection control programs. The Hospital Infections Program of the Center for Infectious Diseases of the CDC has provided a major service by developing a manual entitled, *Guidelines for the Prevention and Control of Nosocomial Infection* (Simmons, 1981). These guidelines relate to the control and prevention of nosocomial urinary tract infections, intravascular infections, surgical wound infections, and respiratory infections. Unfortunately, these guidelines have not been revised since publication in 1981.

The *Joint Commission on Accreditation of Healthcare Organizations (JCAHO)* has become very involved in standards for hospital infection control practice. The JCAHO standards for 1994 require hospital infection control committees to recommend and approve surveillance programs based on previous nosocomial infection findings. The standard also requires the establishment of hospital-wide infection control policies and procedures and regular continuing education for all hospital employees in matters regarding infection control (JCAHO, 1994).

Recently, the *Occupational Safety and Health Administration (OSHA)* has published a regulatory document entitled *The OSHA Bloodborne Pathogen Standard.* This document requires that all employers of health care workers provide employees an environment safe from exposure to bloodborne pathogens (US Department of Labor, 1991). Regulations are also being developed regarding care of patients with tuberculosis.

APIC is the national professional organization for ICPs in the United States. The organization provides resources to its membership in a variety of ways. Educational programs are provided locally and at the national level. In addition, members receive the *American Journal of Infection Control.* The organization has been active in developing practice guidelines for ICPs. A separate board for certification of ICPs has been established. Certification assures that a basic level of knowledge and skill is possessed by those persons certified in the practice of infection control.

STRUCTURE AND ORGANIZATION OF INFECTION CONTROL PROGRAMS

The components of an *infection control program* can be divided into two general categories: surveillance and reporting, and control and prevention. *Surveillance* and reporting activities include data collection, tabulation, and analysis of infections occurring in patients and personnel in the health care institution. Certain areas of the hospital environment may also be monitored. In addition, the infection control program personnel are usually responsible for reporting all communicable diseases to the appropriate health authorities.

Control and prevention activities include teaching and consulting. New employees must be oriented to infection control principles, isolation policies, and appropriate infection control procedures. In addition to formal and informal teaching, the infection control practitioner is often consulted regarding questions pertinent to isolation of a patient or specific procedure guidelines. Teaching and consultation activities do not always occur within the health care institution and may extend to people not employed by the hospital, such as health sciences students or personnel from other health care facilities in the community.

Another aspect of the prevention and control activities pertain to administrative responsibilities. The ICP is usually responsible for the coordination and development of a hospital-wide infection control manual. This manual contains hospital policies and procedures related to infection control. In addition, the ICP may serve on other administrative committees, such as the safety, product standardization, and pharmacy and therapeutics committees. The ICP is recognized as the hospital's expert on infection control matters.

Special studies constitute another component of the prevention and control activities. When surveillance activities detect a problem or when a new procedure or product requires evaluation, special studies may be instituted. The ICP is usually the person coordinating these investigations or evaluations.

According to the JCAHO, a multidisciplinary committee must oversee the program for surveillance, prevention, and control of infection. The *infection control committee* (ICC) is charged with providing structure and direction to the infection control program. During the meetings of the ICC, members review surveillance data, policies and procedures, and any special investigations or studies. The ICC then makes recommendations to appropriate groups or departments in the hospital for action to be taken. At a future meeting, the proposed interventions are then evaluated to determine whether the problem has been resolved or whether further recommendations are necessary.

Committee membership includes representatives from the medical staff, nursing, administration, and the person directly responsible for the management of the infection control program. Representatives from housekeeping, central services, laundry, the dietetic department, the engineering and maintenance department, pharmacy, and the operating room suite may also be members or may serve on a consultative basis.

The ICC is chaired by a person, usually a physician, who possesses credentials that document knowledge and interest or experience in infection control. Chairpersons of infection control committees must have the respect of their peers. It is preferable that the chairperson possess specific training in microbiology, epidemiology, or infectious disease. However, in a hospital where there is no physician with these characteristics, someone who is interested and willing to learn about infection control and has the respect of the medical and nursing staffs, hospital administration, and other hospital personnel can be appointed to chair the ICC.

The minutes of the ICC are forwarded to the medical staff through the executive committee, the chief executive officer of the hospital, the nurse executive, and the person responsible for hospital quality assessment and improvement activities (JCAHO, 1992).

The authority of the committee must be defined in writing and approved by the hospital administration and the medical staff. Usually, this written authority allows the chairperson of the ICC to call for outside help if necessary, discontinue admissions to a facility or service, institute isolation measures, discontinue a procedure associated with a high risk of infection, or implement other control measures when there is reason to believe patients or personnel may be in danger of nosocomial infection.

The ICP is the central figure in infection control programs. ICPs have played the major role in the collection of routine infection surveillance data. In addition, infection control nurses or practitioners spend time researching and developing infection control policies, conducting educational programs, consulting with hospital personnel regarding infection control practice, and assisting in the investigation of outbreaks or clusters of infection. The CDC *Study on the Efficacy of*

Nosocomial Infection Control (SENIC) documented that 42% of the SENIC hospitals had at least one full-time ICP for every 300 beds. The authors of this study were able to demonstrate that having a full-time, equivalent ICP for every 250 occupied beds was an important component of programs designated as very effective (Haley and others, 1980).

The hospital administrator is responsible for the allocation of funds and resources for the infection control activities. Infection control programs have been most successful when there is administrative support. As a key member on the ICC, the hospital administrator is in a position to guide the committee in developing realistic interventions regarding infection control problems and aid in the implementation of policies, programs, and control measures.

Reporting lines for ICPs vary among hospitals. Some ICPs report to the director of nursing, but the majority are accountable to a hospital administrator, the hospital epidemiologist, or the director of the hospital's quality improvement program. Regardless of the ICP's position on the organizational chart, it is imperative that practitioners have clear authority from administration to implement and maintain a consistent infection control program throughout the entire hospital.

SURVEILLANCE AND REPORTING OF NOSOCOMIAL INFECTIONS

The purpose of surveillance is to establish and maintain a data base that describes the endemic rates of nosocomial infections. Knowing the endemic rates allows the ICP and hospital epidemiologist to recognize increased rates of nosocomial infection resulting in clusters or outbreaks (Thompson, 1987). Surveillance data is used to prioritize infection control activities and to identify epidemics as well as trends, such as shifts in pathogens, infection rates, or outcomes of hospital-acquired infections. Elements of surveillance include definitions of nosocomial infections, systematic case findings, tabulation of the data, analysis and interpretation of the data, and reporting of relevant data to individuals and groups for appropriate action.

Before data collection can be initiated, definitions for nosocomial infections must be established. *Nosocomial infections* are defined as infections appearing in hospitalized patients that were not present or incubating at the time of admission. The CDC has developed a set of definitions for surveillance of nosocomial infections in adults and neonates. These definitions combine clinical findings with results of laboratory and other tests (Garner and others, 1988). Definitions must be approved or revised by the hospital ICC for use in their institution. Once established, definitions need to be applied consistently in the collection of surveillance data.

The infection control nurse may use several sources of information to identify cases of nosocomial infection. Sources of data for infection surveillance in health care facilities include microbiology data, the patient's medical record, admission records, staff interviews, unit rounds, temperature records, radiographic and autopsy reports, patient care plans (Kardex), operating room records, and pharmacy reports. ICPs must determine which of these sources of data is most beneficial for the type of surveillance conducted in their institutions.

The ICP in cooperation with the ICC decides what information should be collected about each nosocomial infection. Data collected usually include the demographic information about the patient (name, age, sex, hospital identification number, unit location, and service), date of admission, date of onset of infection, site of infection, microorganism isolated, the antibiotic susceptibility pattern, dates and types of surgical procedures, the operating surgeons, predisposing treatments, and underlying conditions. Each ICC determines which data are necessary for the type of surveillance being conducted in their institution. Data should only be collected if it is going to be included in the analysis for reporting to the ICC, hospital administration, and medical staff.

Prior to collection of data, a data collection instrument must be developed. There are many forms that have been developed for collecting pertinent information. Some ICPs use 3 x 5 file cards, and others use 8½ x 11 sheets of paper. When data are to be entered into a computer, it is often most efficient if the data collection sheet can be organized in the same sequence as the data-entry screens on the computer. A sample of a surveillance tool is illustrated in Fig. 12-1.

Types of surveillance

An important decision to be made by the ICC is the type of surveillance to be conducted in the facility. *Total house surveillance* is one type of system that detects and records all nosocomial infections that occur on every service in every area of the hospital. Total house surveillance is the traditional CDC-recommended surveillance technique. However, total house surveillance is an expensive method due to time and personnel requirements.

Another approach to surveillance that may be selected is a *priority-directed* or targeted *surveillance.* This type of surveillance may be conducted for specific units or areas, specific patient populations, or specific procedures. Surveillance activities may focus on intensive care units or bone marrow transplant units with the rationale being that the patients on these units are the most compromised and therefore the most at risk for nosocomial infection. Surveillance for procedure-related nosocomial infections is another type of targeted surveillance. For example, all patients who have had Hickman catheters inserted as a part of their treatment could be followed for the duration of their treatment to determine the rate of nosocomial infection related to this specific invasive procedure.

A third approach to surveillance is the *problem-oriented* or outbreak response *surveillance* technique. This type of surveillance is conducted to measure the occurrence of specific infection problems. The ICC may also recommend that the investigation be extended to collect comparable data from appropriate control groups to identify statistically significant risk factors for which control measures can be developed (JCAHO, 1992).

An approach developed by Wenzel and his colleagues in 1976 used the nursing care plan (Kardex) found on most hospital units (Wenzel and others, 1976). The surveillance person reviews the Kardex for risk factors associated with nosocomial infection. Using this method the time required for surveillance was cut from 25 to 16 hours per week with a maintenance of 82% to 94% accuracy. More

FIGURE 12-1

INFECTION CONTROL WORKSHEET

AGE:	M\Y:	SEX:	MR#:	NAME:
DX:		ADM DATE:		DC DATE\OUTCOME:
MD:	MD#:	SERVICE:		ROOMS:

URINARY TRACT INFECTION ONSET:<\\> REVIEW:<\\>

Asymp ______ Symp ______ Culture Data ______
Path 01 ______ Path 02 ______ Path 03 ______
Urgency ______ Fever 101* ______ Pyuria ______
Dysuria ______ Cloudy ______ Foley ______
Foley LOS ______ Foley DOI ______ Foley D\C ______

SURGICAL WOUND INFECTION ONSET:<\\> REVIEW:<\\>

Deep ______ Inc ______ Culture Site ______
Culture Date ______ Class 1 2 3 4 5
Path 01 ______ Path 02 ______ Path 03 ______
Surgeon ______________ Service ______
Procedure ______________
Fever ______ Puss ______ Redness ______
Dehis ______ Abscess ______ Drainage ______

BLOOD STREAM INFECTION ONSET:<\\> REVIEW:<\\>

Primary ______ Culture Date ______
Path 01 ______ Path 02 ______ Path 03 ______
Cath Related ______ Culture Date ______ Culture Org ______
10:5 ______ Fever 101+ ______ BP Below 90 ______
Chills ______ Urine Below 20\° ______

PNEUMONIA & OTHER RESPITORY INFECTION ONSET:<\\> REVIEW:<\\>

Culture Date ______ Sput Source Asp ______ Exp ______
BW ______ BB ______
Path 01 ______ Path 02 ______ Path 03 ______
Puru Spru ______ Rales ______ CXR inf ______
Vent ______ Vent LOS ______ Fever 101+ ______
Con ______ PE ______ Vent DOI ______
Broncho Date ______ SP Exp ______ Endo ______
BW ______

ARTERIAL OR VASCULAR CATH INFECTION ONSET:<\\> REVIEW:<\\>

Cath Culture
Path 01 ______ Path 02 ______ Path 03 ______
Colony Count 15+ ______ Cent Line ______ Peri ______
L ______ R ______
Site: ______ S\C ______ Bra ______
Rad ______ Ante ______
IP ______ O ______
Type: ______ TLC ______ Swan ______
PICC ______ Art ______
Epi ______ HICC ______
Cook ______
Other ______________
Fever 101+ ______ Redness ______ Pain ______
Puru Phlebitis ______

OTHER INFECTIONS ONSET:<\\> REVIEW:<\\>

Site ______ Culture Date ______
Path 01 ______ Path 02 ______ Path 03 ______
Symptoms: ______________

Comments: ______________

____

____

Fig. 12-1 Infection control work sheet.

recently Broderick and colleagues at the University of Iowa have developed a computer model for the identification of patients with a high probability of nosocomial infection. The group has identified five variables that independently predict infection. If validated, the model would provide an efficient mechanism to conduct hospital-wide surveillance (Broderick and others, 1990).

Another type of surveillance activity is a prevalence survey, which can be used periodically to validate the routine system used for incidence surveillance data. Prevalence is defined as the proportion of patients in the hospital with infections at given point in time.

An area yet to be developed is that of outpatient and postdischarge surveillance. With the increased number of outpatient procedures and shorter hospital stays, nosocomial infections related to procedures done in the hospital may not manifest until after discharge from the hospital. Telephone surveys of patients and postdischarge surveys of patients or physicians have been used to determine the risk of infection following an outpatient procedure or following discharge after a short hospital stay. Currently, a cost-effective method has not been developed to accurately collect data regarding postdischarge infections.

Analysis and reporting of nosocomial infection data

To achieve the goal of reducing and preventing nosocomial infections, surveillance data must be tabulated and reported to key people including members of the hospital ICC, hospital administrators, physicians, and quality assurance personnel. Data must be relevant and understandable to the persons involved in order for them to use the information to initiate actions that will decrease the nosocomial infection rate.

Most often the data are tabulated and analyzed by the hospital epidemiologist and the ICP. The data are first presented to the members of the ICC. Infection control reports of nosocomial infections are usually tabulated monthly. Traditional hospital rates have been calculated using the number of nosocomial infections as the numerator. Denominators vary from institution to institution but are generally the number of admissions, discharges, or patient days for the time period of the report. These denominator numbers are usually readily available from the hospital medical records department or hospital business office. The number of patients infected in a population at risk is expressed as a rate. In other words, patient infection rates are calculated as follows:

$$\frac{\text{Number of patients with infections (time period)}}{\text{Number of patients at risk (time period)}} \times 100$$

This rate is called a patient infection rate, an attack rate, or an incidence rate, since it is the number of patients who acquire an infection over a specific time period from a population at risk of acquiring infection (see Chapter 3).

Rates can be further broken down by ward, service, and infection site. Fig. 12-2 illustrates a report format for service rates and infection site rates. Information on the organisms involved in nosocomial infections can also be presented to the ICC. All of these various report formats can be used individually or in combination to determine whether the endemic rate is being maintained or whether clusters or epidemic proportions of infections are occurring. Graphics may also be used to present meaningful data.

When information is required about a specific group of infections, a line list may be created. A line list is used to record all information collected through daily surveillance activities. Data are collected on work sheets for each patient

NOSOCOMIAL INFECTION RATES BY SERVICE

SERVICE	# OF INFECTIONS (A)	# OF ADMISSIONS/ DISCHARGES, OR PATIENT DAYS (B)	ATTACK RATE A/B X 100
MEDICINE			
SURGERY			

NOSOCOMIAL INFECTION RATES BY SITE

SITE	# OF INFECTIONS (A)	# OF ADMISSIONS/ DISCHARGES, OR PATIENT DAYS (B)	ATTACK RATE A/B X 100
LOWER RESPITORY			
URINARY TRACT			
BLOODSTREAM			

Fig. 12-2 Nosocomial infection rates by service and by site.

and for each occurrence of nosocomial infection. Line listings are then created from these work sheets and used to periodically review the infections found during the month to determine if there are unusual occurrences in the population being studied.

Several computer programs have been developed for analyzing and tabulating nosocomial infection reports. Some programs have been developed by hospitals to be used with mainframe systems. Other software packages for personal computers are available commercially. Data regarding the individual patients and their infections are entered, and the monthly reports and line lists are then generated by computer.

Another report often generated on a semiannual or annual basis is a surgeon-specific, surgical wound infection rate. Two independent studies have determined that reporting of surgeon-specific, wound infection rates may be effective in the reduction of nosocomial surgical wound infections (Cruse and others, 1980; Haley and others, 1985b).

The traditional rates used for reporting nosocomial infections do not adjust for specific infection risks, and therefore do not lend themselves to interhospital comparison. The CDC recently published a report describing new methods for calculating infection rates, including device-associated infection rates, device-day–infection rates for intensive care units and high-risk nurseries, and the use of the *National Nosocomial Infections Surveillance (NNIS)* surgical wound infection risk index (CDC, 1991). Because the crude overall infection rate (total number of nosocomial infections over admissions, discharges, or patient days) does not consider underlying risk or severity of illnesses, interhospital comparisons are not valid. Site-specific nosocomial infection rates by service also do not adjust for intrinsic and extrinsic infection risk factors. If interhospital infection rates are to be meaningfully compared, the numerator should represent the number of infections that occur in patients exposed to a common extrinsic factor, and the denominator should be the number of patient days of exposure to that risk factor (see incidence density, Chapter 3). For example, bloodstream infections associated with central lines should be reported as follows (CDC, 1991).

$$\frac{\text{Number of bloodstream infections associated with a central line}}{\text{Number of patient days of exposure}} \times 1000$$

Central lines may need to be further defined by determining whether they are umbilical lines, triple lumen lines, or others. The challenge facing ICPs in calculating these rates is the lack of available denominator data. Data, such as the number of IV line, central line, ventilator, and foley catheter days, are not easily accessible in many hospitals. If device data is available the formula for *device-associated infections* is:

$$\frac{\text{Number of device-associated infections}}{\text{Number of device days of exposure}} \times 1000$$

This rate provides the number of infections associated with a particular device for a specific nosocomial infection site for every 1000 device days.

Surgical wound infection rates are most meaningful if procedures and patients are stratified by risk factors. The most widely used classification system for surgical wounds categorizes wounds as clean, clean-contaminated, contaminated, or dirty, as defined by the National Research Council (Haley, 1985). Definitions for these classifications are as follows:

Clean	Clean wounds are those in which neither the gastrointestinal tract, respiratory system, genitourinary tract, or pharyngeal cavity are entered. No inflammation is found during surgery. These are also cases in which no breaks in aseptic technique have occurred.
Clean-contaminated	Clean-contaminated wounds are those in which the gastrointestinal tract, respiratory system, or genitourinary tract are entered, but significant spillage has not occurred during the procedure.
Contaminated	Wounds in this category include surgical procedures in which (1) there has been a major break in aseptic technique, (2) gross spillage from a contaminated system has occurred, or (3) acute inflammation without pus is encountered. Fresh trauma wounds also fit in this category.
Dirty	Dirty wounds include old traumatic wounds, wounds with pus, or a perforated viscus.

Incidence rates of wound infections are calculated using the number of infections in each group as the numerator and the number of operations performed in each category as the denominator. In a 10-year study of surgical wound infections, Cruse and others (1980) reported the rates for each group as follows: clean—1.5%; clean-contaminated—7.7%; contaminated—15.2%; and dirty—40% Cruse and others, (1980).

The CDC has indicated that reporting surgical wound infections in the traditional manner of clean, clean-contaminated, and dirty, does not include a measure of intrinsic patient risk factors. The NNIS surgical wound infection risk index includes the following elements:(1) the patient's wound class was contaminated or dirty; (2) the patient was assigned an American Society of Anesthesiology score of three, four, or five by the anesthesiologist prior to the operative procedure; and (3) the procedure lasted longer than T hours (where T is the approximate 75th percentile of the duration of surgery for the various operative procedures reported to the NNIS data base). A patient's risk category is determined by adding the number of risk factors present. Therefore a patient's risk score may range from zero to three (CDC, 1991). Investigators believe the NNIS surgical wound infection index is a better indicator of patients at risk for surgical wound infection than wound class alone (Culver and others, 1991). Another surgical wound index was developed based on the SENIC study results and includes whether the patient's wound class is contaminated or dirty, whether the duration of surgery is greater than 2 hours, whether the operation is abdominal or thoracic, and whether the patient has three or more discharge diagnoses. However, the SENIC risk index does not stratify risks by individual operative procedures (Haley and others, 1985a).

As can be determined from the preceding discussion, the use of epidemiologic principles to monitor the occurrence of nosocomial infections is well established. However, continual refinement of the process is essential. Crude overall rates do not sufficiently adjust for the individual risk factors to permit meaningful interhospital comparison. The challenge facing hospital infection control and hospital epidemiology is to measure adverse outcomes, adjusting for the potential confounding variables, such as severity of underlying illness.

Use of the surveillance data in outbreak investigations

The ICP must use the monthly surveillance report to recognize situations in need of investigation, change patient care practices, and reduce endemic rates of nosocomial infection. Routine nosocomial infection surveillance data are used to determine the endemic or the usual level of nosocomial infections occurring in the hospital. A threshold is then established. The threshold is often set at one or two standard directions from the mean. An example of a 12-month graph of nosocomial pneumonia per 100 ventilator days is illustrated in Fig. 12-3. The mean and threshold level is drawn on the graph to aid in monthly review of the findings. When the monthly report indicates a number of infections above the established threshold, an investigation is conducted to determine if an outbreak is occurring. Once again, the ICP uses epidemiologic methods to investigate the increased number of infections. The steps used to investigate a nosocomial infection cluster

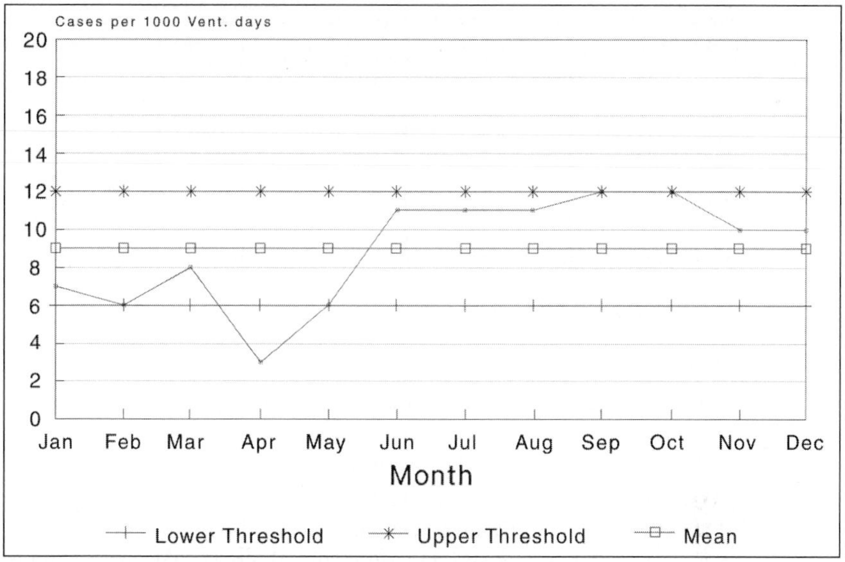

Fig. 12-3 Ventilator-related nosocomial pneumonia.

or outbreak are the same as the steps in any other epidemiologic investigation. Those steps include: (1) establish or verify the diagnosis of cases and identify the agent responsible; (2) confirm that an outbreak exists; (3) search for additional cases; (4) characterize cases by person, place, and time; (5) formulate a tentative hypothesis; (6) test the hypothesis; (7) consider control measures and institute those control measures that are most appropriate; (8) evaluate the efficacy of control measures; and (9) write a report (see Chapters 4 and 7).

The primary goal of an outbreak investigation is prompt control of the spread of the infection. In most hospitals, the key people involved in outbreak investigations are the ICP and the chairperson of the ICC or the hospital epidemiologist. Other key people include those representing the areas affected by the outbreak.

The first step in an outbreak investigation is to develop a working definition of a case. This definition is usually a combination of clinical and laboratory data and should fulfill the person-place-time criteria. For example, a case definition might be an inpatient on the surgical ICU between October 1 and October 18 who developed a temperature higher than 38.5°C (100.4°F), and has a purulent Hickman catheter site and positive Hickman site culture for *Pseudomonas maltophilia.*

After the case is defined, thorough case finding must be conducted. Data are collected on all of those persons who would fit the person-place-time criteria defining the case. The data collected on the hypothetical case presented above would include the collection of demographic data and information regarding the insertion and care of the Hickman catheter. Other information needed would include risk information about the patient, including the length of time the person was on the unit before infection appeared, number, date, and type of invasive pro-

PATIENT NAME	DATE OF INSERTION	DATE OF INFECTION	WARD	ORGANISM
B.J.	9/15	10/1	ICU	Ps. maltophilia
J.S.	9/30	10/5	ICU	Ps. maltophilia
S.S.	9/4	10/8	ICU	Ps. maltophilia
L.C.	9/10	10/11	ICU	Ps. maltophilia
C.B.	10/1	10/18		

Fig. 12-4 Line list of Hickman site infections with *Pseudomonas maltophilia.*

cedures, underlying diseases, and antibiotic therapy before the appearance of the infection.

It must be confirmed that the problem observed is new. Therefore information on past infections related to this site and organism should be reviewed. Preferably, data from the previous year should be reviewed to establish the frequency of Hickman line site infections with the particular organism identified. A line listing of all cases should be prepared. A sample line listing can be found in Fig. 12-4.

Using the information collected, an epidemic curve can be plotted by date of onset. Attack rates are then calculated. To compare previous experience to the current episodes, rates rather than numbers are used. The epidemic and endemic rates are compared to verify that an outbreak is truly present. Verifying the existence of an outbreak by using these epidemiologic methods is extremely important. Sometimes these initial steps determine that an outbreak really does not exist. Temporary increases in the number of cases may be due to intrinsic or extrinsic patient risk factors. Establishing the true existence of an outbreak can prevent investigation of a pseudoepidemic.

Based on the data collected from the above activities, a hypothesis on the likely reservoir, source, and mode of transmission of disease can be formulated. The hypothesis should explain the majority of cases. In the previous example, the hypothesis may be that the antiseptic solution used to cleanse the skin prior to insertion of the Hickman lines was contaminated with *P. maltophilia.*

At the same time, reasonable control measures should be instituted. For example, if contaminated solution is suspected, the existing solution should be identified in terms of company and lot number and reported to the company and the Food and Drug Administration. Samples should be sent to the microbiology laboratory for testing. In addition, the ICP might review Hickman line insertion techniques and site care procedures.

Whenever an investigation is underway, it is very important to include the microbiology laboratory. It is preferable that one person in the laboratory be identified as a key person with a clear understanding of the nature of the outbreak and the role that the laboratory might play in the investigation. In some situations, the laboratory may need to make special preparations. For example, the laboratory may need to order additional or special culture media to accommodate the testing required for the investigation.

It is always wise on the part of the ICP to alert the hospital public relations department that an investigation is underway. News of the outbreak may reach the community and the media, and public relations personnel should be prepared to respond if inquiries occur.

Many times, problems resolve with the institution of control measures. Occasionally outbreaks are not so easily resolved and, despite institution of control measures, the outbreak continues. At this time, the process is repeated with the formulation of a new hypothesis, and new investigation approaches established. When a nosocomial infection epidemic continues despite control measures, a case control study may be conducted.

At the conclusion of an epidemic investigation, all persons involved must be informed that the problem has been resolved and the infection rate has returned to an established endemic rate. Although the precise cause of an outbreak is often not determined, a written report must be prepared and presented to the ICC, appropriate department heads, and administrative staff. It is the responsibility of the ICC to disseminate conclusions and recommendations resulting from an outbreak investigation. The committee must also evaluate measures instituted as a result of an epidemic.

In the absence of an outbreak, the ICP may choose to review the endemic nosocomial infection rates and set a goal to reduce the rate of a specific infection site. In 1984, Haley introduced the concept of surveillance by objectives (Haley, 1985). Haley encouraged setting outcome objectives to decrease morbidity, mortality, and hospital costs to patients by using process objectives to reduce the endemic rate of infection. For example, an outcome objective might be to reduce the surgical wound infection rate by 7% by using process goals, such as reporting surgeon-specific, wound infection rates and changing policies and procedures that are not optimal for wound healing.

The ICP must also use epidemiologic methods and surveillance findings to evaluate current infection control practice. Many infection control guidelines historically have been based on common sense, expert consensus, and tradition rather than scientific inquiry. With increased sensitivity to the economics of health care, the merits of these guidelines are being questioned. Data need to be collected and analyzed to determine which of the infection control procedures are cost-effective in preventing morbidity and mortality of nosocomial infections. For example, the benefits of the various types of isolation systems have never been scientifically proven. Whether the traditional category system of isolation or the newer proposed body substance isolation is most effective in preventing infection transmission has yet to be determined. In addition, many new products come on the marketplace with claims that the product will significantly impact the nosocomial infection rate. These products require scientific investigation for evidence of efficacy and cost-effectiveness. Likewise, scientific data do not exist to establish what type of surveillance system is most efficient and cost-effective. Surveillance systems need to be evaluated in terms of sensitivity and specificity in relation to the resource requirements for the various approaches of surveillance (Goldmann, 1991).

Infection control practice has been established primarily in the acute care setting of hospitals, and therefore existing guidelines for infection control procedures have been developed for patients in hospitals and, to some extent, long-term care facilities. However, guidelines for use by home health personnel are not in existence. As the trend to discharge patients earlier continues, an increasing number of patients with invasive devices will receive care in their home environment. Epidemiologic methods should be used to assess cost-effective but safe practice in the home. Questions, such as how frequently intravascular devices need to be changed and whether indwelling urinary catheters can be disinfected and reused by the homebound patient, are in need of study. As home care expands, guidelines specific to these patients need to be established based on scientifically evaluated practice.

EXPANDED ROLE OF HOSPITAL EPIDEMIOLOGY

Traditionally, epidemiology in hospitals has limited its focus to infectious diseases. Currently the application of epidemiology in hospitals is expanding to activities, such as accident prevention, risk management, transfusion review, use review, and quality assessment. The term hospital epidemiology can now include all of these activities, whether they are organized under one administrative department or spread across several departments. Types of nosocomial problems that may be studied in this expanded role are injuries among hospital personnel (such as needle sticks and back injuries), slips and falls among patients and/or hospital personnel, medication errors, situations commonly requiring an incident report, postoperative complications (such as atalectasis, hemorrhage, return to surgery), patient dissatisfaction, and unexpected death during hospitalizations (Jackson and others, 1985). It is believed that the epidemiologic techniques that have made infection control clinically successful and cost-effective can be used to reduce noninfectious hazards of medical care and enhance the diagnostic and therapeutic benefits of modern medical management. Epidemiology will be involved in the study of the distribution and determinants of desirable practice, leading to optimally achievable health care (Wenzel, 1990).

SUMMARY

The epidemiologic model long used in the field of public health to review illnesses or injuries associated with morbidity and mortality among the general public is well-adapted to the study of the occurrence of adverse events in the hospital setting. The discipline of hospital infection control has established a sound practice base during the last 20 years. However, the rates that are the most meaningful for interhospital comparisons must be firmly established. Scientific data are still needed to determine which infection control policies and procedures are most beneficial in the reduction of nosocomial infections. However, even more challenging is the application of epidemiologic methods to the measurement of noninfectious adverse outcomes affecting patients in today's hospital. By applying the tools of epidemiology, significant adverse outcomes of hospitalized patients can be evaluated for possible intervention and reduction of morbidity and for mortality associated with hospitalization.

Critical Thinking Questions

1. Trace the historic development of hospital infection control programs.
2. Discuss the role of the ICP within a hospital infection control program.
3. Discuss the types of hospital surveillance systems identified in this chapter.
4. To be useful to hospital staff, surveillance data must be relevant and understandable. Explain how infection rates are calculated and how this data might be presented to the staff.

REFERENCES

Broderick A and others: Nosocomial infections: validation of surveillance and computer modeling to identify patients at risk, *Am J Epidemiol* 131:734-742, 1990.

Centers for Disease Control: Infection surveillance and control programs in US hospitals: an assessment, 1976, *MMWR* 27:139-145, 1978.

Centers for Disease Control: Nosocomial infection rates for interhospital comparison: limitations and possible solutions, *Infect Control Hosp Epidemiol* 12:609-621, 1991.

Cruse PJ and others: The epidemiology of wound infection: a 10-year prospective study of 62,939 wounds, *Surg Clin North Am* 60:27-40, 1980.

Culver DH and others: Surgical wound infection rates by wound class, operation, and risk index in US hospitals, 1986-90, *Am J Med* 91(suppl 3B):152-157, 1991.

Dixon RE: Historical perspective: the landmark conference in 1980, *Am J Med* 91(suppl 3B):65-75, 1991.

Eickhoff T: Historical perspective: the landmark conference in 1970, *Am J Med* 91(suppl 3B):3-5, 1991.

Garner JS and others: CDC definitions for nosocomial infections, 1988, *Am J Infect Control* 16:128-140, 1988.

Goldmann DA: Contemporary challenges for hospital epidemiology, *Am J Med* 91(suppl 3B):8S-15S, 1991.

Haley RW: Surveillance by objective: a new priority-directed approach to the control of nosocomial infections, *Am J Infect Control* 13(2):78-89, 1985.

Haley RW and others: The emergence of infection surveillance and control programs in US hospitals: an assessment, 1976, *Am J Epidemiol* 111:574-591, 1980.

Haley RW and others: The efficacy of infection surveillance and control programs in preventing nosocomial infections in US hospitals, *Am J Epidemiol* 121:182-205, 1985a.

Haley RW and others: Identifying patients at high risk of surgical wound infection: a simple multivariate index of patient susceptibility and wound contamination, *Am J Epidemiol* 121:206-215, 1985b.

Jackson MM and others: Applying an epidemiological structure to risk management and quality assurance activities, *QRB* 11:306-312, 1985.

Joint Commission on Accreditation of Healthcare Organizations: *Accreditation manual for hospitals,* Chicago, 1992, The Commission.

Joint Commission on Accreditation of Healthcare Organizations: *Accreditation manual for hospitals,* Chicago, 1994, The Commission.

LaForce FM: Control of infections in hospitals: 1750 to 1950. In Wenzel RP, editor: *Prevention and control of nosocomial infections,* Baltimore, 1987, Williams & Wilkins.

Simmons BP, editor: *Guidelines for the prevention and control of nosocomial infection,* Atlanta, 1981, Centers for Disease Control.

Thompson RL: Surveillance and reporting of nosocomial infections. In Wenzel RP, editor: *Prevention and control of nosocomial infections,* Baltimore, 1987, Williams & Wilkins.

US Department of Labor: Occupational exposure to bloodborne pathogens, *Federal Register* 58 December 6, 1991.

Wenzel RP: Quality assessment: an emerging component of hospital epidemiology, *Diag Microbiol Infect Dis* 13:197-204, 1990.

Wenzel RP and others: Hospital acquired infections. I. Surveillance in a university hospital, *Am J Epidemiol* 103:251, 1976.

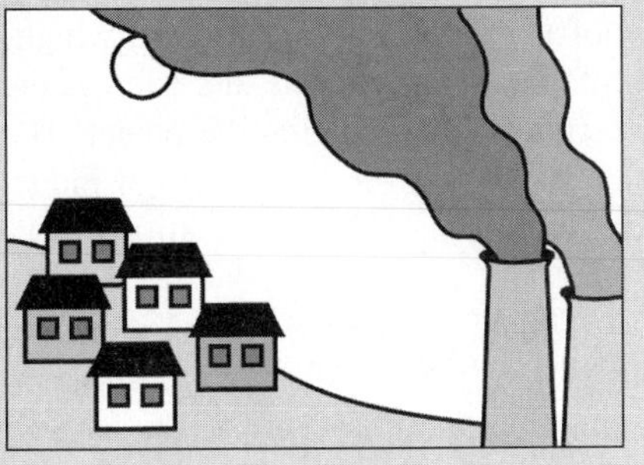

13

Epidemiology in Occupational and Environmental Health

CAROL LOVE

OBJECTIVES

1. State the environmental health objectives for the year 2000.
2. Explain 12 activities that can be initiated that will reduce risk of exposure to environmental hazards.
3. Identify epidemiologic data required to measure the effects of environmental exposure on the nation's health.
4. Discuss activities nurses can initiate that will reduce the exposure of the community to environmental hazards.
5. Interpret the role of the occupational health nurse.
6. Explain six strategies that will result in achievement of the occupational health objectives for the year 2000.
7. Design an epidemiologic surveillance system for occupational health.
8. Explain the process of risk assessment for occupational hazards.

KEY TERMS

environmental health
epidemiologic surveillance
Healthy People 2000
occupational health
occupational health nurse
Occupational Health and Safety Administration (OSHA)
risk assessment

The organization and implementation of the Earth Summit meetings highlight society's demand that the world population recognize and address the political, social, economic, and health effects of contaminating the planet. The long-term use and misuse of the environment's wealth for the process of industrialization has resulted in pollution of the environment and contamination of natural resources.

As one reads the popular literature, the United States is identified as having 5% of the world's population yet is using 25% of the world's energy, thus producing 22% of all carbon monoxide. In contrast, India has 16% of the world's population, uses 3% of the world's energy, and releases only 3% of all carbon monoxide emissions (Elmer-Dewitt, 1992). What do these figures mean? What is their impact on the health care system? How are they derived, and how are they used to make decisions about health care? What are the health effects of global warming, deforestation, maritime pollution, ozone depletion, nuclear energy, and "space waste"? Taken as a whole, these issues are gigantic and seemingly insolvable. On a smaller scale, health care professionals can ask questions, develop hypotheses, gather data, and devise and manage direct interventions.

ENVIRONMENTAL HEALTH

In the document *Healthy People 2000,* specific goals and objectives for *environmental health* have been established. By reviewing hundreds of research studies and epidemiologic data, the authors were able to set very specific goals and objectives. The boxes on pp. 229-230 list the specific objectives on the areas of health status, risk reduction, and services needed. If implemented, these objectives should decrease the incidence of environmentally induced diseases. Environmental and human factors are synergistic; each are central players in the nature and effects of environmental change. The science base for predicting these changes is in its infancy. For example, the effect of particular chemicals and chemical products on the process of human and environmental development is poorly understood.

Knowledge has developed about such issues as toxic waste sites, maritime pollution, and ozone depletion. The challenges for environmental scientists now is to discover the toxic effects and outcomes of exposure to synthetic chemicals. In 1984, the National Academy of Sciences reported that 82% of chemicals currently in use have insufficient data concerning risks for disease induction. These figures have not improved at present. The role of public health and the science of epidemiology will be essential to the development of models for decision-making as health challenges arise.

The science of epidemiology studies the effect of a specific event on a population and helps predict expected risks. Traditionally, epidemiology has been defined as "the study of the distribution and determinants of disease frequency in man (McMahon and Pugh, 1970). Today the principles of epidemiology applied to not only disease but also natural disasters, such as hurricanes, typhoons, earthquakes, as well as industrial disasters, such as air pollution, accidents, nuclear

HEALTHY PEOPLE 2000 ENVIRONMENTAL HEALTH OBJECTIVES—HEALTH STATUS OBJECTIVES

Reduce asthma morbidity, as measured by a reduction in asthma hospitalizations, to no more than 160 per 100,000 people

Reduce the prevalence of serious mental retardation among school-aged children to no more than two per 1000 children

Reduce outbreaks of waterborne diseases from infectious agents and chemical poisoning to no more than 11 per year

Reduce the prevalence of blood lead levels exceeding 15 mg/dl and 25 mg/dl among children age 6 months to 5 years to no more than 500,000 and zero respectively

Reduce human exposure to criteria air pollutants, as measured by an increase to at least 85% in the proportion of people who live in countries that have not exceeded any Environmental Protection Standard for air quality in the previous 12 months

From Healthy People 2000: National Health Promotion and Disease Prevention Objectives, Public Health Service, US Department of Health and Human Services, 1990, pp 105-106.

HEALTHY PEOPLE 2000 ENVIRONMENTAL HEALTH OBJECTIVES—RISK REDUCTION OBJECTIVES

Reduce human exposure to criteria air pollutants, as measured by an increase to at least 85% in the proportion of people who live in countries that have not exceeded any Environmental Protection Agency standard for air quality in the previous 12 months (pollutants measured include ozone, carbon monoxide, nitrogen oxide, sulfur oxide, particulates, and lead)

Increase to at least 40% the proportion of homes that homeowners/occupants have tested for radon concentration and that have either been found to pose minimal risk or have been modified to reduce risk to health

Reduce human exposure to toxic agents by confining total pounds of toxic agents released into the air, water, and soil each year

Reduce human exposure to solid waste-related water, air, and soil contamination, as measured by reduction in average pounds of municipal, solid waste produced per person each day to no more than 3.6 pounds

Increase to at least 85% the proportion of people who receive a supply of drinking water that meets the safe drinking water standards established by the Environmental Protection Agency

Reduce potential risk to human health from surface water, as measured by a decrease to no more than 15% in the proportion of assessed rivers, lakes, and estuaries that do not support beneficial uses, such as fishing and swimming

From Healthy People 2000: National Health Promotion and Disease Prevention Objectives, Public Health Service, US Department of Health and Human Services, 1990, p 106.

HEALTHY PEOPLE 2000 ENVIRONMENTAL OBJECTIVES—SERVICE AND PROMOTION OBJECTIVES

Perform testing for lead-based paint in at least 50% of homes built since 1950

Expand to at least 35 the number of states in which at least 75% of local jurisdictions have adopted construction standards and techniques that minimize elevated indoor radon levels in those new building areas locally determined to have elevated radon levels

Increase to at least 30 the number of states requiring that prospective buyers be informed of the presence of lead-based paint and radon concentrations in all buildings offered for sale

Eliminate significant health risks from National Priority List hazardous waste sites, as measured by performance of clean-up at these sites sufficient to eliminate immediate and significant health threats as specified in health assessments completed at all sites

Establish programs for recyclable materials and household hazardous waste in at least 75% of counties

Establish and monitor in at least 35 states plans to define and track sentinel environmental disease (sentinel diseases include lead poisoning, cadmium, arsenic, and mercury poisoning, pesticides, carbon monoxide poisoning, and other environmental exposures)

From Healthy People 2000: National Health Promotion and Disease Prevention Objectives, Public Health Service, US Department of Health and Human Services, 1990, p 107.

power plant melt downs, oil spills, and accidental release of toxic chemicals. By analyzing data on the number of dead and injured and the resulting survivor morbidity, information is obtained that facilitates long-range planning.

For example, the analysis of data from major earthquakes, such as the 1985 Mexican earthquake, which resulted in 10,000 deaths, initiated the development of new standards for building construction (Zeballos, 1986). The effects of these antiseismic construction codes were well demonstrated by the low casualty rate after the 1989 earthquake in San Francisco. Data collected from the explosion of the nuclear reactor in Chernobyl in 1986 predict that death from cancer in exposed populations will vary from 5000 to 40,000 over the next several decades. These data will help health professionals make not only health decisions but also economic decisions regarding the best use of limited resources.

Still another area of use for epidemiologic data is in the area of mental health. Sudden unexpected disasters, such as floods, mass murders, airline crashes, and natural disasters, have heightened our awareness of a lack of knowledge regarding the long-term psychologic impact on people experiencing major disasters. The resulting physical and psychologic illnesses must be studied in depth in order to develop theraputic health care interventions.

A recent study by Durkin and others (1993), reported a natural experiment where children age 2 to 9 had been tested for selected behavioral problems. Six months later, a flood disaster occurred. Of the previously tested children, 162 were retested. Results showed an increase in enuresis and aggressive behavior in children after the flood disaster. The study findings help to define posttraumatic stress in children as well as contributing to the increasing evidence of the need to develop interventions to assess and evaluate individuals who have suffered major psychologic stress.

Efficient, effective programs to avoid an increase in environmentally induced diseases should be developed through the innovative use of the principles of primary health care: health promotion, health protection, and health surveillance. Epidemiologic data will be essential in making health care decisions concerning the development of scarce resources.

Research needs

Research needs in the area of environmental health have been clearly defined. Accurate data on the actual effects of environmental changes, such as atmospheric warming and ozone depletion, must be compiled. Kilbourne (1989) reports that the daily mortality rate increases 30% to 50% during prolonged heat waves. What are the statistical models that will help us predict changes in mortality and morbidity rates for specific diseases and specific populations as a result of global warming? Reliable information must be obtained and centralized in a common data base to determine the health effects of specific environmental exposure. Such a data base would allow for the development of predictive models that would provide health care professionals the needed information to develop and fund primary prevention programs. The development of a scientific data base that allows for critical decision-making in the area of risk management, cost-effective program development, and cost-benefit analysis of regulatory actions is essential. Researchers must initiate improved surveillance processes for evaluating the effectiveness of mandatory regulations in decreasing environmentally induced diseases. From these data, new health programs can be implemented.

These innovations should lead to a national system for measuring the nation's health in relation to (1) levels of environmental exposure, (2) incidence and prevalence of environmentally induced diseases, and (3) subsequent morbidity and mortality data. A process to critically study a dose-response relationship between environmental exposure levels and resulting disease or lack of disease is needed. From these data a national plan to decrease morbidity and mortality resulting from environmental exposures and environmentally induced disease can be initiated. A national registry that can correlate specific diseases and specific environmental exposures will allow health care professionals to develop primary health care programs and clinical interventions that decrease environmental exposures and resulting diseases in the national population.

Nursing implications

Recognizing that the environment may pose health risks, nurses in the community, schools, and health clinics should identify populations within their own practices who may be at risk for or who are showing effects of toxic exposures. School nurses who see groups of children with similar symptoms and community health nurses who have clusters of clients with similar diseases need to question the likelihood of common environmental exposures. The community population, work sites, dump sites, history of industries within the community, and the local historian are all rich sources of information concerning possible community exposure to specific chemicals. Further investigation into city records, death certificates, and infant morbidity and mortality can help nurses to recognize risks and implement provider outreach services. As expert professionals, nurses are also informed consumers and can initiate proactive planning for environmental safety and conservation. By active involvement in community planning and providing appropriate consultation to decision-makers, community and environmental health will be fostered.

OCCUPATIONAL HEALTH

Closely allied to the science of environmental health is the specialty of occupational health. *Occupational health* studies the effects of occupational exposure—physical, chemical and biological—on the employees. Careful attention is paid to the congruence of the health needs of the working population with the production and economic needs of the business community. There is a strong association between sound management practices in occupational safety and health and a low incidence of occupational illness and injury.

The use of epidemiology as a tool for assessing the hazards of workers has a long and productive history. Sigerist (1936) studied ancient Egyptian papyrus that discussed the hard life of those people who worked. Other early historic publications addressed the hazards of working as a goldsmith. Crafters recognized the health effects of hazardous exposures to metals used in the process of metal-working. Mercury and lead, both neurotoxic metals, were identified as health hazards. Agricola, a physician living in the sixteenth century, devoted much of his professional practice to the study of the hazardous conditions of mines. He documented not only the physical hazard of digging deep into the earth with the ever-present danger of cave-ins but also the physiologic effects of breathing metal fumes and coal dust and exposure to radiation. His studies lead to the development of primitive protective equipment. Bernadino Rammazzini was probably the first physician to clearly recognize the complimentary relationship between a healthy worker and economic productivity. His writings, *The Disease of Workers,* carefully delineate his observations of workers in the trade. The box on p. 233 lists many of the occupations he observed. Reading his manuscript, a true appreciation of the art of clinical observation, assessment, and decision-making is developed. Information was not obtained by use of laboratory tests, microscopic analysis, x-ray films, or nuclear imagery. Rather, diagnoses—very accurate ones—were made by skilled history-taking and perceptive observation.

Occupational health nursing

There are more than 110 million men and women in the American work force. Premature death, occupational disease, injury, and disability have become national health problems. New technologies, computers, robotics, automation, and new chemicals add increased health risks to the working population. Lung disease, musculoskeletal injuries, occupationally induced cancer, traumatic injuries, cardiovascular disease, disorders of reproduction, neurotoxic disorders, hearing

OCCUPATIONS RECORDED AND DISCUSSED BY RAMMAZZINI

Miners of metals	Bathmen
Gilders	Salt workers
Healers by injunction	Workers who stand
Chemists	Sedentary workers
Potters	Jews
Tinsmiths	Runners
Glassmakers	Horsemen
Painters	Porters
Sulfur workers	Athletes
Blacksmiths	Workers in mines
Plasterers and lime workers	Voice trainers and singers
Apothecaries	Farmers
Cleaners of cesspits	Fishermen
Fullers	Soldiers
Oilmen, tanners, cheese makers	The learned
Lute string makers	Printers
Corpse bearers	Confectioners
Midwives	Weavers
Wet nurses	Coppersmiths
Vinters and brewers	Carpenters
Bakers and Millers	Razor and lancet grinders
Starch makers	Brick makers
Corn-sifter and measures	Well diggers
Stone cutters	Sailors and rowers
Laundry workers	Hunters
Hemp flax and silk workers	Soap makers

Rammazzini B: *The diseases of workers (demorbis artificum),* Library of the New York Academy of Medicine, New York, 1964, Hafner, pp 1-25.

loss, occupational dermatitis, and mental health disorders are some of the health issues that confront the *occupational health nurse* (OHN). The box on p. 234 lists the 10 most common occupational illnesses. The goal of the occupational health team is to decrease the incidence and prevalence of these occupationally related disorders and to gather the epidemiologic data that will predict future health problems. The OHN is the key player on this team, since the scope of nursing practice includes the assessment and evaluation of the workers.

The position of the OHN was established early in the nineteenth century. The goal of management was to employ a nurse who could care for the ill and injured at the work site thus increasing productivity and decreasing costs. Today the role has expanded. The OHN is responsible for the evaluation of the worksite, recognition of health hazards, preemployment evaluation of workers, evaluation and treatment of occupational illness and injury, development of health screening programs specific to the industry, implementation of safety programs, development

TEN LEADING OCCUPATIONAL ILLNESSES

Occupational lung disease
Musculoskeletal injuries
Occupational cancers
Severe occupational traumatic injuries
Occupational cardiovascular disease
Disorders of reproduction
Neurotoxic disorders
Noise-induced hearing loss
Dermatologic conditions
Psychologic disorders

From Healthy People 2000: National Health Promotion and Disease Prevention Objectives, Public Health Service, US Department of Health and Human Services, 1990, p 65.

of health promotion and wellness programs, coordination of cost-effective health care, and collection and analysis of epidemiologic data to identify and predict risks. The OHN is usually the only health professional on site. The role description requires that the nurse be skilled not only in health promotion and health screening, but also in responding immediately to life-threatening situations that may arise at the work site.

Interdisciplinary teamwork is the core of a productive occupational health program. The members of the team should develop a comprehensive occupational health program for the employees. The team includes nurses, physicians, industrial hygienists, safety officers, union representatives, management staff, and others. Health promotion and health protection are key concepts to the success of any occupational health program. Pender (1987) defines health as a manifestation of the ever-evolving interaction of people with the environment. The definition is particularly well-suited to the occupational health setting. The goal of any occupational health program is to interface people with the work setting in such a way as to maximize individual health and production schedules. To accomplish these goals, the concepts of health promotion and health protection must be woven into the fabric of the occupational health program. Pender (1987) defines health promotion as being "directed toward decreasing the probability of experiencing illness by active protection of the body against pathologic stresses or detection of illness in the asymptomatic stage. Health promotion is directed toward increasing the level of well-being and self-actualization of a given individual or group" thus moving toward health.

Epidemiologic surveillance

A concept essential to an occupational health program is that of health surveillance. The need to carefully monitor both the employee and the work environment to detect any health risk and thereby be able to initiate health protective be-

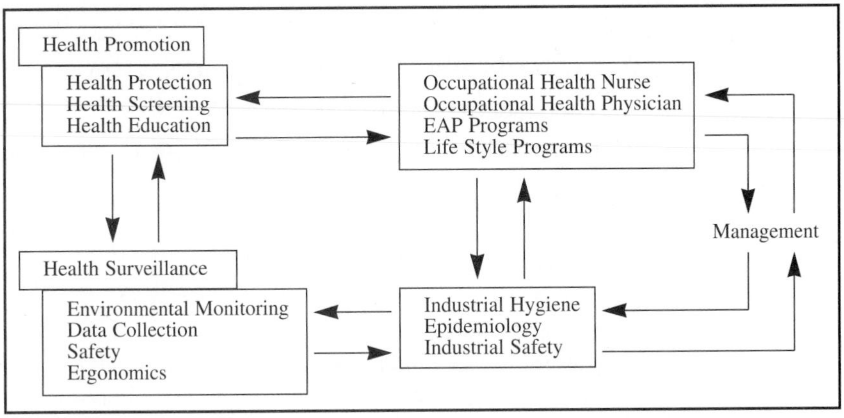

Fig. 13-1 Interdisciplinary model for occupational health.

haviors is critical. Fig. 13-1 illustrates the relationship of these three concepts within the context of the occupational health team.

Historically, occupational disease has been thought of as an acute illness resulting directly from an immediate exposure to a hazardous substance in the workplace. This is no longer true. Data from epidemiologic studies now reveal that long-term, low-level exposure to some substances may have a major impact on worker health and longevity. The boxes on pp. 236-238 identify the health status, risk reduction, and health protection objectives as promulgated by Healthy People 2000. Examination of these objectives clearly demonstrates the variety of illnesses and injuries related to the workplace. Although daily exposure may be perceived as minimal, the physiologic effects may be insidious. Active symptomatic disease may not be recognized until much later in a worker's life or even into retirement. This long latent period is especially true of many chemicals known to have carcinogenic properties and those affecting reproductive outcomes. The box on p. 238, top, lists unfavorable reproductive outcomes related to occupational exposure. The May 13, 1992, Occupational Safety and Health Letter reports the National Institutes for Occupational Safety and Health estimate that more than 11 million workers are exposed to occupational carcinogens. The relative risk for the development of cancer in a wide range of organ systems following exposure to occupational carcinogens is excessive when compared to the general population.

The goals of epidemiologic studies in the area of occupational health are to (1) identify if a relationship exists between a specific exposure and the incidence of disease, (2) predict and prevent occupational diseases, (3) determine safe levels of exposure to harmful substances for the worker population, and (4) provide data that will facilitate the establishment of standards for occupational safety and health. Retrospective case-control epidemiologic studies are effective tools for gathering data to evaluate the relationship of exposure and disease. Once these data are collected and analyzed, care must be taken in interpretation. Some data

HEALTHY PEOPLE 2000 OCCUPATIONAL HEALTH OBJECTIVES—HEALTH STATUS OBJECTIVES

Reduce deaths from work-related injuries to no more than 4 per 100,000 full-time workers

- Special population targets
  - Mine workers
  - Construction workers
  - Transportation workers
  - Farm workers

Reduce work-related injuries resulting in medical treatment, lost time from work, or restricted work activity to no more than 6 cases per 100 full-time workers

- Special population targets
  - Construction workers
  - Nursing and personnel care workers
  - Farm workers
  - Transportation workers
  - Mine workers

Reduce cumulative trauma disorders to an incidence of no more than 60 cases per 100,000 full-time workers

- Special population targets
  - Manufacturing industry workers
  - Meat product workers

Reduce occupational skin disorders or disease to an incidence of no more than 55 per 100,000 full-time workers

Reduce hepatitis B infections among occupationally exposed workers to an incidence of no more than 1250 cases

From Healthy People 2000: National Health Promotion and Disease Prevention Objectives, Public Health Service, US Department of Health and Human Services, 1990, pp 104-105.

will provide a firm base for initial changes in productive processes or protective behavior; other data may be subject to multiple interpretations. Changes should occur only when the evidence is overwhelmingly in favor of that change.

To accomplish these goals, an *epidemiologic surveillance* program should be established. The epidemiologist must have access to records that document individual health and work histories and company processes. The results of any epidemiologic study will be only as good as the record-keeping system of the unit being studied. Each occupational health program must maintain scrupulous records in relation to environmental exposures, personal exposures, and accident and illness reports. The box on p. 238, bottom, lists types of information needed for occupational exposure records. Occupational exposures must be documented, including all substances used in each work area, the air concentration known, and suspected hazardous substances.

HEALTHY PEOPLE 2000 OCCUPATIONAL HEALTH OBJECTIVES—RISK REDUCTION OBJECTIVES

Increase to at least 75% the proportion of work sites with 50 or more employees that mandate employee use of occupant protection systems

Reduce to no more than 15% the proportion of workers exposed to average daily noise levels that exceed 85 dBA

Eliminate exposure that results in workers having blood lead concentrations greater than 25 mg/dl of whole blood

Increase hepatitis B immunization levels to 90% among occupationally exposed workers

From Healthy People 2000: National Health Promotion and Disease Prevention Objectives, Public Health Service, US Department of Health and Human Services, 1990, p 105.

Once an epidemiologic program has been developed that allows the accumulation and analysis of data concerning factors affecting the work force, studies can be designed to provide data for decision-making. Questions about the incidence of cancer in the total plant population by age, sex, and race, as well as the

HEALTHY PEOPLE 2000 OCCUPATIONAL HEALTH OBJECTIVES—SERVICES AND PROTECTION OBJECTIVES

Implement occupational safety and health plans in 50 states for the identification, management, and prevention of leading work-related diseases and injuries within the state

Establish in 50 states exposure standards adequate to prevent the major occupational lung diseases to which worker populations are exposed (bysinosis, asbestosis, coal workers' pneumoconiosis, and silicosis)

Increase to at least 70% the proportion of worksites with 50 or more employees that have implemented programs on worker safety and health

Increase to at least 50% the proportion of worksites with 50 or more employees that offer back injury prevention and rehabilitation programs

Establish in 50 states either public health or labor department programs that provide consultation and assistance to small businesses to implement safety and health programs for their employees

Increase to at least 75% the proportion of primary care providers who routinely elicit occupational health exposures as a part of patient history and provide relevant counseling

* From Healthy People 2000: National Health Promotion and Disease Prevention Objectives, Public Health Service, US Department of Health and Human Services, 1990, p 105.

POTENTIAL REPRODUCTIVE OUTCOMES RESULTING FROM OCCUPATIONAL OR ENVIRONMENTAL EXPOSURES

Sexual dysfunction
Abnormal sperm
Decreased sperm count
Early fetal loss (28 weeks)
Late fetal loss (still birth)
Intrapartum death
Low birth weight
Altered gestational age
Altered sex ratio
Multiple births
Birth defects
Chromosome abnormalities
Infant death
Childhood morbidity
Childhood cancer

incidence of cancer at specific work sites can be answered. The relationship of work exposure to a hazardous substance and incidence of respiratory disease can be determined. Again, these data can be further broken down into age-specific rates or site-specific rates. At the present time, the *Occupational Safety and Health Administration (OSHA)* requires that occupational records be maintained for 40 years. Data sets accumulated over that time frame will allow for determination of attack incidence and morbidity and mortality rates of many different occupational exposures to hazardous substances. These rates can be compared to standardized rates for age, sex, and ethnicity to identify the relationship of exposure to specific disease and/or symptomology.

Risk assessment

Health care costs are a major economic concern in the United States, and industry bears a major portion of the cost of occupational injuries and illness. The oc-

OCCUPATIONAL EXPOSURE INFORMATION

All chemicals used in the plant
Specific chemicals to which specific workers were exposed
The quantity of the exposure
The length of the exposure
Known health effects of chemicals
Toxicity of specific chemicals
Sampling techniques used

RISK ASSESSMENT PROCESS

I. Focus of the risk assessment
   A. What is the purpose?
      1. Identification of needs
      2. Clarification of problem
      3. Analysis of desire (desire for an exercise program)
      4. Identification of resource
      5. Use of resource
   B. What is the scope of the program?
      1. What do you intend to accomplish?
      2. How large is the employee population?
      3. Do you have the needed expertise?
      4. Is the time available?
      5. What is the cost/benefit ratio?
II. Areas of assessment
   A. Employees
   B. Work environment
   C. Organizational resources
   D. Health effects
   E. Economic impact

cupational health nurse uses data from epidemiologic studies of major health problems, both occupational and nonoccupational, to determine the scope of the occupational health program. The goal is to identify risks, assess them, and plan a program that will reduce risk in a cost-effective manner (see box above). The purpose of a *risk assessment* is to carefully determine if a risk exists and what can be done to reduce it. The box above outlines the process of a risk assessment. The risk assessment is performed to identify specific health needs, clarify problem areas, determine feasibility of a program, and identify company resources and use. The scope of the assessment will be determined by the number of employers, availability of a health professional, time available, and cost of the program. The assessment should include data from the epidemiologic surveillance program discussed earlier.

Personal histories must also be maintained. It is essential to accumulate as much data as possible in an individual health history as well as demographic variables on each worker. At the same time, the issue of confidentiality of workers must be addressed. The box on p. 240 lists the types of data needed to determine individual exposure as well as those variables that may affect the development of disease. Accident and illness records are essential data for a well-designed epidemiologic surveillance program. Records from worker compensation claims, disability insurance, health insurance companies, occupational safety and health reports, health maintenance organizations, and death certification are primary sources of data.

PERSONAL EXPOSURE FACTORS

Current and past work history
Nature of jobs
Demographic data (age, sex, race, educational level)
Habits (smoking, drinking, recreational drug use, diet)
Family health history
Health history (chronic illness, genetic predisposition)
Results of multiphasic screening programs
Results of periodic health evaluations

Risk assessments provide management personnel with carefully analyzed data that can be used to make decisions. Occupational health nurses use these data to validate the importance and effectiveness of a program. For example, in 1990, the U.S. Department of Labor reported that repetitive motion disorder accounted for the majority of the cases' increase in the nation's job-related illnesses. About 32,000 new cases of cumulative trauma disorder (CTD) occurred. CTDs now account for 48% of all workplace injuries, up from only 18% in 1980 (Fletcher, 1990). The exposure and eventual injury from CTDs have been reported across a variety of industries including data processing, meat processing, and automotive work. Siebenater (1992) reports that in meat processing alone, the incidence of CTD has risen from 10 reports per 10,000 to 668 reports per 10,000.

The occupational health nurse in a plant employing workers at risk for CTD can now plan a program that decreases the risk to the worker and is cost-effective to the company. Employer costs are both direct and indirect. Direct costs include medical and rehabilitation costs, insurance premiums, and worker compensation payments for lost workdays. Indirect costs include worker replacement and training, decreased productivity, lower morale, and worker turnover (Locke, 1990). Degostino (1989) reports that surgically treated cases of CTD can cost between $5000 and $20,000 depending on the geographic area. Total costs, both direct and indirect, can cost a company $20,000 to $200,000 per case (Katz, 1988). What, then, does the occupational health nurse do with these data? Based on the epidemiologic data and goals of Healthy People 2000 regarding CTD, the nurse can make a good case for changes in company procedures for employees at risk for CTD. For example, assume that the company has 50 workers at risk for CTD and that 10% of these workers develop CTD this year. The following details the cost in health care and worker compensation. (This does not include indirect costs.)

50 employees at risk: 10% (or 5) develop CTD

1. $5000 per employee in avoidable medical costs

   5 Employees × $5000 = $25,000

2. Lost work time

   $10/hour × 8 hours/day = $80
   20 Workdays × 5 employees = $8000

3. Disability payments:
   Average disability: \$1600/month × 5 Employees = \$8000
4. Total dollar cost
   \$41,000 (Low estimate)
   \$116,000 (High estimate)

By developing a program to reduce CTD, the occupational health nurse could save the company between \$40,000 and \$116,000 per year. This example does not account for indirect costs to the company or the very real costs to the employees. Other programs for control of cardiac disease, cancer screenings, fitness programs, back health, respiratory disease, musculoskeletal injuries, and many others can be detailed in this same manner. Epidemiologic data provide the base for an in-depth risk assessment of medical costs. This assessment can lead to changes in the occupational environments that will decrease health risks to the worker and increase productivity.

Accurate and complete data will allow the occupational health team to maintain a complete assessment of the number, causes (internal and external), severity, and other characteristics of occupational illness and injury. Data will also facilitate the identification of high-risk populations within the workplace and permit comparison by demographic and geographic variables. A sound data base is needed in gathering specific data as to the incidence of diseases and the development of predictive models for identifying populations at risk. Epidemiologic research will provide information that leads to the identification of new stressors and the development of reliable and sensitive measurements that will evaluate exposure levels and physiologic response.

This information allows the occupational health professional to make decisions about new programs, additional technology, use of protective equipment, and necessary alteration of the plant or processes that protect the workers and provide a safe and healthful work environment.

SUMMARY

The use of epidemiologic data, both in the environment and occupational settings, to predict health risks to the population is the focus of occupational health. Sources of epidemiologic data for occupational health can be found in the box on p. 242. The establishment of an epidemiologic surveillance program that provides the necessary data is essential. This includes the use of incidence rates, attack rates, and morbidity and mortality data for health care decision-making. The occupational health nurse has a substantial role in analyzing data and developing risk assessments.

CRITICAL THINKING QUESTIONS

1. List three specific community health nursing activities that would have an impact on the environmental health of a given population.
2. The role of the nurse in occupational health includes several distinct areas of practice; identify seven of these areas.

SOURCES OF EPIDEMIOLOGIC DATA FOR OCCUPATIONAL AND ENVIRONMENTAL HEALTH

American Association of Occupational Health Nurses 50 Lennox Pointe NE Atlanta, GA 30324 404-262-1162

American Industrial Health Council 1330 Connecticut Avenue, NW Washington, DC 20036 202-659-0060

Annual Survey of Occupational Injuries and Illnesses US Department of Labor 200 Constitution Ave NW Washington, DC 20210 202-219-6411

Centers for Disease Control and Prevention Public Health Service US Department of Health and Human Services 1600 Clifton Road, NE Atlanta, GA 30333
404-639-3311 (Center for Infectious Diseases)
404-329-3771 (National Institute for Occupational Safety and Health)

Environmental Protection Agency 401 M Street SW Washington, DC 20460 202-260-2090

National Clearinghouse for Mental Health National Institute of Mental Health Parklawn Building 5600 Fisher's Lane Rockville, MD 20857 301-443-4513

National Safety Council 1121 Spring Lake Drive Itasca, IL 60143 708-285-1121

Occupational Safety and Health Administration US Department of Labor 200 Constitution Avenue NW Washington, DC 20210 202-219-8151

Office of Disease Prevention and Health Promotion Department of Health and Human Services 200 Independence Avenue SW Washington, DC 20201 202-205-8611

Public Health Foundation 1120 L Street NW Suite 350 Washington, DC 20005 202-898-5600

3. Discuss the role of the epidemiologist in occupational health surveillance.
4. Describe the process of risk assessment for a hypothetic occupational setting.

REFERENCES

Aldana S, Stone W: Employee physical activity: how does it compare to the nation, *AAOHN J* 40(4):167-172, 1992.

Barlow R, Handelman E: OSHA's final bloodborne pathogen standard, *AAOHN J* 41(1):8-15, 1993.

Degostino M: Carpel tunnel syndrome, an industrial epidemic, *Safety & Health* 11(3):37-39, 1989.

Durkin M and others: The effects of a natural disaster on child behavior: evidence for post traumatic stress, *Am J Public Health* 83(11):1549-1553, 1993.

Eisenbud M and others: *J Indust Hygiene* 31(5):282, 1949.

Elmer-Dewitt P: Summit to save the earth: rich vs poor, *Time* 139(22):43, 1992.

Fletcher M: Cumulative trauma disorders repetitive motion cases costs billions annually, *Business Insurance* 10(6):1-3, 1990.

Frederick L: Cumulative trauma disorders: an overview, *AAOHN J* 40(3):113-116, 1992.

Gold D and others: Rotating shift work, sleep, and accidents related to sleepiness in hospital nurses, *Am J Public Health* 82(7):1011-1013, 1993.

Grady M and others: Occupational exposure to bloodborne diseases and universal precautions, *AAOHN J* 41(11):533-450, 1993.

Haag AB, Glazner LK: A remembrance of the past, an investment for the future, *AAOHN J* 40(2):56-60, 1992.

Hall L: Breast self-examination, *AAOHN J* 40(4):186-191, 1992.

Katz J, Liang M: CTS and the workplace: epidemiologic and management issues, *Int Med Special* 9(5):11-16, 1988.

Kilbourne EM: *Heatwaves: the public health consequences of disasters,* Atlanta, US Department of Health and Human Services, Centers for Disease Control, 46-52, 1989.

Kritz-Silverstein D, Wingard DL, Barrett-Connor E: Employment status and heart disease risk factors in middle-aged women: the Rancho Bernardo study, *Am J Public Health* 82(2):215-218, 1992.

Lechat MF: The epidemiology of health effects of disasters, *Epidemiol Rev* 12:192-195, 1990.

Locke A: Control of disability claims, *Business* 7(24):16-20, 1990.

McMahon B, Pugh T: *Epidemiology principles and methods,* Boston, 1970, Little, Brown, p 1.

Monson RR: *Occupational epidemiology* Boston, 1990, CRC Press, p 105-114.

National Research Council: *Toxicity testing: strategies to determine needs and priorities,* Washington, DC, 1984, National Academy Press, p 18-25.

Occupational carcinogenises: *Occupational Health and Safety News* 5(13):10, 1989.

Office of Cancer Communication: *Cancer of the prostate research report,* NIH Publication No. 89-528, National Cancer Institute, 1989.

Pender, N: *Health promotion in nursing practice,* ed 2, Norwalk, CT, 1987, Appleton & Lange, pp 1-13.

Public Health Service: *Health promotion and disease prevention,* DHHS Pub No. (PHS) 88-1591, Hyattsville, MD, 1988, US Department of Health and Human Services, p 18-36.

Public Health Service: *Healthy People 2000: National Health Promotion and Disease Prevention Objectives,* DHHS Publication No. (PHS) 91-50212, Washington, DC, 1990, US Department of Health and Human Services, pp 318-332.

Rammazzini B: *The diseases of workers (demorbis artificum),* Library of the New York Academy of Medicine, New York, 1964, Hafner, pp 1-25.

Siebernater MJ, McGovern P: Carpel tunnel syndrome, priorities for prevention, *AAOHN J* 40(2):62-71, 1992.

Sigerist HE: Historical background of industrial and occupational disease, *Bull N Y Acad Med* (2nd series) 12:597-609, 1936.

Sorenseon G and others: Work-site nutrition intervention and employees' dietary habits: the Treatwell program, *Am J Public Health* 82(6):877-881, 1992.

Wicher C: AIDS and HIV: the dilemma of the health care worker, *AAOHN J* 41(6):282-288, 1993.

Zeballos TL: Health aspects of the Mexico earthquake—19th September, 1985, *Disasters* 10:141-149, 1986.

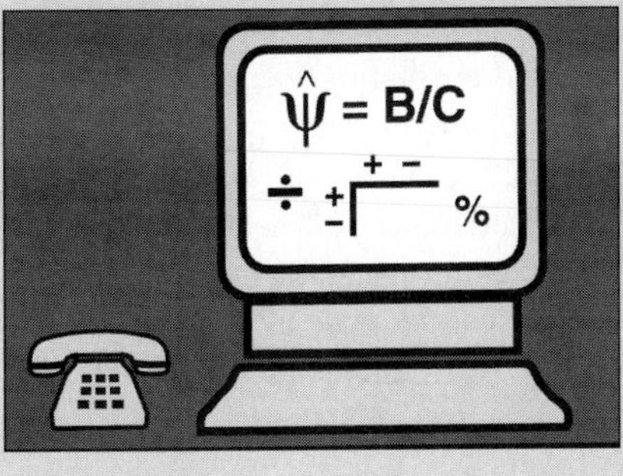

14

Epidemiology in Health Planning and Health Policy

MARIE V. ROBERTO

Objectives

1. Apply epidemiologic methods to concepts of health planning and health policy development.
2. Define the role of nursing in health policy and health planning.
3. Define core functions of public health and the basis for health planning.
4. Use public health concepts and epidemiologic methods in developing capacity building intervention strategies.
5. Explore the concept of planned change, including the interrelationships of the scientific method, nursing process, epidemiology, and health care planning.
6. Develop a basic understanding of small-area analysis as a method in health planning at the local level.
7. Define health policy and a framework for evaluating policy.

Key terms

cost-benefit analysis
distributive policies
health planning
health policy
inputs
outputs
planned change
population-based planning
redistributive policies
regulative policies
small-area analysis

Health services research and health policy development are dependent on epidemiologic data. For example, planning and evaluating medical and health care rely on ascertaining appropriate data on the patients being served by a program, services received, quality of those services, and outcomes. Data about populations is then used to plan for health services and to set new health policy. Fig. 14-1 illustrates the interrelationships among epidemiologic data, health planning, health policy, and health programs. Epidemiologic data serve as foundations for planning and implementing health programs and for policies that eventually affect the health status of populations and health services delivered to populations. For example, patient classification systems begin with information on the kinds of patients being seen in a hospital, doctor's office, clinic, or home care agency. Who are they, and what are their problems? The emphasis is on the aggregate and not on an individual patient.

In 1862, Florence Nightingale proposed that data be collected on individual patients and aggregated for the purposes of defining mortality for the hospital as a whole and for individual wards (Nightingale, 1863). She proposed collecting data on diagnoses, operations, complications, and demographic information, such as age, sex, and occupation. She also was interested in the length of stay of the patient and proposed collecting information on the dates of admission, discharge or death. Thus Florence Nightingale contributed to today's interest in patient classification systems and diagnosis-related groupings. Both are basic to health services planning and policy and are areas where nurses have contributed much research.

NEW DIRECTIONS FOR PUBLIC HEALTH

Because of a national concern with the public's health and the system for delivery of public health services in the United States, the Institute of Medicine (IOM) initiated a study of the future of public health in the United States (Committee for

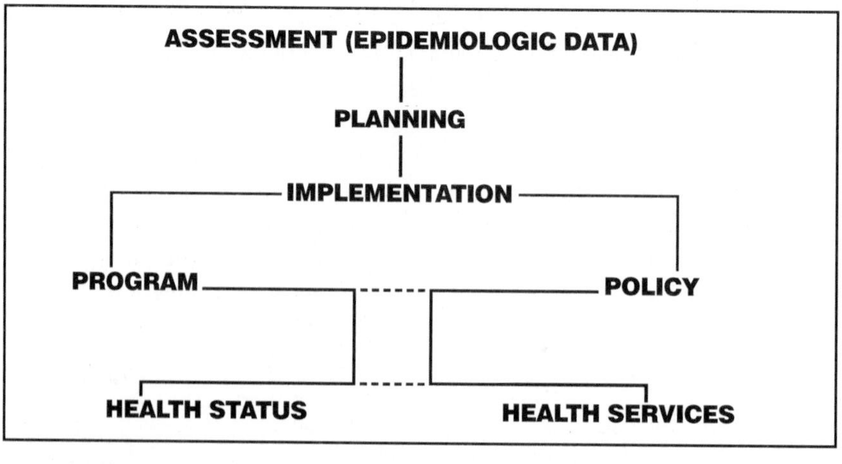

Fig. 14-1 Relationships between epidemiologic data, health planning, policy, and program development.

the Study of the Future of Public Health, 1988). This study is referred to as the IOM report on *The Future of Public Health.* The mission of public health is defined in this report as promoting the interest of society to guarantee that conditions exist so that people can be healthy (Committee, 1988). Fulfilling this mission involves both the public and private sectors working together to apply current scientific data to prevent disease and promote health.

Why is it important to define public health and understand the mission of public health? Public health is the arena in which planning efforts and policy decisions are made. These decisions influence not only how health services are delivered in the United States, but also how the effects of prevention and promotion strategies impact the health of the collective whole.

For purposes of this discussion, the definition of public health by C.E.A. Winslow, as quoted in the IOM report, will serve as the basis for health planning and policy (Committee, 1988):

> "Public health is the science and the art of (1) preventing disease, (2) prolonging life, and (3) organized community efforts for (a) the sanitation of the environment, (b) the control of communicable infections, (c) the education of the individual in personal hygiene, (d) the organization of medical and nursing services for the early diagnosis and preventive treatment of disease, and (e) the development of the social machinery to ensure everyone a standard of living adequate for the maintenance of health, so organizing these benefits as to enable every citizen to realize his birthright of health and longevity."

Public health, then, is concerned with organized, planned approaches to fulfilling the activities outlined by Winslow.

Lillian Wald understood the need to activate the "social machinery" to make lasting changes in the health of the population. As the founder of the Henry Street Settlement and Visiting Nurse Service of New York in 1893, Wald worked actively for better social conditions and better health care for the immigrant families of the Lower East Side of New York (Daniels, 1989). That meant active involvement in the politics of the times, planning for funding for her operations, and more importantly, planning for the delivery of services to the community she served. As a reformer of the social order of the day, and of the health care system, Wald had to be more than an idealist. She gave substance to her ideals by employing an understanding of the political system and developing pragmatic plans to achieve her ends.

As the mission of public health in the United States for the year 2000 and beyond is rethought, there is a need to review Wald's views, ideas, and strategies for building the capacity to address modern-day public health concerns, including those in the environmental and mother-child health arenas. A working knowledge of the principles and methods of epidemiology applied to the problems of prevention and health promotion is the framework for action, as it was for Wald, in solving health care problems for this decade and into the next century.

The IOM report on *The Future of Public Health* ascribes three core functions to government's role in public health: assessment, policy development, and assurance. These core functions are similar to three of the problem-solving techniques underlying the nursing process: (1) assessment to define the problem; (2)

intervention through the development of relevant public policy, which includes mobilizing the appropriate resources to address the problem; and (3) assurance (evaluation) that services were delivered and outcomes achieved.

The issue of health care access for the uninsured in the United States has become an important issue for candidates for public office and members of the health care industry. How do we provide for the "working poor" who do not receive health benefits through their employer? How do we provide for workers who have preexisting conditions (health care problems that existed before employment or application for health insurance) that make them ineligible for insurance because of the high risks they impose to insurers? Assessing who the uninsured are requires data on employment and health care status. Financing as a barrier to health care access is being explored to determine the appropriate intervention (solution) to the problem. Such a discussion raises issues of access to health care for all Americans regardless of economic status and the need for a reform of the health care agenda for the nation.

The American Nurses Association (ANA) spearheaded a plan to address the need for health care reform in the United States (ANA, 1991). This plan incorporates a public/private initiative using elements of planned change to foresee health service needs that correlate with the changing national demographics (ANA, 1991). It proposes as an outcome a cost-effective, accessible, and federally defined core service package. The system for care is envisioned as preventive, emphasizing primary care, health promotion, and disease prevention. A new health care policy for the United States is the goal. Perhaps a modern version of Lillian Wald's and Florence Nightingale's activism through efforts of organized nursing has been witnessed. The outcome will be decided through the political process.

If the public health system needs reform, what strategies are suggested to build the capacity to strengthen the core functions of assessment, policy development, and assurance? In January 1991, the Public Health Service of the United States proposed several strategies (U.S. Public Health Service, 1991).

To assess the health needs of the nation, quality health information (data) is essential. Assessment must include epidemiologic data, including demographic information (natality and mortality statistics). Identifying the gaps in the data that are available is important. Need cannot be defined and progress cannot be tracked without (1) measures of evaluation, such as measures of health status (morbidity, mortality, risk factors) and health services (the existing structure for provision of care, public or private); (2) measuring ways in which health care is delivered and the performance of providers; and (3) measuring outcomes or the effects of clinical care.

When scientists defined a new disease, acquired immunodeficiency syndrome (AIDS), new policies for prevention, education, and equal protection under the law (confidentiality of the data) were developed. At the same time, gaps in services were identified. Reviews of sectors of the health care delivery system, including practices of clinical providers resulted in the initiation of new recommendations, such as the adoption of universal precautions by health care personnel. As a result, new health care concerns, citizen agendas, and political policies emerged. Planning and policy related to AIDS and the human immunodeficiency virus (HIV) were based on the epidemiology of the disease and its etiologic agent.

Health policy, when based on science and public health knowledge, will use strategic health planning as the vehicle for realizing goals for public health. Epidemiology drives both the health planning and health policy process.

EPIDEMIOLOGY: BASIS FOR ASSESSMENT

Epidemiology is not a new science. In London in 1662, John Graunt analyzed data on births and deaths and described patterns of infant and childhood mortality and causes of adult deaths (see Chapter 1). Epidemiology originated in England with record-keeping. The records on births and deaths provided the mechanism for monitoring statistics on death and illness (Rothman, 1981). Is it no wonder, then, that the environment was conducive to the analyses that Florence Nightingale conducted nearly 200 years later?

Note that both Graunt's and Nightingale's analyses were nonexperimental in nature. They derived their conclusions from using secondary data, the recorded episodes of events. They applied the scientific method to systematically review and analyze the data that they collected. They did not conduct clinical trials or experiments but rather used data to help describe what they were encountering, make inferences, and, for Nightingale, intervene in the process of health care delivery based on conclusions from the data.

From the early 1600s to the present day, epidemiology has been the methodology used to describe risks from various sources. As Rothman (1981) notes, we can point to epidemiology for information that led to the identification of an association between the quality of water and spread of cholera, between cigarette smoking and lung cancer, and between diet and cardiovascular disease.

Today epidemiologists are concerned with risks from different sources. For example, the health effects of low-level radiation and toxic wastes are being examined. Occupational exposures to toxins in the workplace and its relationship to cancer incidence are being investigated. The relationship between effectiveness of immunizations among children and outbreaks of infectious diseases that are preventable are being studied. As the United States grapples with the high infant mortality rates in some cities, epidemiologists continue to track and monitor trends in infant deaths and risk factors affecting birth outcomes. Whether it is infectious disease, chronic disease, environmental causes of disease, or risks related to mother-child health, epidemiologists contribute to changes in health care delivery by analyzing and interpreting the epidemiologic data derived from demographic information, vital statistics, and small-area studies. Epidemiologic methods can help identify new health problems and contribute to solutions to solve these problems.

Epidemiologic methods describe phenomena occurring in groups or populations through statistical analysis and interpretation of findings. The aim of epidemiology is to define the risks associated with various states of health, identify clues to disease causation, and support the need for health care services to ameliorate specific conditions. For example, women residing in defined, high-risk, geographic areas can be provided with better access to prenatal care. Epidemiologic methods also emphasize the capacity to predict which variables are more significantly associated with the problem under study. For example, education, race, sex, religion/ethnicity, or age may be a significant predictor of use of family planning services in a given community.

Traditionally, epidemiology has been concerned with describing the health status of a given population. It includes information on the agent, host, and environmental interaction. The personal characteristics of the host include demographic data, such as age, sex, and socioeconomic and marital status. Environmental factors include information on toxins from the macrosystem (water and air) or from occupational exposures in the workplace. The agent is the etiologic factor(s) responsible for the disease or health condition.

A more recent use of epidemiology is in the area of health services. Health services may be viewed as either a factor affecting the health status of a population (independent variable) or the outcome of a planning and policy process (dependent variable). A researcher may be interested in the effect of the availability of mammography screening on breast cancer detection. In this situation, examining the need for mammography screening, coupled with the demand for services, would affect the outcome or availability of services within a given community. The cost of those services would be of interest from a planning and policy perspective. In addition, the effect of services on breast cancer detection would close the loop between health status and health services. Ibrahim (1985) states this relationship as follows:

> "Concerns of medical care research and health policy analysis have largely been process oriented. That is, their focus has been on the efficiency of health services rather than the efficacy and effectiveness. The epidemiologic approach, with its primary concern on changes in health conditions of populations, adds an important element to the shaping of health policy. Considering health services as 'another' factor in determining health states would place the provision of these services within their proper context: a means to an end rather than an end in itself."

EPIDEMIOLOGY: METHOD FOR PLANNED CHANGE

Thus far, the relationship of epidemiology to the field of public health and, specifically, to the core functions of government in public health that include policy development has been examined. The application of epidemiologic methods to the definition of a population's health status and the impact of health services research on the planning and policy process was explored. A brief review of the elements of change that define change as planned and not happenstance is important before we consider the planning process in detail.

What does the term *planned change* mean? As defined by Chin and Benne (1969) changes that are the result of a thoughtful, deliberate, conscious process are considered planned. What does this mean for nursing? Any change that consciously uses scientific knowledge to cause a modification or alteration in a nursing plan of care is considered planned. It means nurses are not acting solely from an intuitive perspective when assessing patient or population needs. Instead, nurses use the data at hand or information from the literature and research studies to alter their practices. Nurses act as change agents when planning to alter the care for patients. The need to change or alter patient behavior to affect healthy life-styles is of special interest. Such change demands of the nurse a knowledge of behavior and how such behavior may need to be altered to allow a person to assume the maximal posture for a healthy life-style.

Three strategies for change have been described. These strategies are (1) empirical-rational, (2) normative-reeducative, and (3) power-coercive (Chin and Benne 1969). Empirical-rational strategies use epidemiologic methods for creating change. Health education interventions are based on the normative-reeducative strategies employed in health-planning programs aimed at attitudinal/behavioral changes. Health policy is embodied in the power-coercive strategy for change.

Empirical-rational model

The empirical-rational model allows for change based on scientific interpretation of phenomena and application of scientific knowledge to problem solving. This chapter is mainly concerned with the use of the empirical-rational model for affecting change in health planning and health policy. Epidemiologic data applied to the determination of the health status of a given population and to the definition of need for health services can stimulate need for change. When information is available about the causes of infant mortality, such as the risk factors contributing to low birth weight and adequacy of prenatal care, a picture can be drawn of the health of a given population. At the same time, if information on the accessibility and acceptability of prenatal services available to women is obtained, information that can lead to planning new approaches to reach women at risk can also be gathered. This information can also be used to identify needed services, set policy for creating new services, develop new supportive efforts to connect women at risk with those services, and seek new funding sources.

Several approaches can be used to affect change in specific situations. Both the epidemiologic and nursing processes are variations of the scientific method and therefore contribute to the empirical-rational model. A comparison of these two processes is found in Chapter 1. The application of the nursing process in the community resembles the epidemiologic process. Public health nurses (1) assess the health conditions of a population, including the physical environment, beliefs, values, and attitudes of the community; (2) collect data from appropriate sources, including governmental and health agencies; (3) mobilize the community to help determine the appropriate plan of care, such as working with community action groups or interested residents for housing for the elderly; (4) implement the plan in the community, such as instituting a program for follow-up of active tuberculosis in elderly residents or initiation of support groups for at-risk mothers; and (5) evaluate the outcomes of interventions by developing specific measures of accomplishments.

Normative-reeducative model

Normative-reeducative strategies are based on the belief that changes in values and behaviors are changes at the personal level that account for societal and individual change. The individual or group of clients must be involved in their own reeducation. They should be involved in the planning process to affect lasting change. It is not enough for professionals to design systems of care; they also should involve the affected individual, their family, and the community in the design of the necessary change. For example, nurses should involve the individual and appropriate groups when designing or suggesting changes in the individual's nursing care plan or when planning for community-based services, such as prenatal home visits or well-child clinics. The client(s) may determine their needs to be different than the professional's assessment.

Power-coercive model

Power-coercive strategies employ political and economic incentives for change. Such change is derived from health policy initiatives based on analysis of the problems being reviewed. For example, government can determine what services will be paid for by public dollars. Special-interest groups and other power brokers will advocate for the "public good" as they determine it to be for their constituencies. The administration of President George Bush had prevailed on removing federal support from family planning clinics where abortions were an option. That federal policy left the states to determine their level of support for the full range of family planning services, only one of which was an abortion option. Such policies are coercive in nature, because they determine who can and cannot receive full-range health services. These policies also influence the nature of a health provider-patient relationship, whether a plan of care for an individual is developed or programs are developed for groups of women seeking services.

EPIDEMIOLOGY AND HEALTH PLANNING

In this section, three issues will be explored: (1) the benefits of health planning; (2) key elements in the planning process, including the relationship of planning to the scientific method and nursing process; and (3) key concepts in assessment of need, the analysis, design, and implementation of programs, evaluation, and health planning.

Benefits of health planning

Why should nurses be concerned about *health planning*? One basic reason is the current concern with costs of health care and access to health care. Can a community afford the health services that individuals want or need? Are there enough health care professionals, including nurses, available in a given community to address the health care concerns of the public? Planning is essential if we are to address which form of health insurance is the least costly and delivers an agreed-on benefit package. It is hoped that planning will be conducted before health services are instituted. Evaluation of cost-effectiveness should be a part of that planning process. Planning will prepare agencies before they meet with regulatory bodies that include cost-containment commissions.

Planning is the difference between crisis management and rational management of an organization. Does a nurse administrator respond to the current crisis only, or does one assess the nursing needs of patients in the institution, determine how to best meet those needs, and implement a strategy for change? Implementing change takes time and a well-thought-out approach to affect the change desired. Planning encompasses the rational approach to management. Dealing only with crises is not productive when change is desired. Moving from one crisis to another does not permit an individual to assess a situation accurately or design appropriate intervention strategies.

Project management involves the planning process. To reach the objectives for any project the necessary steps must be outlined to meet the objectives and evaluate whether the objectives were met and if so, to what degree or quality. If a nurse teaches group diabetic classes, objectives should be developed, content to be taught or reviewed should be determined, and outlines should be developed for each session. This lesson plan is just that—a planning document. Rational answers to health care dilemmas cannot be expected unless the problem is approached systematically.

Components of the planning process

What, then, are the key elements of the planning process (Fig. 14-2)? According to Herman (1968), there are four steps in program planning: (1) definition of the problem and resources; (2) formulation of a practical objective; (3) selection and implementation of a course of action; and (4) evaluation. These elements closely resemble elements of the nursing process and scientific method. Tools are available for implementing the proposed plan. Some implementation strategies are found in the literature related to time management. The methods worth exploring include use of program evaluation and review techniques (PERT) charts, program planning and budgeting (PPB), and operations management and budgeting (OMB).

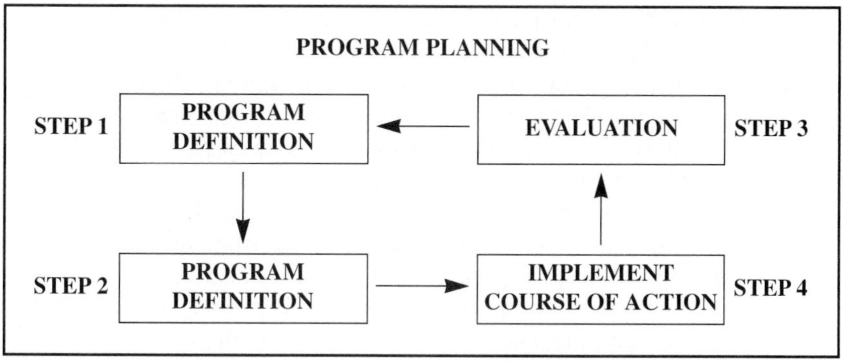

Fig. 14-2 Program planning.

Traditionally, planning focuses on outcomes at several levels (Shonick, 1980). Planning is an integral part of health care institutions. The focus is on the goals, objectives, and needs of the institution and its clients. Hospitals, health maintenance organizations (HMOs), and home care agencies use planning principles to remain viable institutions for the communities they serve.

Program planning is often related to grant administration and the outcomes required of the grantee for changes in the population affected. For example, a health agency may receive state or federal dollars to implement a screening program for high blood pressure. The outcomes may be defined as the number of people screened and the number of positive findings including plans for follow-up of individuals. In this case, the plan for the health agency (program plan) would be based on goals already determined by the granting agency.

Population-based planning

Population-based planning is of particular interest to epidemiologists. As stated previously, epidemiology is more concerned with the health states of populations rather than the states of individuals. Therefore planners interested in affecting changes in populations need to use epidemiologic methods in their deliberations.

Population-based planning often refers to planning for access to health care services. Emphasis is placed on methods to determine the needs and demands (desires) of the public for services. One cannot determine needs of a population for services without information about that population (demographics). In addition, data about the health status of the population derived from epidemiologic investigations, should be the basis of need studies. Without that data as a basis for planning, any determination of services or resources that are needed may be made on false assumptions. How can it be determined if a new mammography facility is necessary without knowing the demographics of the area in which the facility is to be located? Information about the number of women in the targeted risk groups, incidence of breast cancer among the risk groups, and current level of available services is critical to the decision-making process.

Assessment of need

DeBella (1986) aptly defines the components of assessment. DeBella defines need as a health deficiency, or a perceived difference between a desired health outcome and an existing state of health. Such a definition usually is derived from professional interpretation. However, demand can be either professionally or consumer-determined. Consumers demand services based on their wants. Wants often drive the policy process even if the planning process determines that there is no need in a given community for designated health services. Providers of health care can also drive demand, based on the economic survivability of the provider's services. Both are less than adequate methods of determining demand for services.

Where, then, can more objective data be obtained to help in determining the need of a given population? The answer lies in the use of health data that measures the disease/disability index for a given community. Donabedian (1979) has written extensively on the topic of assessment of need and can be referenced for additional understanding of this topic.

What data are used for determining health status and therefore needed for health care interventions or services? Basic epidemiologic data include: (1) demographics, (2) mortality data, (3) morbidity data, (4) natality data, and (5) information on absence of risk factors and sense of well-being (as a measure of a "healthy state"). Community planners cannot know what to recommend to policy-makers without a thorough knowledge of the effects of these data on their community. How can services for prevention and treatment of strokes be designed without knowing the number of people who die from strokes in the community, description of who is suffering from this disease, levels of disability of survivors, and psychosocial and economic effects on the survivors?

A good example of how this type of data is generated for use by state agencies is a health profile produced by the Centers for Disease Control and Prevention. This health profile compares each state with the nation as a whole. The intent is to make state agencies cognizant of their status on major health indicators as compared to the nation and profile areas in which they need to focus interventions and apply resources to better the health of the population in the state. An example is the Connecticut Health Profile for 1991 (CDC, 1991). Demographic information compares Connecticut with the nation on the following factors: median age, percentage of population below the poverty level, percentage of population residing in rural areas, racial distribution of the population, and median years of education for persons 25 years and older. Some information is based on census data. Information is also provided on (1) mortality (leading causes of death, years of potential life lost, and work-related injury/deaths); (2) infectious disease trends (AIDS, salmonellosis, syphilis, and tuberculosis); (3) health and safety of young people (infant mortality, injury fatalities, and measles); and (4) health-promotion strategies (smoking, fluoridation, mammography). Connecticut agencies are using these mortality, natality, and other population data bases to address the health needs of the population of the state as a whole.

Traditionally, epidemiology focuses efforts on person, place, and time when seeking information on a disease and its etiology. Data is produced on several levels: national—to determine health status of the nation; state—to identify major problems affecting the health status of a given population within legally defined borders; and smaller areas of determination of health status, such as cities or rural districts. The application of newer geographic mapping strategies is of interest and importance today. Such action can determine the health of people residing within census tracts of cities or even neighborhood blocks.

Small-area analysis. Why is *small-area analysis* important? Due to the composition of a state or city, wide variations may exist in available resources, use of health care services, and expenditures for support of health care services. For example, screening services may vary, widely based on the geography of a region, availability of medical care services, and public funding for screening. Small-area analysis attempts to define the health needs of a population within a given area.

Small-area analysis allows a planner to compare the needs of a high-risk population to the area as a whole. For example, in some urban centers, infant mortality rates are higher than the state's overall rate. How should policy-makers allocate resources to address the areas of greatest risk? Is it enough to allocate additional resources to the city as a whole? Are there certain areas of the city where infant mortality rates are higher? What programs should be developed to reverse those trends? Small-area analysis, using epidemiologic and other socioeconomic data, can help to pinpoint areas of greatest need and reasons for the negative health indicators. This is truly a public health approach to planning and intervention.

Analysis and design

When designing an intervention, planners consider the impact of the intervention on health status, the acceptability of the intervention to the population, and, an economic evaluation. The economic evaluation is often used to justify the use of resources allocated for a new program. This evaluation can take many forms.

Drummond (1987) identified the components of an economic evaluation. They include *inputs* (resources consumed) and *outputs* (health improvement determined by health effects and benefits). Inputs are measured in costs that include direct, indirect (production losses), and intangible costs passed along to the family, health care, or insurance sectors. Outputs are measured by health data, such as mortality data, years of potential life gained, and incidence of newly diagnosed cases. Outputs are defined by epidemiologic data. Those data concern measures of changes in physical, social, and emotional functioning, quality of life, and use of health care resources.

One of the most interesting areas for further study is the one Drummond (1987) calls quality-adjusted life year, a measure of cost-utility. It is an economic evaluation that focuses on the quality of the health outcome caused or prevented by a health program or treatment. When quality of life is the outcome of interest, cost-utility analysis is a preferred method of economic evaluation. It would seem that nursing can make use of this methodology, since nursing interventions are aimed at improving the quality of life and not just the quantity of life. For example, nurses can support the survival of a stroke victim but more importantly, are concerned with improving the quality of life for the individual. Quality of life can encompass physical functioning (mobility), role functioning (self-care), emotional functioning (adaptation to illness), and other health problems related to adequate functioning, such as hearing deficits that would affect quality of life.

Cost-benefit analysis is currently used in health planning to determine the appropriate amount and levels of health services needed by a given population. To determine the benefit of a given nurse/population ratio, a planner would have to consider the costs to educate and employ a nurse. The benefits would have to be defined as the value of the improved health outcome due to the nursing interventions. Nursing needs to continually consider and measure the effectiveness of nursing interventions in producing healthy outcomes for groups of patients and communities. This type of analysis continues to be a fertile field for nursing research and development.

Implementation

Once a situation has been assessed and analyzed and a plan has been devised, the next step is implementation of the plan. Implementation can take several forms.

Policies can be devised imposing new methods of operating on the public and provider communities. Administrative changes may need to be adopted by an agency, such as a health department, to merge programs serving the same populations. Planned change also includes those affected by the change. Therefore individuals at the operating level of the agency should be involved in the implementation of change. Tools, such as project management, Gant charts, bar charts, and PERT charts can be employed to actualize the implementation strategy. Using graphic displays of the process for implementation is a good management tool; nurses should become comfortable with the diagramming process. The diagram or chart will help in evaluating progress.

Policy development is an intervention strategy. The following discussion examines how epidemiologic data can be applied to policy decisions. The following issue was presented at a health policy forum at George Washington University: *Minority Health: Breaking Down the Barriers.* The purpose of the forum was the examination of successful strategies that have been used in addressing some of the critical health problems that are impacting both quality of life and length of life of minorities, particularly minority youth. The stated policy agenda item to address the noted disparity between majority and minority health status was (The George Washington University, 1991):

> " . . . ultimately, there will most likely be a complete overhaul of the delivery and payment systems, one that is based on primary care and health promotion rather than on acute, episodic care that offers no follow-up beyond the emergency room and no continuity of care for patients whose health problems may be chronic or who otherwise need a more stable, secure source of care."

What data were used to determine the disparity between majority and minority health status? Infant mortality rates were examined to find that the death rate for black babies was more than double that of white babies (17.6 versus 8.5 deaths per 1000 live births in 1988). Many minority babies also suffered long-term disabilities due to the mother's poor nutritional state or drug use. Minority youth were more adversely affected by deaths secondary to violence. Homicide was a leading cause of death of teenage minority men, largely due to substance abuse and the need for channeling aggressive behavior. The life expectancy rates between black and white men showed consistent disparity (72.3 years for whites; 64.9 for blacks).

Such epidemiologic data form the basis for implementation strategies to reverse the disparities. The government's response to an issue at this policy level was the creation of the Office of Minority Health, an administrative division in the Department of Health and Human Services. Creating the administrative agency provides the structure for leveraging public resources to address the issue. Demonstration grants have been awarded to improve outreach and coordinate services for minority males. Some efforts have been put into place to reach minorities through educational programs. However, true reform of the health care delivery and financing system remains a task facing the nation into the twenty-first century. The research agenda must include all epidemiologic considerations, including the effects of socioeconomic status, cultural and life-style patterns, as well as genetic differences when defining strategies for reversing the trends of poor health outcomes for minorities.

Evaluation

The impact of evaluation on selecting an implementation strategy has been discussed. Health outcomes describe the change in health status of a population resulting from an intervention, such as a screening program for prostate cancer. Epidemiologic data are used to define those outcomes. Evaluation then is the final step in a planning process. However, as has been shown, evaluation is also an ongoing process throughout the entire planning project. Assessment and evaluation are key to epidemiologic data and methods. Such information adds to the objective bases for evaluation, making it less subjective in nature.

EPIDEMIOLOGY AND HEALTH POLICY

What is meant when speaking of health policy? What is policy? Webster's New World Dictionary (1991) defines policy as "a principle, plan, or course of action, as pursued by a government, organization, individual, etc."; also "wise, expedient, or prudent conduct or management." Notice the attributes ascribed to the policy process that include planning. Policy has already been defined as an implementation strategy in the planning process. Therefore epidemiologic data should lead to a planning process and should be the foundation of good health policy, especially public health policy.

Politics often defines policy. Why? Politics is the method used by government when fashioning a public policy. The politics of any organization can affect the policy adopted by that organization. For example, the opinions of a medical staff and the principles of an institution may promote or hamper the types of procedures performed at the institution and the levels of care acceptable to a given institution. The method of organization for the delivery of nursing services becomes a policy of a given institution. Whether primary nursing becomes the method of delivery of nursing care in an institution or another form of management is adopted is as much the result of the politics within the nursing leadership of the institution as it is of the planning process.

Another perspective of policy is proposed by Crichton (1981). She suggests that the policy process is concerned with employing a new intervention or maintaining a current activity. Policy, then, is the end result of making a decision. It is hoped that the decision is based on problem solving, a rational approach. However, rationality is tempered by the art of compromise. Compromising is often used as a method of gaining support for one's position. Thus the art of politics becomes a reality when health policy is developed. Where does scientific knowledge play a part? Epidemiologic knowledge can be substituted for scientific knowledge.

Scientific knowledge should define the outer boundaries for policy development, beyond which irrationality predominates. This latter situation occurs when too much is compromised. For example, in encouraging individuals to assume more responsibility for their health, incentives may be given to individuals who adopt health-promotion activities. They may receive reductions on their insurance premiums, a positive outcome of a policy. However, a policy may penalize individuals who become sick by limiting future coverage or taxing that individual. Such a policy would be punitive and not reflect what is known about disease, etiologic factors, aging, and environmental effects.

Policy analysis is used to study how policies began and their desired effects versus actual effects. Such analysis is conducted by policy analysts, many of whom are political scientists. Such analysis usually operates within a given policy framework. As capricious as policy development may appear on the surface, analysts can determine how policies came to be and whether they were the result of action or inaction. Several policy frameworks or conceptual models for policy analysis exist.

Policy framework

Marmor (1973) describes three models for policy analysis: the rational actor model, the organizational process model, and the bureaucratic politics model.

Rational actor model. The rational actor model is the most common model for policy analysis used in the United States. In this model it is assumed that government acts in a purposeful way. The persons in positions to make policy act in a rational way. Decisions are made after defining the goal of the policy and reviewing the alternatives. The focus of this approach is on the strategy chosen by the governmental agency in making its decision. The central concepts include the government as the major player. As the focal point for decision-making, the government sets the goals, defines the solutions, determines the course of action, and evaluates the consequences. These steps should sound familiar. The steps in the problem-solving process and nursing process parallel this model. Goals and objectives are set, assessment of the situation takes place, plans to address the situation are defined, a policy is developed as an implementation strategy, and finally, the policy is analyzed or evaluated. When setting health policy, the content areas of demography and epidemiology are essential. Marmor further describes this rational actor model and the role of government. He states that government is viewed as acting rationally. Government personnel describe the policy needed, define the problem, hypothesize an effect, and evaluate the effect (Marmor, 1973). Epidemiologic methods are important for predicting effects of health care interventions.

Organizational process model. The second model of analysis, the organizational process model, is used when the behavior of an organization is the unit of analysis. The emphasis in this model is on process—how an organization behaved when policy was being made. The major emphasis is on how the organization regularly behaved, its standard operating procedures, its capacity for handling incremental change, its information systems, and its viewpoint as an organization (Marmor, 1973). To understand how a policy was developed the actions of the different organizations or governmental units involved would need to be analyzed. For example, when setting a federal policy for long-term care many organizational units need to be analyzed. These include the Department of Health and Human Services, especially the Health Care Financing Administration that administers the Medicare and Medicaid programs; the Veteran's Administration that provides for elderly veterans' needs and for their families; the Housing and Urban Development Agency, for housing needs for the elderly; the Department of Transportation, for support for elderly transportation services; and the Public Health Service that supports primary care through community health centers and programs training geriatric nurse practitioners. Concepts from epidemiology may not be as immediately useful for this model of analysis.

Bureaucratic politics model. The final model, the bureaucratic politics model, examines the art of compromise defined earlier. The outcome or policy results from bargaining between the key players whether they are governmental employees or lobbyists. This model presumes that the players are of unequal position on the issue. Therefore bargaining and compromise are the methods by which a policy is derived. The difference between this model and the rational actor model is evident. In the rational actor model policy is selected based on data and determining the best solution to a given problem. In the bureaucratic politics model, the art of compromise and "pork barrel politics" or backroom politics is the method for policy determination. When the ANA developed its proposal for health care reform in 1991 it sought support of many nursing organizations for the purpose of increasing its bargaining position and power. When ANA speaks for health care reform, it represents approximately 1,000,000 nurses through the endorsement of the many nursing organizations that signed onto the agenda. That number represents a significant block of votes for members of Congress to consider.

Different models of analysis can be chosen based on the policy under discussion. Many begin with data on the issue but approach the process of analysis differently. Three types of policies apply to the implementation of any public policy: distributive, regulative, and redistributive (Marmor, 1973). *Distributive policies* attempt to hand out benefits to interested parties. *Regulative policies* set parameters around a situation that all parties must adhere to, for example, licensure of home care agencies in order to participate in public reimbursement for services. *Redistributive policies* attempt to reallocate resources among disadvantaged groups, such as small group insurance reform to address the needs of the uninsured or working poor. Different types of policies are derived from the problem needing resolution.

Governmental policies are the cornerstones of important government interventions. When citizens are dissatisfied with the circumstances surrounding an issue, government is expected to act to make matters right. The government uses a policy-making process when making public policy.

Policy-making process

According to Kelman (1987) the policy process is comprised of five steps: (1) policy idea, (2) political choice, (3) production, (4) final government actions, and (5) real-world outcomes. The idea for a policy is the first step. Someone proposes a change they believe the government should initiate. For example, a proposal may be made to expand mother-child health services to women who are at

185% of the poverty level rather than at the poverty level. Such a proposal affects a mother's eligibility and may mean more women and children would be eligible for health services and would expand the access to health care. Such a policy idea would also increase government's financial support to a greater number of individuals, using more tax dollars.

If the decision is made to expand eligibility for mother-child health services, a political choice has been made. Such a choice formally commits government to a certain course of action. The political portion of the action occurs when people disagree with the decision, but the majority prevails. Action through the legislative process may be a mechanism for enacting policy or through fiat (regulation) from a bureaucratic agency of government.

Production means that policies must be put into place or carried out by government organizations. At the federal level, that may be a department such as Health and Human Services or the National Institutes of Health. At the state level, a Department of Health Services may be empowered by a state legislature to implement the political decision.

Final government actions refer to the actual implementation of programs at the local level. The people intended to receive the services actually begin receiving benefits. For example, in any given community, outreach workers actually would begin to enroll individuals eligible for mother-child health services under an expanded eligibility program, and these individuals would receive needed health services.

Real-world outcomes are the end results of the political process. Did the appropriate individuals receive the services needed? Did those services make a difference to the individuals involved? Did more mothers deliver normal weight, full-term infants, or was there no change in the incidence of low birth weight babies? Access to prenatal care should assist in producing normal outcomes.

Steps in the policy-making process are familiar. They approximate steps in the problem-solving and nursing processes from a statement of the problem to assessment, diagnosis, implementation of plans to address the problem, and evaluation. Epidemiologic information would be essential in the example of expanded eligibility of mother-child health services. Data on low birth weight incidence, incidence of infant mortality, and late or absent prenatal care would be important information to enter into the assessment process and evaluation of outcomes.

A state health department is in a position to develop a framework for its policy development. It is important that any policy framework be cognizant of national initiatives in public health and supportive of the policy directives of the executive branch of state government. Similar to Kelman's five-step process for making policy, the Connecticut Department of Health Services has defined five steps in its articulation of health policy (Connecticut Department of Health Services, 1991). They include (1) the definition of the goal of a systematic and standardized policy development process, (2) an agreed on definition of policy, (3) a rationale for a centralized system of policy development, (4) the development of a standard set of criteria for evaluating policy proposals, and (5) an outline of the process used by the department for policy development.

Implementation includes a checklist for approval by various administrative agents of the department and a summary outline to be used by anyone proposing a policy idea.

The mission of the department—to prevent and suppress disease and to protect, preserve and enhance the public's health—is implemented through programs, regulation, policy, and planning. The basis for planning includes health surveillance, priority setting, policy analysis, and coordination. Efforts include the collection, analysis, and interpretation of data to identify areas of morbidity and mortality as well as community planning activities, program initiatives, and interaction with local health departments.

Policy development is a basic responsibility of government in public health as defined in the IOM report, *The Future of Public Health* (Committee, 1988). The committee recommends that every public health agency be involved in the development of comprehensive public health policies by using its scientific (epidemiologic) data base in decision-making about public health and that it should take the lead in determining public health policy. This statement forms the belief system underlying policy development by the Connecticut Department of Health Services. It is further recognized that "policies provide guidance to programs, help define the specific role of the department, and help to provide present and future direction." (Connecticut, 1991). A suggested set of criteria for developing and evaluating policy are proposed in the box that follows. These policy criteria exemplify what Kelman has defined as steps in the policy-making process.

As the United States faces policy decisions for implementing changes in its health care delivery system, a policy promoting health should be considered. Such a policy would encompass health promotion and disease-prevention strategies. Milio (1981) proposes a policy that would encompass minimizing health-damaging circumstances and minimizing or eliminating both excesses and deficits of health-promoting resources, such as selected food and energy supplies.

CRITERIA FOR DEVELOPING AND EVALUATING POLICY

What is the problem to be addressed?
What is the scope of the problem (i.e., incidence and prevalence, severity and urgency, etc.)?
What data have been used to identify the problem (e.g., epidemiologic, surveillance, or program data)?
Does the department have the legal authority to implement the proposed policy?
How will the effectiveness be measured?
How will policy be enforced?
What is the fiscal impact for the department, state, and consumers affected institutions, etc.?
What are the specific program activities to be implemented?
Who will be responsible for the implementation?

Primary prevention would take precedence over secondary prevention (detecting illness and treating). Equity of risks would be the goal of a national health policy. Such a policy then would be heavily dependent on accurate data—epidemiologic data measuring health status through tracking marker health indices. Milio proposes health policy that encompasses the environmental influences on health risks and health-promoting behavior. Environment would also include economic influences on health status.

Because epidemiology focuses on describing changes in health states of populations and provides answers to the effects of certain interventions on the health status of populations, it is clear that epidemiology is the basis for health policy. Shapiro (1991) challenges epidemiologists to carry out the traditional roles of research, surveillance, and monitoring and to develop new methodologies to evaluate the results of planned interventions. Epidemiologists should concentrate on identifying the responsible agents, health care factors that can be favorably changed, outcomes desired (the benefits to be achieved), types of interventions that will yield the most change, and resources required (Shapiro, 1991).

Epidemiologic data and methods are of increasing importance in the development of public health policy. Information on functional status, morbidity, mortality, rates of disease (incidence, prevalence), and trends in health status and health care use patterns should be used to make policy decisions. Epidemiologic methods should also be used to assess the effects of service programs on health outcomes. These health care services can be viewed as determinants of health conditions of populations. Therefore epidemiologic principles and methodologies form the basis for legislative, regulatory, or programmatic public policy.

EPIDEMIOLOGY AS A BASIS FOR CLINICAL DECISIONS AND HEALTH POLICY

In an article in the *New England Journal of Medicine* (Hulley, 1980), the association between triglyceride and coronary heart disease was examined. The purpose was to determine whether screening and treatment of healthy persons for elevated triglyceride levels should be promoted as a medical care policy. To address the concerns raised by this policy question, the authors conducted a review of the literature examining epidemiologic data relating the two variables, triglyceride levels and coronary heart disease. The examination of epidemiologic evidence was the first step in the policy process. The published studies identified that triglycerides have not been proven to be an independent risk factor when multivariate analytic techniques were used to adjust for a full set of major risk factors (Hulley, 1980). Triglycerides alone, then, were not the only cause of coronary heart disease.

The second step in defining policy was analyzing data from one research study. Relative risks were determined, yet the analysis still demonstrated that neither body mass nor triglyceride was determined to be an independent risk factor. Therefore a practical implication for health policy to prevent coronary heart disease would be to develop and/or fund programs aimed at weight reduction rather than lowering triglycerides (Hulley, 1980). Therefore the policy proposed by the authors does not call for screening for triglyceride in the general population. Treatment of asymptomatic hypertriglyceridemia is not recommended. Rather, the authors encourage a preventive medicine approach of weight loss or sugar/alcohol restriction.

SUMMARY

Nurses can become involved in the health care planning and decision-making processes. Nurses are respected for their knowledge of the health care delivery system. They understand not only the needs of clients and communities but also the supports and constraints of the health care delivery system in meeting needs of clients and communities. Nurses should use the nursing process with an emphasis on the assessment of wide-ranging health problems. The body of epidemiologic knowledge about health states and its use contribute to the nursing process, providing the basis for health planning and health policy.

CRITICAL THINKING QUESTIONS

1. Give specific examples of how epidemiologic knowledge would be used in assessing the health needs of a population.
2. Discuss the relationship of small-area analysis to health planning at the local level.
3. Give specific examples of how epidemiologic knowledge would be used to design interventions for a health program.
4. Apply the rational actor model of policy analysis to a selected health policy.

REFERENCES

American Nurses Association: *Nursing's agenda for health care reform,* Kansas City, MO, 1991, The Association.

Centers for Disease Control: *Connecticut health profile 1991,* Department of Health and Human Services, Public Health Service, 1991.

Chin R, Benne KD: General strategies for effecting changes in human systems. In Bennis WG, Benne KD, Chin R, editors: *The planning of change,* New York, 1969, Holt, Rinehart and Winston.

Committee for the Study of the Future of Public Health, Division of Health Care Services, Institute of Medicine: *The future of public health,* Washington, DC, 1988, National Academy Press.

Connecticut Department of Health Services, Center for Policy Development: *Draft health policy process,* Hartford, CT, 1991, The Department.

Crichton A: *Health policy making,* Ann Arbor, MI, 1981, Health Administration Press.

Daniels DG: *Always a sister,* New York, 1989, The Feminist Press.

DeBella S, Martin L, Siddall S, editors: *Nurses' role in health care planning,* Norwalk, CT, 1986, Appleton-Century-Crofts.

Donabedian A: *Aspects of medical care administration,* Cambridge, MA, 1979, Harvard University Press.

Drummond MF, Stoddart GL, Torrance GW: *Methods for the economic evaluation of health care programmes,* Oxford, 1987, Oxford University Press.

Herman H, McKay ME: *Community health services,* Washington, DC, 1968, International City Managers' Association.

Hulley SB and others: Epidemiology as a guide to clinical decisions, *N Engl J Med* 302:1383-1389, 1980.

Ibrahim MA: *Epidemiology and health policy,* Rockville, MD, 1985, Aspen Systems Corp.

Kelman S: *Making public policy,* New York, 1987, Basic Books.

Marmor TR: *The politics of medicare,* New York, 1973, Aldine Publishing.

Milio N: *Promoting health through public policy,* Philadelphia, 1981, FA Davis.

Moroney RM and others: The uses of small-area analysis in community health planning, *Inquiry* XIII:145-151, 1976.

Nightingale F: *Notes on hospitals,* ed 3, London, 1863, Longman, Green, Longman, Roberts, and Green.

Rothman KL: The rise and fall of epidemiology, 1950-2000 AD, *N Engl J Med* 304:10:600-610, 1981.

Shapiro S: Epidemiology and public policy, *Am J Epidemiol* 134:1057-1061, 1991.

Shonick W: Health planning. In *Maxcy-Rosenau public health and preventive medicine,* New York, 1980, Appleton-Century-Crofts.

US Public Health Service: A plan to strengthen public health in the United States, *Public Health Reports,* vol 106, suppl 1, January 1991.

The George Washington University: *Minority health: breaking down the barriers,* National Health Policy Forum, Washington, DC, Issue Brief No. 575, 1991.

Webster's New World Dictionary, ed 3, New York, 1991, Simon & Schuster.

Appendix

CONSTRUCTING TABLES, GRAPHS, AND CHARTS

TABLES

A table is a set of data, arranged in rows and columns, that is used for organizing and communicating information. Tables are useful for demonstrating patterns, exceptions, differences, and other relationships.

I. Preparation
   A. Tables should be as simple as possible. Two or three small tables, each focusing on a different aspect of data, are easier to understand than a single large table that contains many details.
   B. Tables should be self-explanatory. If the table is taken out of its original context, it should still convey all information necessary for the reader to understand the data.
      1. Use a clear and concise title that describes the what, where, and when of the data in the table.
      2. Label each row and column clearly and concisely, using the units of measurement for the data.
      3. Show totals for rows and columns. When using percentages, show the total (100%).
      4. Explain codes, abbreviations, or symbols in a footnote.
      5. Note any exclusions in a footnote.
      6. Note the source of the data in a footnote if the data are not original.

II. One-variable table: The most basic table in descriptive epidemiology is a frequency distribution with only one variable (Fig. A-1).
   A. The first column shows values or categories of the variable represented by the data, such as age, sex, or ethnicity.
   B. The second column shows the number of persons or events that fall into each category.

Adapted from Centers for Disease Control and Prevention: *Principles of Epidemiology,* ed 2, Atlanta, GA, 1992, Public Health Practice Program Office, US Department of Health and Human Services, Public Health Service, pp 206–268.

Responses* to health-related quality-of-life question — Behavioral Risk Factor Surveillance System, 1993†

Question	Response	Respondents‡ (n=44,978) No.	(%)
Self-rated health			
	Excellent	10,764	(24.0)
	Very good	15,328	(34.2)
	Good	12,162	(27.1)
	Fair	4,654	(10.4)
	Poor	1,961	(4.4)
Recent physical health			
(No. days when physical	0 days	29,914	(67.6)
health was not good during	1–2 days	5,010	(11.3)
the 30 days preceding the survey.)	3–7 days	4,402	(9.9)
	≥8 days	4,919	(11.1)
Recent mental health			
(No. days when mental	0 days	30,308	(68.5)
health was not good during	1–2 days	4,373	(9.9)
the 30 days preceding the survey.)	3–7 days	4,708	(10.6)
	≥8 days	4,833	(10.9)
Recent activity limitation			
(No. days when poor physical	0 days	36,130	(81.1)
or mental health kept you from doing	1–2 days	3,081	(6.9)
your usual activities during the 30	3–7 days	2,472	(5.5)
days preceding the survey.)	≥8 days	2,886	(6.5)

*Responses to the last three questions were recorded in actual number of days but are summarized in this table in four response groupings.
†Unweighted data from Alaska, Arkansas, Colorado, Delaware, District of Columbia, Georgia, Idaho, Illinois, Kentucky, Massachusetts, Minnesota, Montana, Nebraska, Oklahoma, Pennsylvania, South Carolina, Tennessee, Utah, Vermont, Virginia, Washington, and West Virginia.
‡Numbers may not add to sample size because persons with missing values were excluded from this analysis.

Fig. A-1 One-variable table. (From Centers for Disease Control and Prevention: Quality of life as a new public health measure—Behavioral Risk Factor Surveillance System, *MMWR* 43(20), 1994.)

C. The third column may be used to list the percentage of persons or events in each category.
   1. The total percent should be 100%, even with rounding.
   2. Differences due to rounding can be explained in a footnote.

III. Two- and three-variable tables
   A. Data can be cross-tabulated to show counts by a second variable. A two-variable table with cross-tabulated data is also known as a *contingency table*.
   B. Contingency tables are often used to display data for calculating measures of association and tests of statistical significance.
   C. Two-by-two tables are contingency tables in which each of the two variables has two categories.
      1. These are useful in studying the association between an exposure and an outcome, where persons with and without exposure are compared to those with or without the outcome.
      2. Disease states are indicated along the top of the table.
      3. Exposure status is indicated along the side of the table.

Percentage of adults who reported having no major risk factors for coronary heart disease,* by age group, education level, and sex — Behavioral Risk Factor Surveillance System, 1992

	Men			Women		
Characteristic	Sample size	% With no risk factor	(95% CI†)	Sample size	% With no risk factor	(95% CI)
Age group (yrs)‡						
18–34	12,202	24.5	(±1.3)	14,647	22.7	(±1.1)
35–49	11,652	12.6	(±0.9)	13,955	17.9	(±1.0)
50–64	6,598	9.4	(±1.0)	8,515	11.6	(±0.9)
≥65	5,601	13.4	(±1.2)	10,488	9.2	(±0.8)
Education (yrs)§						
<12	4,961	10.4	(±1.5)	7,145	8.5	(±1.2)
12	11,577	14.6	(±0.9)	16,941	15.9	(±0.8)
>12	19,515	25.4	(±0.9)	23,519	26.9	(±0.8)

*Risk factors: current cigarette smoking (smoked at least 100 cigarettes in their lifetime and now smoking), physical inactivity (no or irregular leisure-time physical activity), overweight (body mass index ≥27.3 for women and ≥27.8 for men), high blood pressure (told more than once by a health professional he/she has high blood pressure or is currently taking antihypertensive medications), high blood cholesterol (ever told by a health professional he/she has high blood cholesterol), and diabetes (ever told by a doctor he/she has diabetes).
†Confidence interval.
‡Age comparisons were standardized for education and race by using 1980 U.S. Bureau of the Census data.
§Number of years completed; education comparisons were standardized for age and race by using 1980 U.S. Bureau of the Census data.

Fig. A-2 Three-variable table. (From Centers for Disease Control and Prevention: Prevalence of adults with no known major risk factors for coronary heart disease—Behavioral Risk Factor Surveillance System, *MMWR* 43(4), 1994.)

D. Addition of a third variable to a table may show a set of data more completely. Three variables represent the maximum complexity that should be presented in any table (Fig. A-2).

IV. Tables of other statistical measures

Tables can also contain means, rates, ratios, relative risks, and other statistical measures. The basic rules for preparation apply.

V. Table shells

Table shells are complete tables except for entry of the data. They are prepared in advance to organize the data collection process and expedite analysis once the data are collected.

GRAPHS

Graphs are illustrations of quantitative data using a system of coordinates. It is a statistical "snapshot" that helps identify patterns, trends, similarities, and differences in the data.

I. Preparation

A. In epidemiology, coordinate graphs are common. They consist of two lines, one horizontal and one vertical, that intersect at right angles. These lines are referred to as the horizontal axis (x-axis) or the vertical axis (y-axis).

B. The horizontal axis usually shows values of the independent variable (x) that is the method of classification.

C. The vertical axis shows the dependent variable (y) that, in epidemiology, is usually a frequency measure, such as the number of cases or rate of an outcome.
D. Label each axis, and mark a scale of measurement along the line(s).

II. Arithmetic-scale line graphs (Fig. A-3)
A. Created to show patterns or trends, often over time.
B. A set distance along an axis represents the same quantity anywhere on that axis.
C. Make the x-axis (horizontal axis) longer than the y-axis (vertical axis), but in good proportion.
D. Always start the y-axis with 0.
E. Select an interval size that will provide enough intervals to show the data in enough detail.
F. If there is a range of values with no data, a scale break in the graph can be created. It should stop at the point where the gap begins and starts again where the gap ends.

III. Semilogarithmic-scale line graphs (Fig. A-4)
A. Semilog graphs are useful when a wide range of values need to fit on a single graph. Semi-log paper is available commercially.

Death rates* from leading causes of death among men aged 25-44 years, by year — United States, 1982-1992†

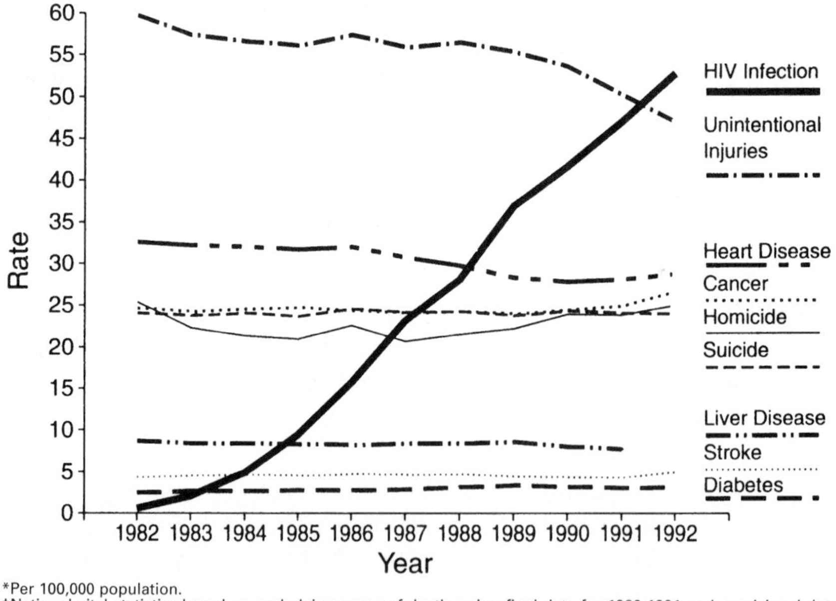

*Per 100,000 population.
†National vital statistics based on underlying cause of death, using final data for 1982-1991 and provisional data for 1992. Data for liver disease in 1992 are unavailable.

Fig. A-3 Arithmetic-scale line graph. (From Centers for Disease Control and Prevention: Update: Mortality attributable to HIV infection among persons aged 25-44 years—United States, 1991 and 1992, *MMWR* 42(45), 1993.)

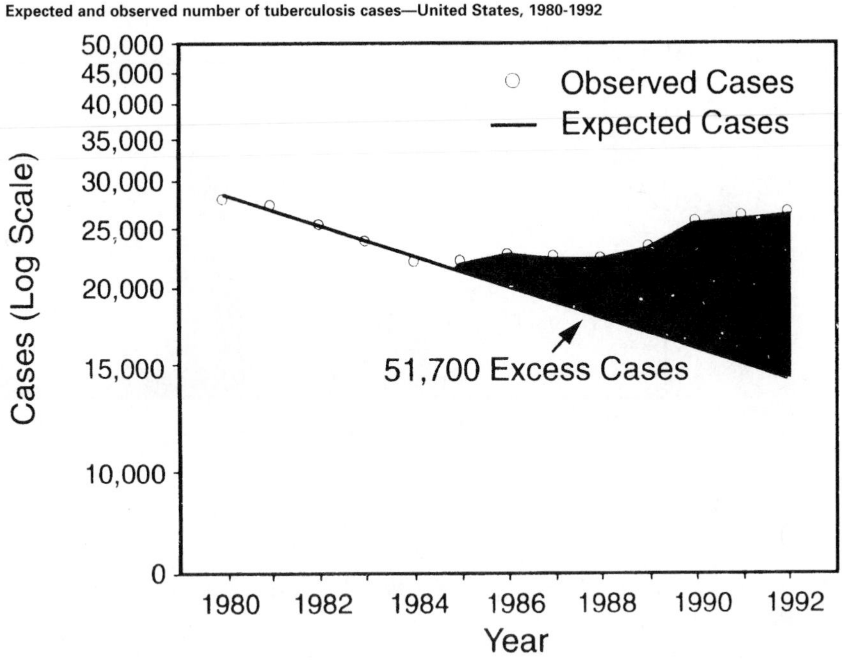

Fig. A-4 Semilogarithmic-scale line graph. (From Centers for Disease Control and Prevention: Tuberculosis morbidity—United States, 1992, *MMWR* 42(36), 1993.)

B. The divisions on the y-axis are logarithmic rather than arithmetic.
C. Cycles covering equal distance on the y-axis represent one order of magnitude greater than the one below it. Equal distances on the y-axis represent an equal percentage of change.
D. Within a cycle are 10 tick-marks, with the space between the tick marks becoming smaller and smaller as they move up the cycle.
E. The axis covers a large range of y-values that would have been difficult to show clearly on an arithmetic scale.
F. To interpret the graph:

    1. A sloping straight line indicates a constant rate of increase or decrease in the values.
    2. A horizontal line indicates no change.
    3. The slope of the line indicates the rate of increase or decrease.
    4. Two or more lines following parallel paths show identical rates of change.

IV. Histograms (Fig. A-5)
  A. A histogram is a graph of the frequency distribution of a continuous variable.
  B. Adjoining columns represent the number of observations for each class interval in the distribution.

Number of measles cases, by date of rash onset and location—St. Louis County, Missouri, and Jersey County, Illinois, April 4-May 17, 1994

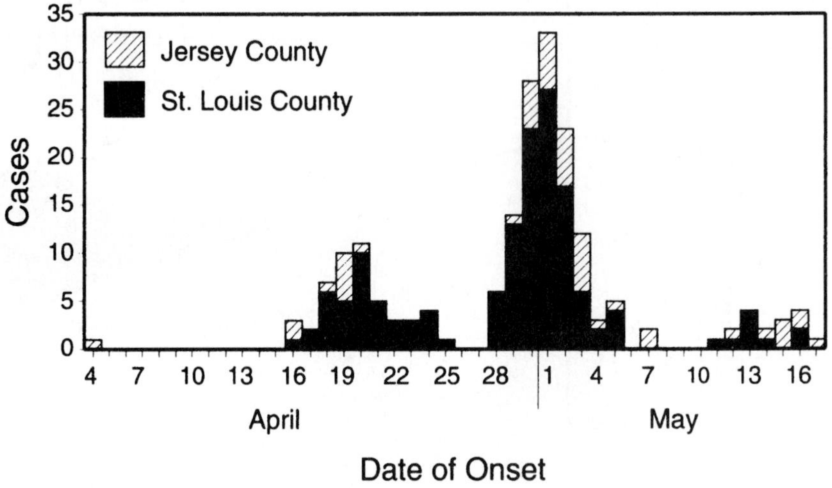

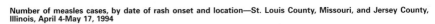

Fig. A-5 Histogram. (From Centers for Disease Control and Prevention: Outbreak of measles among Christian Science students—Missouri and Illinois, 1994, *MMWR* 43(25), 1994.)

C. The area of each column is proportional to the number of observations in that interval.
D. Scale breaks are not recommended.
E. The most common x-axis variable is time; epidemic curves are histograms that show cases of disease during an outbreak by date of onset.

V. Frequency polygons (Fig. A-6)
A. A frequency polygon is also a graph of a frequency distribution of continuous data.
B. The number of observations within an interval are marked with a single point placed at the midpoint of the interval, and points are connected with a straight line.
C. A frequency polygon of a set of data must enclose the same area as a histogram of that data.
D. Two or more sets of data can be presented on the same set of axes.
E. A frequency polygon must be closed at both ends to be representative of the data.

VI. Cumulative frequency and survival curves (Fig. A-7)
A. A cumulative frequency curve plots the cumulative frequency rather than the actual frequency for each class interval of a variable; useful for identifying medians, quartiles, and other percentiles.
B. The x-axis records the class intervals, the y-axis shows the cumulative frequency in actual numbers or proportions of 100%.

Number of reported cases of influenza-like illness by week of onset

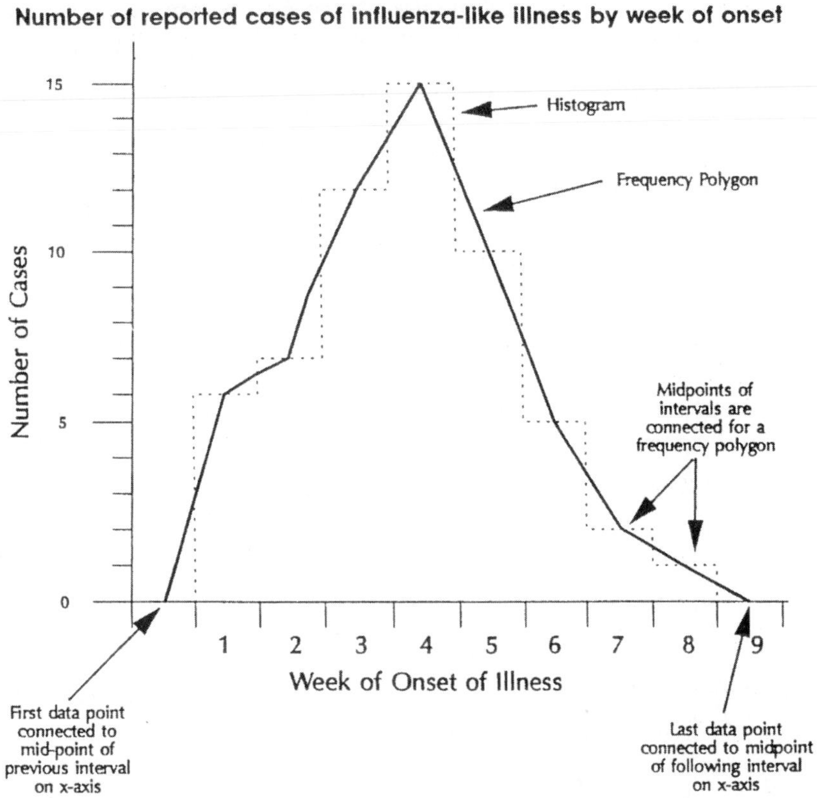

Fig. A-6 Frequency polygon. (From Centers for Disease Control and Prevention: *Principles of epidemiology,* ed 2, Atlanta, GA, 1992, Public Health Service, p. 244.)

C. Cumulative frequency is plotted at the upper limit of the interval, rather than the midpoint.
D. A survival curve is used with follow-up studies to display the proportion of one or more groups still alive at different time periods.

VII. Scatter diagrams

A. A scatter diagram (scattergram) is used for plotting the relationship between two continuous variables.
B. The x-axis represents one variable, and the y-axis the other.
C. Data must include a pair of values for every person, group, or other entity in the data sate, one value for each variable.
D. A point is placed on the graph where the two values intersect.
E. A compact pattern indicates a high degree of correlation. Widely scattered points indicate little correlation. A more quantitative measure of the relationship between the variables can be identified using formal statistical methods, such as linear regression.

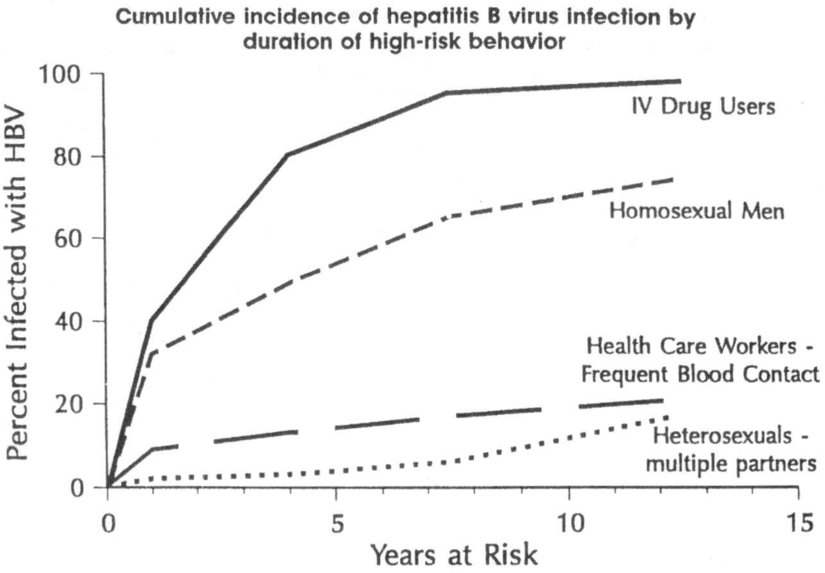

CDC (1994). Outbreak of measles among christian science students – Missouri and Illinois, 1994. MMWR, 43(25), 463.

Fig. A-7 Cumulative frequency curve. (From Centers for Disease Control: *Principles of epidemiology,* ed 2, Atlanta, GA, 1992, Public Health Service, p. 244.)

CHARTS

Charts illustrate statistical information using only *one* coordinate. They are most appropriate for comparing data with discrete categories.

I. Bar charts
   A. Variables in bar charts are either discrete and noncontinuous, or are treated as though they are such.
   B. Each value or category of the variable is represented by a bar.
   C. Bars can be presented either horizontally or vertically.
   D. The length or height of each bar is proportional to the frequency of the event in the category.
   E. The bars of a bar chart are separated, in contrast to a histogram where the bars are joined.
   F. Grouped bar charts illustrate data from two or three variable tables, when an outcome variable has only two categories. Bars within a group are usually joined (Fig. A-8).
   G. Stacked bar charts show categories of a second variable as components of the bars that represent the first variable (Fig. A-9).
   H. Deviation bar charts illustrate deviations in a variable, both positive and negative, from a baseline (Fig. A-10).

Percentage of children aged 1-5 years with blood lead levels ≥10μg/dL, by urban status,* household income, and race/ethnicity—National Health and Nutrition Examination Survey III-Phase 1, United States, 1988-1991

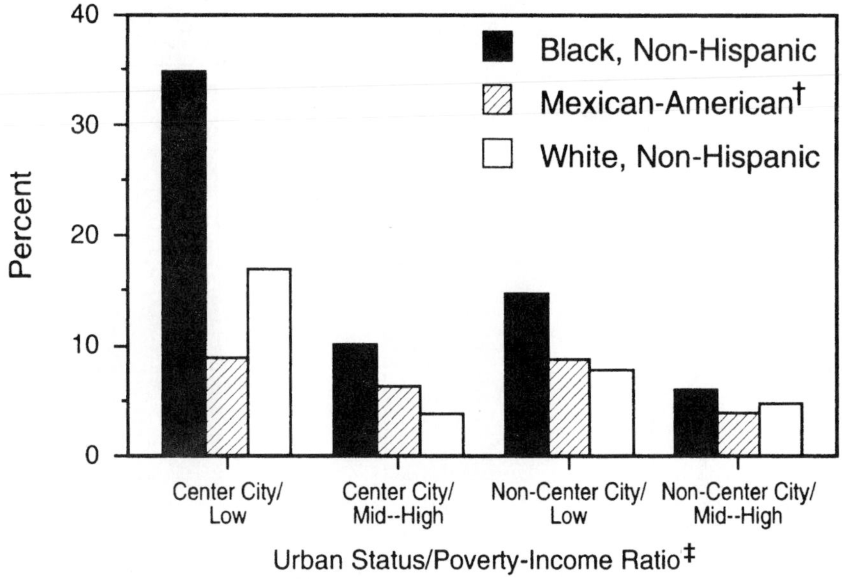

*Urban status: center = living in central city of a standard metropolitan statistical area.
†Persons residing in survey-sample households who reported their national origin or ancestry as Mexican/Mexican-American.
‡Poverty-income ratio: low = household income <1.3 times the proverty level; mid-high = household income ≥1.3 times the poverty level.

Fig. A-8 Grouped bar chart. (From Centers for Disease Control and Prevention: Blood lead levels—United States, 1988-1991, *MMWR* 43(30), 1994.)

I. 100% component bar charts (proportional bar charts) show the components as percents of the total rather than as actual values. All bars are the same height. This type of chart is useful for comparing the contribution of different components to each of the categories of the main variables (Fig. A-11).

II. Preparation of bar charts
   A. Arrange the categories that define the bars, or groups of bars, in a natural order, such as alphabetical or by increasing age, or in an order that will produce increasing or decreasing bar lengths.
   B. Position the bars either vertically or horizontally. Deviation bar charts are usually positioned horizontally.
   C. Make all of the bars the same width.
   D. Make the length of bars in proportion to the frequency of the event. Scale breaks are not used, because it could lead to misinterpretation in comparing the size of different categories.
   E. Show no more than three bars within a group of bars.
   F. Leave a space between adjacent groups of bars, but not between bars within a group.

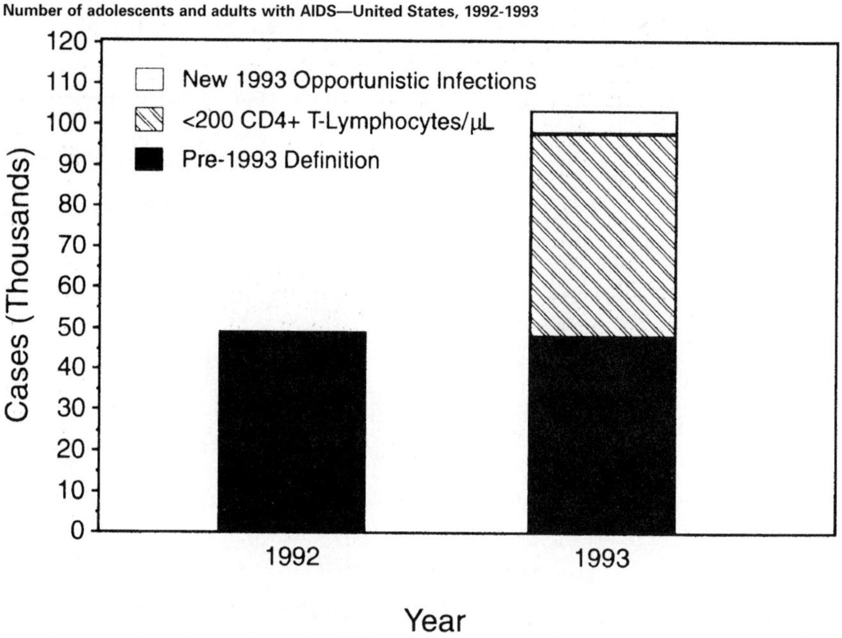

Fig. A-9 Stacked bar chart. (From Centers for Disease Control and Prevention: Update: impact of the expanded AIDS surveillance case definition for adolescents and adults on case reporting—United States, 1993, *MMWR* 43(9), 1993.)

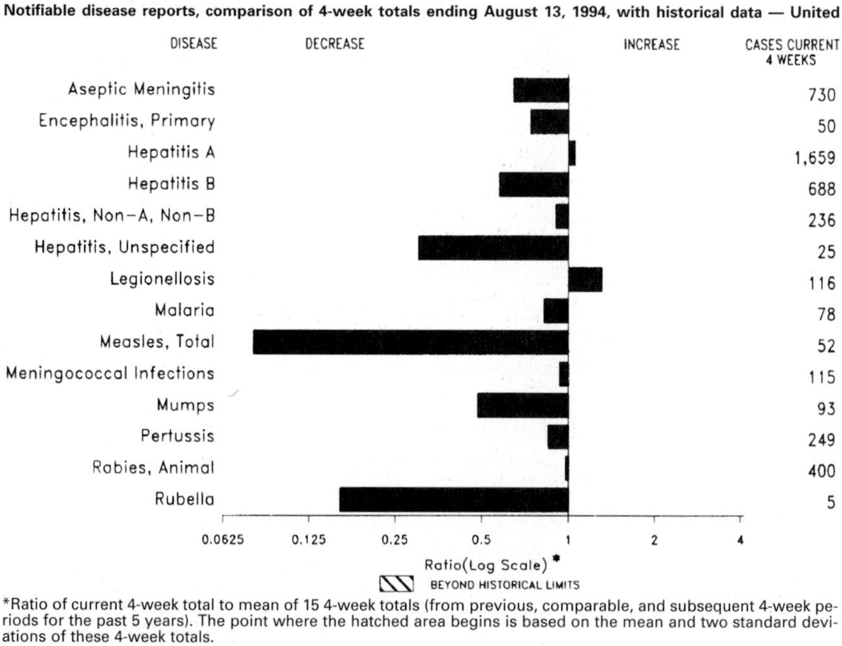

Fig. A-10 Deviation bar chart. (From Centers for Disease Control and Prevention: Current trends, *MMWR* 43(32), 1994.)

Percentage of states reporting involvement in oral health policy-development activities, by level of involvement — United States, 1993

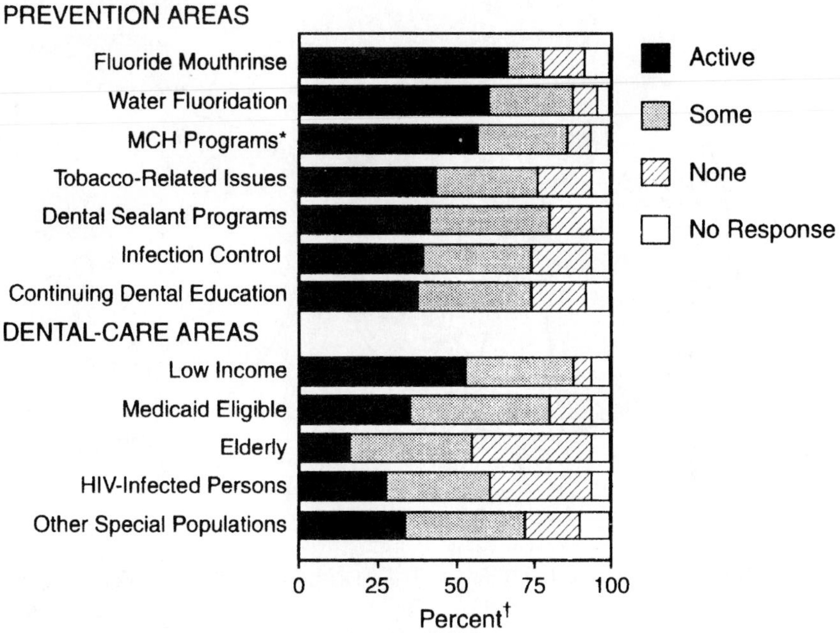

*Maternal and child health programs for prevention of oral diseases.
†Percentage of 50 states and the District of Columbia.

Fig. A-11 100% component bar chart (proportional bar chart). (From Centers for Disease Control and Prevention: Core public health functions and state efforts to improve oral health—United States, 1993, *MMWR* 43(11), 1994.)

G. Code different variables by differences in bar color, shading, cross-hatching, etc. and include a legend that interprets the code.

III. Pie charts (Fig. A-12)

A. Pie charts are useful for showing the components parts of a single group or variable. Size of the slices show the proportional contribution of each component part.

B. Indicate on the chart what 100% represents, and indicate what percentage each slice represents either inside or near each slice.

IV. Maps (geographic coordinate charts)

A. Maps are used to show the location of events or attributes (Fig. A-13).

B. Spot maps use dots or other symbols to show where an event took place or a disease condition exists. Actual numbers, not rates are used.

C. An area map uses shaded or coded areas to show either the incidence of an event in subareas or the distribution of some condition over a geographic area. Numbers or rates can be used.

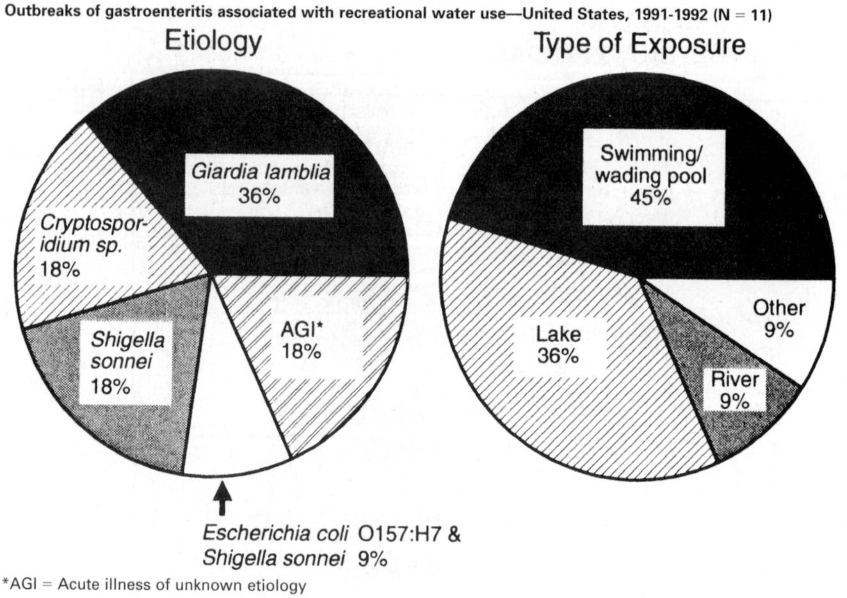

Fig. A-12 Pie chart. (From Centers for Disease Control and Prevention: Surveillance for waterborne disease outbreaks—United States, 1991-1992, *MMWR* 42(SS-5), 1993.)

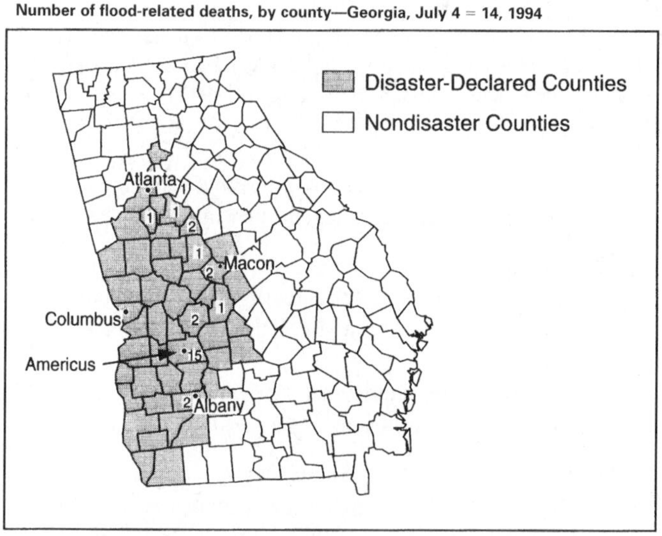

Fig. A-13 Geographic coordinate chart (map). (From Centers for Disease Control and Prevention: Flood-related mortality—Georgia, July 4-14, 1994, *MMWR* 43(29), 1994.)

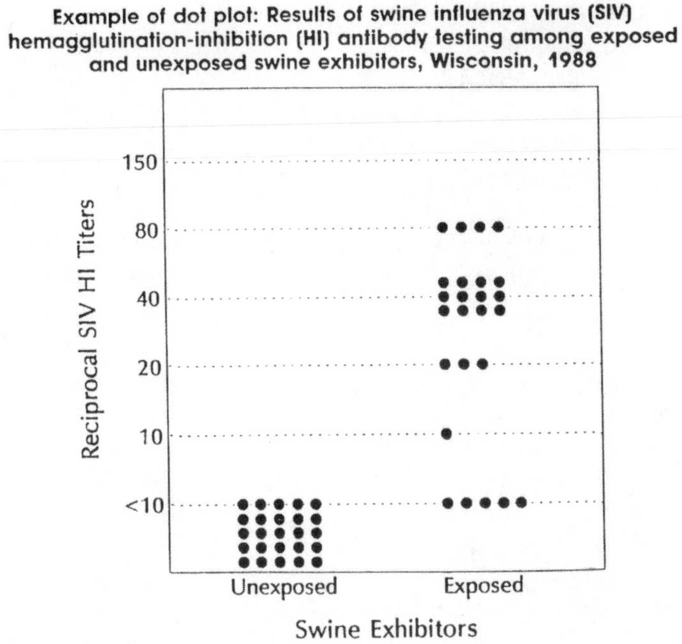

Fig. A-14 Dot plot. (From Centers for Disease Control: *Principles of epidemiology,* ed 2, Atlanta, GA, 1992, Public Health Service, p. 257.)

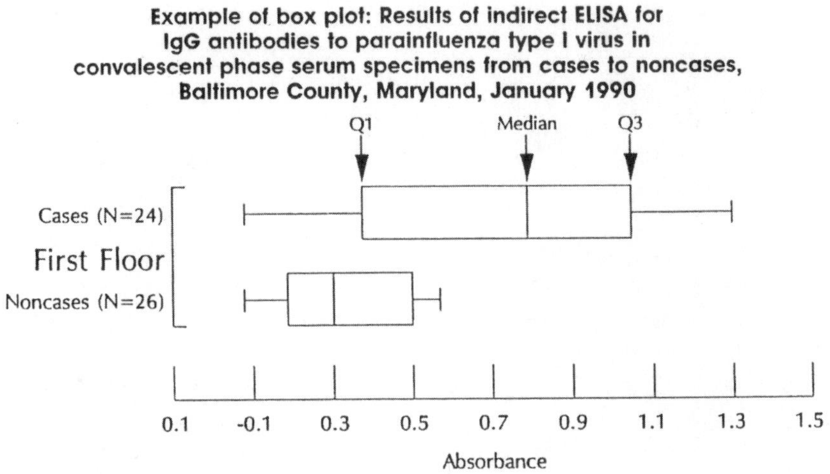

Fig. A-15 Box plot. (From Centers for Disease Control: *Principles of epidemiology,* ed 2, Atlanta, GA, 1992, Public Health Service, p. 258.)

V. Dot Plots and Box Plots
   A. A dot plot is similar to a scatter diagram because it plots one variable against another (Fig. A-14).
   B. The x-axis is not continuous; rather it represents discrete categories of a noncontinuous variable.
   C. Box plots are used to compare the distributions of noncontinuous variables (Fig. A-15).
   D. The box illustrates the middle 50% or interquartile range of the data, and the “whiskers” extend to the minimum and maximum values.

Glossary

active surveillance Ongoing search for episodes of illness or health states.

actual causes of death Underlying causes of death that are due to life-style choices. These are considered modifiable and include such activities as tobacco use, dietary patterns, drug and alcohol use, sexual behavior, and seat belt use.

adjusted rates A process of removing the effects of differences in the composition of a population when calculating rates.

airborne transmission Dissemination of particles suspended in air and containing microorganisms (droplet nuclei).

analytic studies Research studies that focus on identification of the determinants associated with variations in states of health.

association A statistical dependence between two or more variables.

attack rate A cumulative incidence rate observed for limited periods of time and under special circumstances; often used in the surveillance of infectious disease.

attributable risk Rate of an illness in exposed individuals that can be attributed to the exposure; excess risk from exposure beyond that which would normally be found.

Behavioral Risk Factor Surveillance System (BRFSS) A national surveillance system established to collect, analyze, and interpret state-specific behavioral risk factor data that could be used to plan, implement, and monitor health promotion and disease prevention programs; national surveillance system for monitoring health behaviors, such as obesity, lack of physical activity, smoking, and seat belt use.

bias Any factor that produces study results that differ systematically from true values.

biologic vector-borne Transmission of an infectious agent through the bite (inoculation) of a vector; multiplication and development of the infectious agent occurs in the arthropod before it can transmit the infective form of the agent to humans.

case-finding Search for illness that occurs as a part of a client's periodic health examination.

case reports Study of unusual occurrences of single individuals or of a group of people with the same condition.

case-control studies Retrospective studies involving the investigation of a group of people that has a specific health problem (cases) and another group that does not have the health problem (controls). Cases are chosen based on the fact that the outcome or dependent variable has already occurred. Data collection goes back in time to look for factors related to exposure in both cases and controls.

CDC Centers for Disease Control and Prevention. A branch of the Public Health Service whose primary responsibility is to conduct surveillance of the health of the U.S. population.

chemical agents Biochemical and chemical substances that can cause cellular injury; highly toxic substances are known as poisons.

chronic illness Encompasses diseases or conditions that produce signs and symptoms within variable periods of time, are long-lasting, and are often associated with some degree of disability.

clinical trials Therapeutic trials.

cohort studies Prospective, longitudinal studies that investigate a group or groups of people that are classified according to exposure (independent variables) and followed forward in time to determine the onset of outcomes (dependent variables).

colonization Presence of an organism without a clinical or subclinical disease.

common-source epidemic Outbreak characterized by exposure to a common, harmful substance.

communicable disease An infectious disease or infestation that is transmitted from one person or animal to another, directly or indirectly.

community assessment Process of gathering data about community health problems and community health strengths and resources.

community health nursing A specialty of nursing practice that synthesizes principles of nursing and public health to promote and maintain the health of populations.

comorbidity Presence of more than one illness or abnormal condition.

confounding variables Additional, extraneous factors that result in the observation of differences when they do not exist (Type I error) or the observation of no differences when they do exist (Type II error). These variables need to be controlled either in the research design or by statistical procedures.

correlation coefficient Measures the extent of association between two variables, or the extent to which changes in exposure are related to an increase or decrease in adverse health outcomes. Values range from +1 (direct relationship) to -1 (inverse relationship).

correlational studies Research studies that examine the variation between characteristics (variables) under investigation.

cost-benefit analysis Evaluation of financial requirements according to the benefits that would be derived when planning health services for a given population.

cross-sectional studies Surveys that produce prevalence data.

crude rates Measurement of the experience of the entire population in a designated geographic area in regard to the health problem or condition being investigated.

demography The study of the size, distribution, and characteristics of human population groups.

demographic transition Change in population profile of a specified geographic area; reflects movement from high birth and high death rates and a primarily young population to low death rates and low birth rates and a stable older population.

demos People.

dependent variable Outcome variables.

device-associated infection Infections associated with the use of invasive devices.

direct contact Transmission of an infectious agent from a reservoir to a portal of entry into a susceptible host; occurs through touching, biting, kissing, sexual intercourse, or by droplet spray.

distributive policies Policies that distribute benefits to interested parties.

dose-response As the exposure increases, there is a corresponding rise in the occurrence of the outcome.

double-blind study An experiment where neither the subjects or data collectors know who is assigned to the experimental or control group.

droplet nuclei Particle residues resulting from evaporation of fluid from droplets disseminated by an infected person. Particles containing microorganisms become suspended in air, and airborne transmission may occur.

environmental health An aspect of community health that is concerned with conditions in the surroundings that influence health and well-being.

EPA Environmental Protection Agency.

epi Upon.

epidemic A significant increase in the number of new cases of a disease or illness than past experience should have predicted for that place, at that time, among a specified population; an increase in incidence beyond that which is expected.

epidemic curve A graph that plots the distribution of cases by the time of onset of the infectious disease.

epidemiologic descriptive studies Research studies designed to acquire more information about the occurrence of states of health, such as characteristics of person, place, and time.

epidemiologic process Systematic study of the distribution and determinants of states of health and illness in human populations; evolved from the problem-solving process.

epidemiologic triad Model that posits that health status is determined by the interaction of characteristics of the agent, host, and environment, not by any single factor.

epidemiology Study of the distribution and determinants of states of health and illness in human populations.

experimental population The actual group of people that is being sampled.

external validity Degree to which results of a study can be generalized to other populations or settings.

extraneous variables Confounding variables.

Hawthorne effect Change in the behavior of subjects, because they are subjects in a study and not because of the intervention; reactivity.

health planning A process of health program definition, determination of objectives, implementing a course of action, and evaluating the results.

health policy An implementation strategy that addresses health issues in the planning process.

health promotion Defined by the World Health Organization as the process of enabling people to increase control over and improve their own health.

Healthy People 2000 National Health objectives to be accomplished by the year 2000.

herd immunity The presence of a large proportion of immune individuals in a community that decreases the chances of contact between any infected people and susceptible individuals; an entire population need not be immune to prevent an epidemic of a disease.

historical cohort study Prospective study where a group of people who were exposed at some time in the past can be identified and followed from that point in time to determine whether a disease or condition develops.

hospital epidemiology Study of the distribution and determinants of health events in hospital settings. In addition to infection control activities, hospital epidemiology is expanding to include accident prevention, risk management, quality assessment, and types of noninfectious, hospital-associated problems.

hypothesis Statement of predicted relationships between the variables being investigated.

immunogenicity Ability of the agent to produce specific immunity within the host.

inapparent infection Relationship between the agent and host has been limited to an immune response that can only be detected by laboratory means or a positive reaction to a skin test; subclinical infection.

incidence density Use of a person-time denominator in the calculation of rates; a person-day reflects one person at risk for 1 day, and a person-year represents one person at risk for 1 year.

incidence rate Measure of the probability that people without a certain condition will develop the condition over a period of time. Calculated by dividing the number of new conditions or events occurring in a period of time by the population at risk during the same period of time (often midyear), and multiplying by a base multiple of 10.

incubation period Time period between initial contact with the infectious agent and the appearance of the first signs or symptoms of the disease.

independent variable Exposure variables.

indirect association Exposure and outcomes are associated, because both are related to one or more common underlying conditions.

indirect contact Transmission of infectious agents through contaminated substances or objects (vehicles), and animals or arthropods that are carriers of infectious agents (vectors).

infection control committee (ICC) A multidisciplinary committee that oversees the infection control program.

infection control practitioner (ICP) Practitioners, usually nurses, who are responsible for obtaining surveillance data, developing infection control policies, conducting educational programs, consulting with hospital personnel, and assisting with the investigation of outbreaks.

infection control program Process of surveillance and reporting, and control and prevention of hospital-associated infections.

infection rate Incidence rate that measures clinical and subclinical infections. The number of documented infections is included in the numerator, not the number of people infected, (because one person may have more than one infection).

infectious disease Presence and replication of an infectious agent in the tissues of a host, with manifestation of signs and symptoms.

infectivity Ability of the agent to invade the host and replicate; varies with the route of entry, source of the agent, and host susceptibility.

infestation Arthropods on the surface of the body; considered communicable diseases.

internal validity Extent to which the results of a study reflect reality, and not the effects of confounding variables.

JCAHO Joint Commission on Accreditation of Healthcare Organizations.

latency period Long length of time between initial exposure to the agent(s) and the development of illness; more common with noninfectious diseases.

lifetime prevalence Proportion of persons who have ever experienced specific conditions up to the date of assessment.

logistic regression A type of multivariate regression analysis used when the outcome is categoric and the independent variables are not normally distributed within the populations.

logos Thought.

longitudinal study Cohort study; data is collected at more than one point in time.

long-term change Fluctuations in time surrounding health problems that extend over decades and reflect gradual changes.

mass screening Procedures applied to entire populations; screening for phenylketonuria (PKU) testing of newborns is an example.

mechanical vector-borne Transmission of an infectious agent that is located on the surface of the vector to food, water, or other surfaces; multiplication of the infectious agent within the carrier is not required.

morbidity Departure from a state of physiologic or psychologic well-being.

morbidity rate The probability of developing a health problem among the entire population in a designated geographic area.

mortality Death.

mortality rate The probability of death from any cause among the entire population in a designated geographic area.

multiphasic screening A variety of procedures or tests are applied to the same population on the same occasion; preoperative examinations and preadmission procedures use multiphasic screening procedures.

NNIS National Nosocomial Infection Surveillance system.

nosocomial infection Hospital-associated infection.

nurse-managed center Health care facilities, managed by nurses, that have a primary goal of provision of nursing services; services include case management, health assessment, health promotion, screening, and health teaching.

nursing process Organizational framework for the practice of nursing that evolved from the problem-solving process; includes assessment, analysis (diagnosis), planning, implementation, and evaluation.

occupational health Promotion and maintenance of the optimum level of health for employees.

occupational health nurse Practitioner responsible for health assessment of workers, evaluation of the work site, recognition of health hazards, evaluation and treatment of occupational illness and injury, the development of health screening programs, implementation of safety programs, provision of health promotion programs, and coordination of cost-effective health care.

odds ratio Estimation of the relative risk ratio. The ratio of the odds of exposure among cases to the ratio of the odds of exposure among controls. Used primarily to analyze data from case-control studies.

OSHA Occupational Safety and Health Administration.

outbreak An epidemic.

P-value Probability that the obtained results occur from chance alone; probability of committing a Type I error.

pandemic An epidemic that occurs over a wide geographic area, often world-wide.

passive surveillance Information regarding illness or health states is reported on standardized report forms to local and state health officials; primarily instituted for infectious disease.

pathogen Microorganism capable of producing an infection or infectious disease; an infectious agent.

pathogenicity Ability of the agent to produce an infectious disease in a susceptible host.

period prevalence A prevalence rate that indicates the existence of a condition during a period or an interval of time, often a year.

periodic change Seasonal or cyclic fluctuations in time surrounding health problems.

physical agents Environmental agents that can cause cellular injury, including temperature extremes, changes in atmospheric pressure, radiation, trauma, noise, and prolonged vibrations.

placebo effect Tendency for study subjects to report favorable responses to any intervention, whether the intervention is beneficial or not.

planned change Changes that are the result of a thoughtful, deliberate, conscious process.

point prevalence A prevalence rate that indicates the existence of a condition at a specific point in time.

polar-area diagram Graph invented by Florence Nightingale to dramatize the needless deaths in British military hospitals during the Crimean War, 1854-1856.

population at risk Groups of people who have specific characteristics, or risk factors, that increase the probability of developing health problems.

population-based planning Assessing needs and planning for access to health care services.

power Ability to detect existing relationships among variables in a study.

predictive value Measure of the frequency that test results correctly identify the health problem among those who are screened.

prevalence rate A calculation that measures the number of people in a given population who have an existing condition at a given point in time. Calculated by dividing the number of existing conditions or events occurring in a period of time by the population at risk during the same period of time, and multiplying by a base multiple of 10.

preventive trial Experimental study that seeks to reduce the risk of acquiring a specific health condition among a group of people who do not have that health condition at the onset of the study.

primary health care Direct care, first contact service for diagnosis and treatment of minor, acute, and chronic conditions, and the delivery of health promotion and disease prevention activities.

primary prevention Activities that prevent a disease from occurring.

priority-directed surveillance Activities that focus on surveying specific units, areas, patient populations, or procedures.

problem-oriented surveillance Surveillance system that focuses on investigation of specific infectious problems.

propagated epidemic Outbreak resulting from direct or indirect transmission of an infectious agent from an infected person to a susceptible host.

proportion Type of ratio that includes the quantity in the numerator as a part of the denominator; a relationship of a part to the whole.

proportional mortality ratio A ratio that compares deaths from a specific illness to deaths from all other causes.

prospective Going forward in time.

prospective study Cohort study.

quasi-experimental trial An experimental design that manipulates the independent variable but may not involve randomization or may not be able to exert control over confounding variables that could affect the validity of the study.

random assignment Assigning previously selected subjects to either the intervention or control groups based on chance alone.

random selection Choosing subjects for participation in a study based on chance alone.

rate Primary measurement used to describe either the occurrence or the existence of a state of health or illness. Calculated by dividing the number of conditions or events occurring in a specific period of time by the population at risk during the same period of time, and multiplying by a base multiple of 10.

ratio Fraction that represents the relationship between two numbers; obtained by dividing one quantity by another quantity.

redistributive policies Reallocation of resources among disadvantaged groups.

reference population Target population; the entire group of people to whom the results of intervention studies are expected to apply. Represents the scope of the public health impact of the intervention under investigation.

regulative policies Establishment of rules and regulations that set parameters around a situation that all parties must adhere to; licensure of home care agencies to receive reimbursement is an example.

relative risk ratio Ratio of the incidence rate in a group of exposed people and the incidence rate in a group of nonexposed people.

reliability Degree of consistency and repeatability of findings.

reportable disease Communicable disease that must be officially reported to the state health department when it occurs.

reservoir Location where an infectious agent is normally found, where it lives and reproduces under normal circumstances.

retrospective Going backward in time.

retrospective study Case-control study.

risk A probability that an event will occur.

risk assessment Appraisal of the health status of individuals and groups with a focus on identified risk factors for specific illnesses.

risk factor Characteristics that increase the probability that a health problem will develop; disease precursor.

sampling error Difference between the statistics generated from analyzing information from the sample and the true population parameters.

screening Process of active, presumptive detection of unrecognized disease, illness, or deficit in asymptomatic, apparently healthy individuals; strategy for secondary prevention of disease in populations.

secondary prevention Activities designed to detect disease and provide early treatment.

selective screening Procedures applied to specific high-risk populations; use of exposure devices to monitor personnel working with radiation is an example.

SENIC Study on the Efficacy of Nosocomial Infection Control conducted by the Centers for Disease Control and Prevention.

sensitivity Ability of a test to correctly identify people who have a health problem; the probability of testing positive if the health problem is truly present.

sentinel surveillance Random samples of physicians' offices or health care clinics are contacted and asked to report occurrences of illness on a regular basis; identifies trends in frequently occurring conditions.

short-term change Fluctuations in time surrounding health problems that are measured in hours, days, weeks, or months.

source Location from which the infectious agent is immediately transmitted to the host.

small-area analysis A comparison of the needs of a high-risk population to the area as a whole to be used in decisions regarding resource allocation.

special surveillance Surveys that track special problems, such as the emergence of antibiotic-resistant organisms and prevalence of behavioral risk factors.

specific rates Rates calculated for population subgroups; used for understanding the distribution of various health-related conditions by age, sex, race, and other demographic characteristics.

specificity Ability of a test to correctly identify people who do not have a health problem; the probability of testing negative if the health problem is truly absent.

spectrum of health Continuum of states of wellness and illness.

statistical significance Results obtained from analysis of data are unlikely to have been caused by chance; stated by the P value.

surveillance A continual dynamic method for gathering data about the health of the general public for the purpose of primary prevention of illness.

tertiary prevention Treatment, care, and rehabilitation of people with acute and chronic illnesses.

therapeutic trial Clinical trial; experimental study designed to determine the ability of interventions to decrease or prevent recurrence of symptoms and to improve the outcomes for individuals with a specific state of health.

total house surveillance System that detects and records all nosocomial infections that occur on every service in every area of the hospital.

toxicology Science dealing with the detection, characteristics, effects, and antidotes for substances toxic to humans.

Type I error Observation of differences between study groups when differences do not exist.

Type II error Observation of no differences between study groups when differences do exist.

variable A characteristic or attribute of a person or object that varies within the population being studied.

vector Animals or arthropods that are carriers of infectious agents; transmission to humans can occur through indirect contact.

vehicle Substances or objects that have become contaminated with infectious organisms; transmission to humans can occur by indirect contact.

virulence The severity of the infectious disease that results from exposure to the agent.

web of causation An epidemiologic model that depicts the interrelationships between multiple factors that contribute to the occurrence of an illness.

zoonoses Infections acquired from infected animals that serve as reservoirs for human infection. Humans are not a part of the life cycle or reservoir of the agent.

Index

E

P

T